Emerging Therapies in Thoracic Malignancies

Editors

USMAN AHMAD
SUDISH C. MURTHY

SURGICAL ONCOLOGY CLINICS OF NORTH AMERICA

www.surgonc.theclinics.com

Consulting Editor
TIMOTHY M. PAWLIK

October 2020 • Volume 29 • Number 4

ELSEVIER

1600 John F. Kennedy Boulevard ● Suite 1800 ● Philadelphia, Pennsylvania, 19103-2899

http://www.theclinics.com

SURGICAL ONCOLOGY CLINICS OF NORTH AMERICA Volume 29, Number 4
October 2020 ISSN 1055-3207, ISBN-13: 978-0-323-75941-0

Editor: John Vassallo (j.vassallo@elsevier.com)
Developmental Editor: Julia Mckenzie

Surgical Oncology Clinics of North America (ISSN 1055-3207) is published quarterly by Elsevier Inc., 360 Park Avenue South, New York, NY 10010-1710. Months of publication are January, April, July, and October. Business and Editorial Offices: 1600 John F. Kennedy Blvd., Ste. 1800, Philadelphia, PA 19103-2899. Customer Service Office: 3251 Riverport Lane, Maryland Heights, MO 63043. Periodicals postage paid at New York, NY and additional mailing offices. Subscription prices are $309.00 per year (US individuals), $562.00 (US institutions) $100.00 (US student/resident), $352.00 (Canadian individuals), $711.00 (Canadian institutions), $100.00 (Canadian student/resident), $422.00 (foreign individuals), $711.00 (foreign institutions), and $205.00 (foreign student/resident). Foreign air speed delivery is included in all *Clinics* subscription prices. All prices are subject to change without notice. **POSTMASTER**: Send address changes to *Surgical Oncology Clinics of North America*, Elsevier Health Science Division, Subscription Customer Service, 3251 Riverport Lane, Maryland Heights, MO 63043. **Customer Service: 1-800-654-2452 (US and Canada). 314-447-8871 (outside US and Canada). Fax: 314-447-8029. E-mail: journalscustomerservice-usa@elsevier.com (for print support); journalsonline support-usa@elsevier.com (for online support).**

Reprints. For copies of 100 or more, of articles in this publication, please contact the Commercial Reprints Department, Elsevier Inc., 360 Park Avenue South, New York, New York 10010-1710. Tel. 212-633-3874; Fax: 212-633-3820; E-mail: reprints@elsevier.com.

Surgical Oncology Clinics of North America is covered in *MEDLINE/PubMed (Index Medicus)* and *EMBASE/ Excerpta Medica, Current Contents/Clinical Medicine, and ISI/BIOMED.*

Contributors

CONSULTING EDITOR

TIMOTHY M. PAWLIK, MD, MPH, PhD, FACS, FRACS (Hon.)
Professor and Chair, Department of Surgery, The Urban Meyer III and Shelley Meyer Chair for Cancer Research, Professor of Surgery, Oncology, Health Services Management and Policy, The Ohio State University, Wexner Medical Center, Columbus, Ohio, USA

EDITORS

USMAN AHMAD, MD, FACS
Staff Surgeon, Assistant Professor of Surgery, Department of Cardiothoracic Surgery, Heart, Vascular and Thoracic Institute, Cleveland Clinic, Cleveland, Ohio, USA

SUDISH C. MURTHY, MD, PhD, FACS
Staff Surgeon, Professor of Surgery, Chief of Thoracic Surgery, Daniel and Karen Lee Endowed Chair in Thoracic Surgery, Department of Cardiothoracic Surgery, Heart, Vascular and Thoracic Institute, Cleveland Clinic, Cleveland, Ohio, USA

AUTHORS

USMAN AHMAD, MD, FACS
Staff Surgeon, Assistant Professor of Surgery, Department of Cardiothoracic Surgery, Heart, Vascular and Thoracic Institute, Cleveland Clinic, Cleveland, Ohio, USA

MEHMET ALTAN, MD
Assistant Professor, Department of Thoracic/Head and Neck Medical Oncology, The University of Texas MD Anderson Cancer Center, Houston, Texas, USA

FEREDUN AZARI, MD
Department of Surgery, Hospital of the University of Pennsylvania, Philadelphia, Pennsylvania, USA

AMIT BHATT, MD
Director of Endoscopic Submucosal Dissection, Co-director of Endoluminal Surgery Center, Department of Gastroenterology and Hepatology, Digestive Disease Surgical Institute, Cleveland, Ohio, USA

ALEJANDRO C. BRIBRIESCO, MD
Department of Thoracic and Cardiovascular Surgery, Cleveland Clinic, Cleveland, Ohio, USA

ALESSANDRO BRUNELLI, MD
Consultant Thoracic Surgeon and Honorary Clinical Associate Professor, Department of Thoracic Surgery, St. James University Hospital, Leeds Teaching Hospitals NHS Trust, Leeds, United Kingdom

TINA CASCONE, MD, PhD
Assistant Professor, Department of Thoracic/Head and Neck Medical Oncology, The University of Texas MD Anderson Cancer Center, Houston, Texas, USA

HUMBERTO K. CHOI, MD, FCCP
Respiratory Institute, Cleveland Clinic, Cleveland, Ohio, USA

STEPHEN G. CHUN, MD
Assistant Professor, Department of Radiation Oncology, The University of Texas MD Anderson Cancer Center, Houston, Texas, USA

JENALEE N. COSTER, MD
Division of Thoracic Surgery, Michael E. DeBakey Department of Surgery, Baylor College of Medicine, Houston, Texas, USA

RAJA M. FLORES, MD
Chairman and Ames Professor, Department of Thoracic Surgery, Icahn School of Medicine at Mount Sinai, New York, New York, USA

MICHAEL R. GOOSEMAN, MD
Specialist Registrar, Cardiothoracic Surgery, Department of Thoracic Surgery, St. James University Hospital, Leeds Teaching Hospitals NHS Trust, Leeds, United Kingdom

SHAWN S. GROTH, MD, MS, FACS
Associate Professor of Surgery, Division of Thoracic Surgery, Michael E. DeBakey Department of Surgery, Baylor College of Medicine, Houston, Texas, USA

WAYNE L. HOFSTETTER, MD
Professor and Deputy Chair, Department of Thoracic and Cardiovascular Surgery, The University of Texas MD Anderson Cancer Center, Houston, Texas, USA

JAMES HUANG, MD, MPH
Thoracic Service, Department of Surgery, Memorial Sloan Kettering Cancer Center, New York, New York, USA

SUNEEL KAMATH, MD
Taussig Cancer Institute, Cleveland, Ohio, USA

GREG KENNEDY, MD
Department of Surgery, Hospital of the University of Pennsylvania, Philadelphia, Pennsylvania, USA

KENNETH A. KESLER, MD
Department of Surgery, Division of Cardiothoracic Surgery, Indiana University Melvin and Bren Simon Cancer Center, Department of Surgery, Thoracic Surgery Division, Indiana University, Indianapolis, Indiana, USA

XIUNING LE, MD
Assistant Professor, Department of Thoracic/Head and Neck Medical Oncology, The University of Texas MD Anderson Cancer Center, Houston, Texas, USA

PETER J. MAZZONE, MD, MPH, FCCP
Respiratory Institute, Cleveland Clinic, Cleveland, Ohio, USA

MICHAEL MCNAMARA, MD
Associate Staff, Solid Tumor Oncology, Cleveland Clinic, Cleveland, Ohio, USA

NATHAN W. MESKO, MD
Department of Orthopaedic Surgery, Cleveland Clinic, Cleveland, Ohio, USA

SUDISH C. MURTHY, MD, PhD, FACS
Staff Surgeon, Professor of Surgery, Chief of Thoracic Surgery, Daniel and Karen Lee Endowed Chair in Thoracic Surgery, Department of Cardiothoracic Surgery, Heart, Vascular and Thoracic Institute, Cleveland Clinic, Cleveland, Ohio, USA

CECILIA POMPILI, MD, PhD
Thoracic Surgeon and Senior Research Fellow, Department of Thoracic Surgery, St. James University Hospital, Leeds Teaching Hospitals NHS Trust, Leeds, United Kingdom

SIVA RAJA, MD, PhD
Surgical Director, Center for Esophageal Diseases, Staff Surgeon, Department of Thoracic and Cardiovascular Surgery, Cleveland, Ohio, USA

RAVI RAJARAM, MD, MSc
Department of Thoracic and Cardiovascular Surgery, The University of Texas MD Anderson Cancer Center, Houston, Texas, USA

JESSE M.P. RAPPAPORT, MD
Department of Cardiothoracic Surgery, Heart, Vascular and Thoracic Institute, Cleveland Clinic, Cleveland, Ohio, USA

DANIEL P. RAYMOND, MD
Chief Quality Officer, Department of Thoracic and Cardiovascular Surgery, Cleveland Clinic, Cleveland, Ohio, USA

BORIS SEPESI, MD
Associate Professor, Department of Thoracic and Cardiovascular Surgery, The University of Texas MD Anderson Cancer Center, Houston, Texas, USA

SUNIL SINGHAL, MD
Department of Surgery, Division of Thoracic Surgery, University of Pennsylvania, Perelman School of Medicine, Hospital of the University of Pennsylvania, Philadelphia, Pennsylvania, USA

DAVENDRA SOHAL, MD, MPH
Associate Staff, Solid Tumor Oncology, Assistant Professor, Lerner College of Medicine, Cleveland Clinic, Cleveland, Ohio, USA

AMANDA R. STRAM, MD, PhD
Department of Surgery, Division of Cardiothoracic Surgery, Indiana University Melvin and Bren Simon Cancer Center, Department of Surgery, Thoracic Surgery Division, Indiana University, Indianapolis, Indiana, USA

MONISHA SUDARSHAN, MD, MPH
Thoracic Surgeon, Thoracic Surgery, Cleveland Clinic, Cleveland, Ohio, USA

ANDREW TANG, MD
Resident, Thoracic and Cardiovascular Surgery, Cleveland Clinic Foundation, Cleveland, Ohio, USA

ANDREA S. WOLF, MD, MPH
Associate Professor, Department of Thoracic Surgery, Icahn School of Medicine at Mount Sinai, New York, New York, USA

NICOLAS ZHOU, DO
Department of Thoracic and Cardiovascular Surgery, The University of Texas MD Anderson Cancer Center, Houston, Texas, USA

Contents

Modern surgical practice places increased emphasis on treatment outcomes. There has been a paradigm shift from paternalistic ways of practicing medicine to patients having a major involvement in decision making and treatment planning. The combination of these two factors undoubtedly leaves the surgeon open to greater scrutiny in respect of results and outcomes. In dealing with this it is important that the surgeon, wider multidisciplinary team, and patient appreciate the idea of surgical risk. This article reviews the latest evidence relating to risk assessment in thoracic surgery and suggests how this should be incorporated into clinical practice.

Lung cancer is the leading cause of US cancer-related deaths. Lung cancer screening with a low radiation dose chest computed tomography scan is now standard of care for a high-risk eligible population. It is imperative for clinicians and surgeons to evaluate the trade-offs of benefits and harms, including the identification of many benign lung nodules, overdiagnosis, and complications. Integration of smoking cessation interventions augments the clinical benefits of screening. Screening programs must develop strategies to manage screening-detected findings to minimize potential harms. Further research should focus on how to improve patient selection, minimize harms, and facilitate access to screening.

Lung cancer is the most frequent cause of cancer-related death worldwide. Despite advances in systemic therapy, the 5-year survival remains humbling at 4% to 17%. For those diagnosed early, surgical therapy can yield potentially curative results. Surgical resection remains a cornerstone of medical care. Success hinges on sound oncologic resection principles. Various techniques can be used to identify pulmonary nodules. A challenge is intraoperative assessment of the surgical specimen to confirm disease localization and ensure an R0 resection. The primary tool is frozen section. Understanding the options available enhances the arsenal of thoracic surgeons and leads to better patient care.

Jenalee N. Coster and Shawn S. Groth

Locally advanced non–small cell lung cancer is a heterogeneous group of tumors that require multidisciplinary treatment. Although there is much debate with regard to their management, a multimodal treatment strategy for carefully selected patients that includes surgery can extend survival compared with nonoperative definitive therapy. As the role of targeted therapies and immune checkpoint inhibitors for these tumors becomes better defined, practices will continue to evolve.

Boris Sepesi, Tina Cascone, Stephen G. Chun, Mehmet Altan, and Xiuning Le

Immunotherapy, targeted therapy, and adoptive T-cell therapy have been revolutionary advancements in cancer research. Some of these therapies have become the standard of care for lung cancer and replaced older treatment algorithms; some continue to be studied in clinical trials. This article discusses the current state of novel treatment options for non–small cell lung cancer patients with metastatic and locoregional disease, with focus on immunotherapy, targeted therapy, and adoptive T-cell therapy.

Amanda R. Stram and Kenneth A. Kesler

Primary mediastinal nonseminomatous germ cell tumors represent a rare but important malignancy that occurs in otherwise young and healthy patients. Treatment is challenging and involves cisplatin-based chemotherapy followed by surgery to remove residual disease. Avoiding bleomycin-containing chemotherapy in the treatment of primary mediastinal nonseminomatous germ cell tumors is important. Pre-chemotherapy and postchemotherapy pathology as well as postoperative serum tumor markers are independent predictors of long-term survival.

Jesse M.P. Rappaport, James Huang, and Usman Ahmad

Thymomas are relatively indolent tumors that present with locally advanced disease in 30% of the patients. Thymic carcinoma is a more aggressive histology with shorter disease-free and overall survival. Early-stage tumors are managed best with complete resection. Multimodal therapy is the standard of care for locally advanced tumors and neoadjuvant therapy may help improve respectability. Stage and complete resection are the strongest prognostic factors for long-term survival. Based on early experience, targeted and immunotherapies have shown limited promise in advanced disease.

SURGICAL ONCOLOGY
CLINICS OF NORTH AMERICA

SERIES OF RELATED INTEREST

Surgical Clinics of North America
http://www.surgical.theclinics.com
Thoracic Surgery Clinics
http://www.thoracic.theclinics.com
Advances in Surgery
http://www.advancessurgery.com

THE CLINICS ARE AVAILABLE ONLINE!
Access your subscription at:
www.theclinics.com

Foreword

Emerging Therapies in Thoracic Malignancies

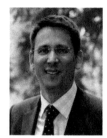

Timothy M. Pawlik, MD, MPH, MTS, PhD, FACS, FRACS (Hon.)
Consulting Editor

This issue of the *Surgical Oncology Clinics of North America* covers the important topic of Emerging Therapies in Thoracic Malignancies. Thoracic cancers include a broad range of malignancies, such as lung cancers, mediastinal tumors, chest wall sarcomas, as well as thymic and tracheal lesions. Similar to the diverse types of cancers contained within the rubric of "thoracic malignancies," the surgical procedures, systemic treatments, staging systems, as well as prognoses of these different diseases are varied. That said, one point of relative consistency has been the dramatic advances in the understanding of these diseases, as well as the progress in surgical and systemic treatments. In addition, successful management of thoracic malignancies is also unified by the need for a well-informed multidisciplinary approach that incorporates an understanding of thoracic anatomy, surgical techniques, oncologic principles, as well as underlying pathogenesis to inform optimal therapy. As such, surgeons need to be well versed in the latest data regarding the diagnostic and treatment options for patients with thorcic malignancies. In light of this need, I am delighted to have Dr Usman Ahmad and Dr Sudish Murthy as the guest editors of this important issue of *Surgical Oncology Clinics of North America*. Dr Ahmad is a throacic surgeon in the Thoracic and Cardiovascular Surgery Department at the Cleveland Clinic, who is recognized for his expertise in the clinical management of patients with thoracic malignancies. Dr Ahmad has a strong interest in cancer outcomes research and has written many peer-reviewed publications and book chapters on thoracic cancer. His research has been presented at the Society of Thoracic Surgeons, American Association of Thoracic Surgery, and the International Thymic Malignancy Interest Group. Joining Dr Ahmad is Dr Murthy, who is the Section Head of Thoracic Surgery and the Daniel and Karen Lee Endowed Chair in Thoracic Surgery at Cleveland Clinic. Dr Murthy is a dedicated researcher and prolific writer. He has authored or coauthored more than 100 scientific articles in leading peer-reviewed medical journals and more than a dozen

Surg Oncol Clin N Am 29 (2020) xiii–xiv
https://doi.org/10.1016/j.soc.2020.07.003
1055-3207/20/© 2020 Published by Elsevier Inc.

chapters in medical textbooks. His research interests include lung cancer, lung transplant, and emphysema. These 2 editors bring a wealth of personal knowledge to this issue of the *Surgical Oncology Clinics of North America* as our invited Guest Editors.

The issue covers a number of important topics, including the workup, as well as medical and surgical management of patients with mediastinal germ cell tumors, esophageal cancer, mesothelioma, chest wall sarcoma, and lung cancer. Dr Ahmad and Dr Murthy have assembled a wide array of expert authors to cover not only the surgical management of thoracic malignancies but also topics such as screening, staging, as well as targeted therapies, immunotherapy, and T-cell therapy. I want to thank all of our authors who contributed to this issue of *Surgical Oncology Clinics of North America*, as well as Dr Ahmad and Dr Murthy for enlisting the help of this great group of authors, who are leaders in the field of thoracic malignancies. As you read this issue, I am convinced that you will experience firsthand the skill and talent of our authors to highlight the most relevant, topical, and up-to-date information relevant to caring for patients with thoracic malignancies. The knowledge contained in this issue of *Surgical Oncology Clinics of North America* will well serve thoracic surgeons, oncologists, trainees, and other health care providers who care for patients with these challenging tumors. Once again, I would like to thank Dr Ahmad and Dr Murthy and all the contributing authors for an excellent issue of the *Surgical Oncology Clinics of North America*.

Timothy M. Pawlik, MD, MPH, MTS, PhD, FACS, FRACS (Hon.)
Department of Surgery
Oncology, Health Services Management and Policy
The Ohio State University
Wexner Medical Center
395 West 12th Avenue
Suite 670
Columbus, OH 43210, USA

E-mail address:
tim.pawlik@osumc.edu

Preface

Updates in Thoracic Surgery and Oncology

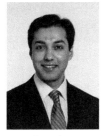 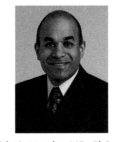

Usman Ahmad, MD, FACS   Sudish C. Murthy, MD, PhD, FACS
Editors

Surgery of the chest, particularly extirpative surgery for malignancy, is uniquely complex. Cancers are aggressive, and resectability is limited by both anatomic constraints and patient performance status. Unfortunately, locoregional as well as systemic recurrences are common with limited salvage options. The last 2 decades has seen tremendous advancements in thoracic oncology. Early detection and screening have reduced mortality for early esophageal and lung cancers. Moreover, locally advanced and systemic disease can be treated with targeted therapeutics and now immunotherapy. Surgical interventions have evolved as well with dissemination and application of minimally invasive approaches for all thoracic malignancies.

This issue of the journal provides a thorough discourse on contemporary issues and advances in thoracic surgery and oncology. The topics range from detection of early-stage cancers through screening to multimodal and immunotherapy for locally advanced and systemic disease. Intraoperative detection of small pulmonary tumors is an exciting area of research, and recent advances are highlighted. Exciting developments are being made in management of early-stage esophageal cancer as well as locally advanced disease and are expertly discussed. Important updates in the fields of pleural mesothelioma mediastinal tumors have also been detailed.

There is little doubt that there are exciting times ahead. Yet, we would be remiss if we didn't pause and acknowledge the giants upon whose shoulders we all now sit and those critical mentors who have so importantly shaped our thought processes and surgical judgment. Though there is simply not enough room to list all, those who stand out in our careers include F. Griffith Pearson, David J. Sugarbaker, Manjit S. Bain, Valerie

Surg Oncol Clin N Am 29 (2020) xv–xvi
https://doi.org/10.1016/j.soc.2020.07.004

W. Rusch, and G. Alexander Patterson. We also very much recognize the support from our families.

Usman Ahmad, MD, FACS
Department of Cardiothoracic Surgery
Heart, Vascular and Thoracic Institute
Cleveland Clinic
9500 Euclid Avenue, J4-1
Cleveland, OH 44195, USA

Sudish C. Murthy, MD, PhD, FACS
Department of Cardiothoracic Surgery
Heart, Vascular and Thoracic Institute
Cleveland Clinic
9500 Euclid Avenue, J4-1
Cleveland, OH 44195, USA

E-mail addresses:
AHMADU@ccf.org (U. Ahmad)
MURTHYS1@ccf.org (S.C. Murthy)

Evaluation of Risk for Thoracic Surgery

Alessandro Brunelli, MD*, Michael R. Gooseman, MD, Cecilia Pompili, MD, PhD

KEYWORDS

- Functional staging • Operative risk • Shared decision making

KEY POINTS

- There should be an attempt, whatever the pathologic status, to discuss all thoracic surgical patients in a multidisciplinary setting.
- A meticulous preoperative physiologic assessment allows the surgeon and wider team to identify those at highest risk.
- The functional assessment can help the surgeon to identify areas for optimization to potentially reduce risk.
- This information should be shared clearly and openly with the patient in a "shared decision making" process.

INTRODUCTION

The surgical decision-making process has undoubtedly changed over the last couple of decades. Traditionally the surgeon, often practicing in relative isolation, would act on intuition, which would have reflected training and previous experience. In the current climate of surgeon outcome reporting, decision making in surgery often reflects not only the surgeon's thoughts but the wider multidisciplinary team and, perhaps more importantly, the patient's views. The decision-making process can therefore become much more complicated than the intended surgical procedure.

There is no doubt that surgery has always been associated with risk. The prediction and assessment of risk is more recent and continues to develop. Historically, when the patient was not considered "fit enough" for a surgical procedure, they may have been referred elsewhere for "conservative" management, which often represented a large and diverse group of nonsurgical treatment strategies. Each surgical procedure has its own recognized profile of risks and complications. It must also be remembered that risk, for both surgeon and patient, is relative. For instance, the thoracic surgeon may quote an operative mortality of 6% to a patient likely to need pneumonectomy

Cardiothoracic Surgery, Department of Thoracic Surgery, St. James University Hospital, Leeds Teaching Hospitals NHS Trust, Leeds LS9 7TF, UK
* Corresponding author.
E-mail address: alex.brunelli@nhs.net

Surg Oncol Clin N Am 29 (2020) 497–508
https://doi.org/10.1016/j.soc.2020.06.001

for non–small cell lung cancer (NSCLC): this will mostly be deemed acceptable. However, what will both surgeon and patient think if a similar rate was suggested for intervention for a middle-aged patient with recurrent pneumothorax?

Although there is no doubt that surgeons have developed risk-prediction models to inform and develop their own practice, it may also be representative of the increasing role of clinical governance in health systems around the world. It is now reasonably common for surgeons to have to defend their own decision making including the major decision to offer a patient surgery. The traditional sense of using one's intuition is difficult to defend when asked if a thorough risk assessment was undertaken to allow for clear objectivity.

Some surgical specialties have little influence over what arrives in their care. However, it is important to remember that in many aspects of thoracic surgical practice, the patient will have been referred after extensive discussion in a multidisciplinary team (MDT) setting. In the United Kingdom it is mandatory that a patient with cancer is discussed in this setting. This well-described approach allows for specialists with different areas of expertise to input their views on a management plan and allow formation of the best treatment plan for a patient. In respect of solid cancers, surgical resection still generally remains the best chance of a relative cure and thus, whatever the potential risk, should be discussed extensively. The traditional view that the decision to not offer someone surgery remains more difficult than the one to proceed with surgery remains relevant.

ESTIMATION OF CARDIOVASCULAR RISK

A major portion of most thoracic surgeons' practice will involve surgical resections for early-stage lung cancer. This patient group will frequently have a significant cigarette smoking history that is itself associated with an increased risk of underlying cardiovascular comorbidity. There is evidence to show that the risk of major cardiac complications including ventricular arrhythmias, pulmonary edema, and cardiac arrest after major anatomic lung resection is approximately 3%.[1,2] There is published guidance that can be consulted by the thoracic surgeon regarding cardiac risk evaluation in patients being considered for lung cancer resection surgery. The 2 major guidelines from the American College of Chest Physicians and the European Respiratory Society/European Society Thoracic Surgeons (ERS/ESTS) joint task force are very similar.[3,4] They are closely based on the American College of Cardiology/American Heart Association (ACC/AHA) 2007 guidelines on perioperative cardiovascular evaluation and care for noncardiac surgery.[5]

Both guidelines recommend the use of a scoring system to estimate the risk of major perioperative cardiac events. In 1999, Lee and colleagues[1] developed the Revised Cardiac Risk Index (RCRI) for patients undergoing major nonurgent surgery. The RCRI, which is a 6-factor cardiac risk index, includes history of coronary artery disease, cerebrovascular disease, insulin-dependent diabetes, congestive heart failure, serum creatinine level greater than 2 mg/dL, and high-risk surgery. All factors are equally weighted.

Brunelli and colleagues[4] refined this and recalibrated the RCRI in a large population of candidates being submitted to major anatomic lung resection, producing the thoracic (Th)RCRI. The aim was to make it more specific to thoracic surgeons and their patients. A simplified weighted score composed of 4 out of the original 6 factors has been shown to be reliably associated with major cardiac mortality. The factors have different weights: history of coronary artery disease, 1.5 points; cerebrovascular disease, 1.5 points; serum creatinine level greater than 2 mg/dL, 1 point; and pneumonectomy, 1.5 points. The recent American College of Clinical Pharmacy (ACCP) guidelines state that a ThRCRI with a score of 1.5 or higher is one of the reasons to refer for a cardiology opinion. At this stage patients should be investigated as per ACC/AHA guidance, which recommends noninvasive investigation including an echocardiogram.[5] The ThRCRI has been clearly validated by numerous studies.[6,7]

PULMONARY FUNCTION

Full spirometry and diffusing capacity provide important information for the thoracic surgeon. The forced expiratory volume at first second (FEV_1) and predicted postoperative (ppo)FEV_1 have been extensively used to stratify risk but should no longer be considered in isolation. There is a significant number of studies demonstrating that a reduced FEV_1 or ppoFEV_1 is associated with increased morbidity and mortality in patients proceeding with lung resection. Licker and colleagues[8] showed that an FEV_1 of less than 60% is an independent risk factor for morality and respiratory morbidity. However, several studies have shown that consideration of an FEV_1 in isolation is not a good indicator of postoperative outcome.[9,10] This is particularly apparent in patients with chronic obstructive pulmonary disease (COPD), which obviously represents a significant portion of any thoracic surgeon's practice.

Ferguson and colleagues[11] first demonstrated the importance of the carbon monoxide lung diffusion capacity (DLCO) as an independent assessment of surgical risk. This study showed that an impaired DLCO was related to the development of postoperative respiratory complications and death. When the DLCO decreased to less than 60%, the complication rate was 50% with a mortality of 20%. Berry and colleagues[12] confirmed similar findings in 2010. Studies have shown that a substantial proportion of patients with normal FEV_1 have a reduced DLCO, and even for non-COPD patients a low DLCO or ppoDLCO is associated with increased risk of pulmonary complications and mortality.[13,14] This evidence supports the concept that DLCO should be measured in all candidates to lung resection regardless of their baseline FEV_1.

EXERCISE TESTS

Exercise testing remains a critical component of a thorough preoperative functional assessment. It has a role in assessing the entire oxygen transport system with a view to the detection of deficit that may manifest as perioperative morbidity or mortality. There is now a wide and informative body of literature analyzing exercise assessment in patients being considered for lung cancer resection surgery. Published guidelines include those from the ERS/ESTS, ACCP, and the British Thoracic Society/Society for Cardiothoracic Surgeons.[3,4,15]

The general consensus is that the cardiopulmonary exercise test (CPET) is the gold standard for functional assessment and risk stratification in patients proceeding to lung resection. However, there is literature showing that the CPET is not always readily accessible.[16] As such, other forms of exercise testing are regularly used including the 6-minute walk test, stair-climbing test, and the shuttle test.

Low-technology testing is used to describe exercise testing not including CPET. The 6-minute walk test has been used since the 1960s and has been extensively studied. Most recently, Marjanski and colleagues[17] demonstrated that patients walking less than 500 m had both increased postoperative morbidity and length of hospital stay. Current clinical guidance recommends that it should not be used in selecting patients for operation.

Conversely, current guidelines do support the use of the shuttle walk test. One of the more recent studies examining this from Fennelly and colleagues[18] showed that patients walking further than 400 m experienced a very low rate of perioperative complications. As such, guidelines suggest that patients who can complete 400 m on the shuttle walk test are fit to undergo surgical resection.[3]

Stair climbing has often been seen practically as an exercise test that the surgeon can directly engage with during the patient's preoperative review. It is well validated as an exercise test. Brunelli and colleagues[19] measured oxygen consumption during stair climbing, whereby 98% of patients climbing more than 22 m had a positive predictive value of 86% to predict a Vo_2 peak of 15 mL/kg/min. As such, current clinical guidance suggests that patients able to ascend greater than 22 m can proceed with lung resection.[3]

CPET provides a detailed and broad physiologic evaluation of the patient that allows for measurement of the maximal oxygen consumption (Vo_{2max}). The Vo_{2max} was the first ergometric measurement found to be related to postoperative morbidity and mortality. In 1995, Bolliger and colleagues[20] showed that patients with a Vo_{2max} of less than 60% of predicted had postoperative morbidity approaching 90%. Brunelli and colleagues[21] demonstrated that the Vo_{2max} is the best predictor of respiratory morbidity. This study showed that a Vo_{2max} of less than 12 mL/kg/min had a mortality rate of 13%, whereas patients with a Vo_{2max} of greater than 20 mL/kg/min had no mortality. As such, patients with a Vo_{2max} greater than 20 mL/kg/min can safely proceed with surgical resection including pneumonectomy and can be classed as low risk. Conversely a Vo_{2max} less than 10 mL/kg/min is now generally regarded as a contraindication to lung resection: case series have shown that patients with Vo_{2max} below this threshold have a very high risk of postoperative mortality.[3]

The pulmonary function and exercise test evaluations have been integrated in an algorithm to guide fitness evaluation (**Fig. 1**[3]).

A Vo_{2max} between 10 and 15 mL/kg/min is associated with an increased risk of postoperative mortality. For patients who fall within this range, the minute ventilation to carbon dioxide output (V_E/Vco_2) slope can be helpful because it has been shown to be an independent predictor of mortality. Brunelli and colleagues[22] demonstrated that patients with a V_E/Vco_2 ≥ 35 were 3 times as likely to develop postoperative respiratory morbidity. Shafiek and colleagues[23] confirmed this value and verified V_E/Vco_2 as a predictor of increased morbidity and mortality.

V_E/Vco_2 slope has not yet been included in guidelines for estimation of fitness before surgery. However, Salati and Brunelli[24] have proposed an algorithm incorporating this parameter to refine the moderate risk group (**Fig. 2**).

Low-technology testing can be safely and efficiently used as a first-line screening exercise test in candidates for lung resection. If the patient is not able to meet the thresholds set out in current guidance, they should ideally be referred for formal CPET.

IMPLICATIONS OF RISK ASSESSMENT

One of the advantages of performing a thorough preoperative functional assessment is to potentially allow for optimization of those patients at higher risk. It does not mean that the option for surgery should be immediately removed. In the setting of lung cancer, there is obviously critical importance in reducing the time to definitive treatment. However, careful consideration must be paid to smoking cessation and completion of a program of pulmonary rehabilitation or "prehabilitation." The problems faced by patients continuing to smoke through lung surgery is well described and recognized in clinical practice. A longer length of preoperative time from smoking cessation has been shown to decrease operative mortality. It is therefore important to try and help the patient engage with smoking cessation services, especially when deemed at increased risk.

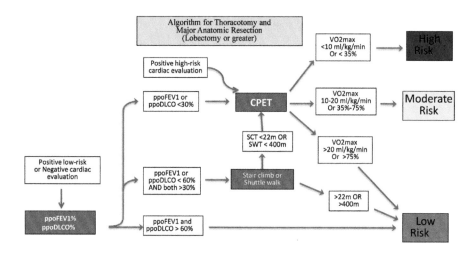

Fig. 1. American College of Chest Physicians functional evaluation algorithm for lung resection candidates. (*Adapted from* Brunelli A, Kim AW, Berger KI, et al. Physiologic evaluation of the patient with lung cancer being considered for resectional surgery: diagnosis and management of lung cancer, 3rd ed: American College of Chest Physicians evidence-based clinical practice guidelines. Chest 2013;143: e166S-90S; with permission.)

The ACCP guidance recommends that high-risk patients should be referred for pulmonary rehabilitation.[3] In the setting of lung volume reduction (LVRS), this has been shown to improve breathlessness, quality of life, an exercise tolerance.[25] In respect of lung cancer resection surgery, one study has shown that a preoperative regimen reduced the patients' length of stay.[26] Pulmonary rehabilitation can present difficult challenges before lung cancer resection surgery, given that time to surgery is critical. However, in the future the format in which pulmonary rehabilitation can be offered is likely to continue to develop. Technology is enabling for app-based programs, meaning that it can be available almost immediately for the patients to use.[27]

Surgical risk-prediction algorithms are now available to help the thoracic surgeon to objectively estimate complications. A thorough preoperative functional assessment before surgery is important because even the apparently "healthy" patient may have undetected but significant cardiorespiratory impairment, which could put the patient at high risk of major perioperative complications.

SPECIAL CONSIDERATIONS
Risk Assessment of Candidates for Pneumonectomy

Pneumonectomy is still associated with a 6% risk of perioperative mortality.[28] This operation is a consistent risk factor for major cardiac events[2] and 30-day mortality.[29] The physiologic burden imposed by such a large lung resection to the cardiorespiratory system warrants a meticulous functional workup. In the authors' institution, all

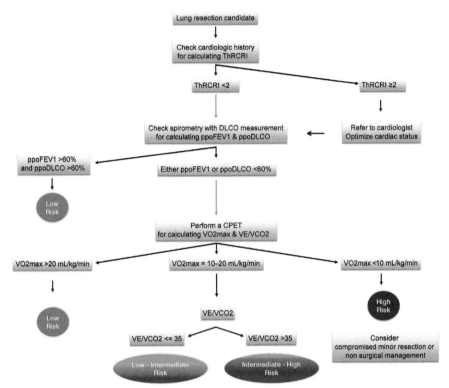

Fig. 2. Functional algorithm incorporating the V_E/V_{CO_2} slope as measure to refine the risk stratification. (*From* Salati, M., Brunelli, A. Risk Stratification in Lung Resection. Curr Surg Rep 2016; 4, 37; with permission.)

candidates for pneumonectomy undergo a quantitative perfusion scan to estimate the ppoFEV$_1$ and are systematically referred to a CPET.

Risk Stratification in Patients Receiving Neoadjuvant Chemotherapy

A recent study from the ESTS database has shown that neoadjuvant chemotherapy was associated with similar rates of 30-day mortality after lobectomy or pneumonectomy compared with matched patients not receiving chemotherapy. However, neoadjuvant chemotherapy was associated with higher cardiopulmonary morbidity and when combined with radiotherapy was associated with a 2-fold higher risk of mortality following pneumonectomy.[30] A similar recent analysis from the National Cancer Database of more than 130,000 patients undergoing lung resection for lung cancer found an increased incidence of 30-day and 90-day mortality after neoadjuvant treatment.[31]

Neoadjuvant chemotherapy has been found to be associated with structural changes in the lung leading to decreased diffusion capacity, which in turn may predispose to development of postoperative respiratory complications.[32–35] The evidence from the literature warrants a re-evaluation of the pulmonary function after completion of the chemotherapy treatment and before lung resection to evaluate possible changes, particularly in diffusion capacity.[3,4]

Does Ability to Undergo Minimally Invasive Surgery Change the Pulmonary Risk Profile?

Minimally invasive thoracic surgery is known to be associated with improved early postoperative outcomes in comparison with thoracotomy. Both robotic and thoracoscopic lung resections have been associated with lower rates of morbidity and mortality.[36–38] The benefits of a minimally invasive thoracic approach are particularly evident in patients with prohibitive pulmonary functions.[39] For this reason, the ACCP guidelines recommend that patients deemed at high risk for resection should be considered for minimally invasive surgery if feasible.[3] At this stage there is no sufficient evidence to suggest a different risk-assessment strategy in candidates for minimally invasive surgery. The advancement in technology, pain management, and enhanced recovery program may contribute in a future to offer lung cancer surgery to an increasing number of patients. Future guidelines should reflect these changes by elaborating the cumulative body of evidence in this field.

SHARED DECISION MAKING

One of the most important intimations of preoperative risk assessment is to provide scientific data to inform the shared decision making (SDM) process with the patient.

Little is known on how to measure patients' participation in SDM in patients with early-stage NSCLC. SDM is a concept defined by the National Institute of Health and Care Excellence (NICE) as a process whereby care or treatment options are fully explored along with their risks and benefits. The NICE document makes clear that persons both receiving and delivering care need to understand what is important to the other person. In the United States, the Institute of Medicine identified engaging patients and supporting patient decision making as an essential component of care, especially during a crisis.[40]

Regarding NSCLC, however, treatment effectiveness guidance is still mainly based on survival data[15,41]; there are no studies adequately comparing treatments' effectiveness in terms of impact on patients' quality of life (QOL).[42,43] Particularly in early-stage lung cancer, the lack of long-term QOL data after treatments has highlighted the importance of understanding whether a truly informed "shared decision" is made when discussing the situation with the patient. To develop SDM guidelines or integrate this concept into the existing decisional algorithms and guidelines, in the last 2 decades an increasing number of studies investigating the overall lack of concordance between physician and patient perceptions of the decisional context has been reported. Most of these studies have shown that concerns and treatment strategies were insufficiently discussed between the patients and physicians.[44,45]

Computerized interactive methods with outcome probabilities tailored to individual patients are new strategies to potentially increase communication, patient engagement, and documentation of consent. Online decision aids for treatment decision making resulted in a positive influence on clinicians' decisions and has been already developed for advanced-stage NSCLC.[46]

The main value of the SDM has been the improvement of patients' knowledge of their treatment trajectory to improve patients' adherence and satisfaction. In recent years, this strategy has been promoted also as a means to reduce health care overtreatment and costs.[47] Indeed, 20% of patients who participate in SDM choose less invasive surgical options and more conservative treatment than do patients who do not use decision aids.[48]

Patients with lung cancer have expressed their aversion to risk acceptance: however, facing the cancer progression and no alternatives for cure, patients are willing to take extremely high risks of postoperative complications and surgery-related death.[49] On the other hand, they are always more demanding about the risks of a permanent and long-lasting disability: the interference of cancer treatment in their daily lifestyle is one of the main treatment outcomes for the patient. Information about residual QOL after surgical treatment become mandatory when medical alternatives have been implemented in a decision-making algorithm, such as stereotactic ablative radiotherapy (SABR) for early-stage lung cancers. The growing size of the older population and the increasing number of lung cancer screening scans are slightly changing the populations facing the surgical decision-making process. Increasing numbers of patients older than 75 years are being diagnosed with thoracic malignancies, and advancements in medical treatments now offer valid alternatives. Most importantly, holistic comprehension of cognitive abilities in older people has to be taken into account by the surgeons explaining the surgical risks. Hopmans and colleagues[44] interviewed in 2015 early-stage NSCLC patients submitted to either SABR or surgery. Guidance by the clinician and conduct of the clinician were found to be the most important factors for the patients during the decision-making process. Both SABR and surgery were only offered to 28.9% of patients. In another recent qualitative article, most patients preferred to not be aware of mortality risks. Surgery was the only treatment discussed for most patients, and they preferred clinicians to make treatment decisions because of the belief that clinicians know best.[45] However, Sullivan and colleagues[50] surveyed 114 patients with early-stage NSCLC 4 to 6 months after radical treatments (either SABR or surgery): more participants valued independence and QOL as "most important" compared with survival or cancer recurrence.

Furthermore, with the shift of health care in involving patients in medical decisions, the burden on patients to understand health-related information so as to make fully informed choices needs to be fully investigated. However, patients who are disadvantaged by poverty, lack of education, or linguistic barriers are also likely to make informed decisions without a real comprehension of risks and benefits. In an ideal health care system, all the people may be able to access the decision aids regardless their social and financial background. In real life, low numeracy also distorts perceptions of risks and benefits of screening, reduces medication compliance, impedes access to treatments, and impairs risk communication.[51]

Patient participation in the SDM may also play a role in increasing the QOL after the treatment. There are insufficient data to confirm this theory in our specialty, but results from the NELSON screening trial, for example, showed that subjects who did not make an informed decision to participate in lung cancer computed tomography screening trial did not experience worse QOL during screening than subjects who did make an informed decision.[52] In breast reconstruction surgery, patients who adopted a more active role, whether using an informed or shared approach, had higher general patient satisfaction and physical component QOL scores compared with patients whose decision making was paternalistic.[53]

SUMMARY

The concept of surgical risk continues to progress. There has been development of surgical risk-prediction models that have been adapted successfully for use in thoracic surgery. A meticulous preoperative physiologic assessment allows the surgeon and wider MDT to identify those at the highest risk. This then enables potential optimization of individuals deemed at high risk in an attempt to reduce this risk and also allows the surgeon and patient to engage in a full and frank discussion regarding treatment planning. However, caution is advised because no risk-prediction model in isolation is the perfect tool, and the clinical acumen and surgical intuition of an expert physician remains of critical importance in this process.

DISCLOSURE

The authors have nothing to disclose.

REFERENCES

1. Lee TH, Marcantonio ER, Mangione CM, et al. Derivation and prospective validation of a simple index for prediction of cardiac risk of major noncardiac surgery. Circulation 1999;100:1043–9.
2. Brunelli A, Varela G, Salati M, et al. Recalibration of the revised cardiac risk index in lung resection candidates. Ann Thorac Surg 2010;90:199–203.
3. Brunelli A, Kim AW, Berger KI, et al. Physiologic evaluation of the patient with lung cancer being considered for resectional surgery: diagnosis and management of lung cancer, 3rd ed: American College of Chest Physicians evidence-based clinical practice guidelines. Chest 2013;143:e166S–190.
4. Brunelli A, Charloux A, Bollinger CT, et al. ERS/ESTS clinical guidelines on fitness for radical therapy in lung cancer patients (surgery and chemo-radiotherapy). Eur Respir J 2009;34:17–41.
5. Fleisher LA, Beckman JA, Brown KA, et al. ACC/AHA 2007 guidelines on perioperative cardiovascular evaluation and care for noncardiac surgery: a report of the American College of Cardiology/American Heart Association Task Force on Practice Guidelines (Writing Committee to Revise the 2002 Guidelines on Perioperative Cardiovascular Evaluation for Noncardiac Surgery): developed in collaboration with the American Society of Echocardiography, American Society of Nuclear Cardiology, Heart Rhythm Society, Society of Cardiovascular Anesthesiologists, Society for Cardiovascular Angiography and Interventions, Society for Vascular Medicine and Biology, and Society for Vascular Surgery. Circulation 2007;116:e418–99.
6. Brunelli A, Cassivi SD, Fibla J, et al. External validation of the recalibrated thoracic revised cardiac risk index for predicting the risk of major cardiac complications after lung resection. Ann Thorac Surg 2011;92:445–8.
7. Ferguson MK, Celauro AD, Vigneswaran WT. Validation of a modified scoring system for cardiovascular risk associated with major lung resection. Eur J Cardiothorac Surg 2012;41(3):598–602.
8. Licker MJ, Widikker I, Robert J, et al. Operative mortality and respiratory complications after lung resection for cancer: impact of chronic obstructive pulmonary disease and time trends. Ann Thorac Surg 2006;81:1830–7.
9. Brunelli A, Al Refai M, Monteverde M, et al. Predictors of early morbidity after major lung resection in patients with and without airflow limitation. Ann Thorac Surg 2002;74:999–1003.
10. Brunelli A, Xiumé F, Refai M, et al. Evaluation of expiratory volume, diffusion capacity, and exercise tolerance following major lung resection: a prospective follow-up analysis. Chest 2007;131:141–7.
11. Ferguson MK, Little L, Rizzo L, et al. Diffusing capacity predicts morbidity and mortality after pulmonary resection. J Thorac Cardiovasc Surg 1988;96:894–900.
12. Berry MF, Villamizar-Ortiz NR, Tong BC, et al. Pulmonary function tests do not predict pulmonary complications after thoracoscopic lobectomy. Ann Thorac Surg 2010;89:1044–51.

13. Brunelli A, Refai MA, Salati M, et al. Carbon monoxide lung diffusion capacity improves risk stratification in patients without airflow limitation: evidence for systematic measurement before lung resection. Eur J Cardiothorac Surg 2006;29(4): 567–70.

14. Ferguson MK, Vigneswaran WT. Diffusing capacity predicts morbidity after lung resection in patients without obstructive lung disease. Ann Thorac Surg 2008; 85(4):1158–64.

15. Lim E, Baldwin D, Beckles M, et al. Guidelines on the radical management of patients with lung cancer. Thorax 2010;65:iii1–27.

16. Charloux A, Brunelli A, Bollinger CT, et al. European Respiratory Society and European Society of Thoracic Surgeons Joint Task Force on Fitness for Radical Therapy. Lung function evaluation before surgery in lung cancer patients: how are recent advances put into practice? A survey among members of the European Society of Thoracic Surgeons (ESTS) and of the Thoracic Oncology Section of the European Respiratory Society (ERS). Interact Cardiovasc Thorac Surg 2009;9:925–31.

17. Marjanski T, Wnuk D, Bosakowski D, et al. Patients who do not reach a distance of 500 m during the 6-min walk test have an increased risk of postoperative complications and prolonged hospital stay after lobectomy. Eur J Cardiothorac Surg 2015;47:213–9.

18. Fennelly J, Potter L, Pompili C, et al. Performance in the shuttle walk test is associated with cardiopulmonary complications after lung resections. J Thorac Dis 2017;9(3):789–95.

19. Brunelli A, Xiume F, Refai M, et al. Peak oxygen consumption measured during the stair-climbing test in lung resection candidates. Respiration 2010;80(3): 207–11.

20. Bolliger CT, Jordan P, Solèr M, et al. Exercise capacity as a predictor of postoperative complications in lung resection candidates. Am J Respir Crit Care Med 1995;151:1472–80.

21. Brunelli A, Belardinelli R, Refai M, et al. Peak oxygen consumption during cardiopulmonary exercise test improves risk stratification in candidates to major lung resection. Chest 2009;135:1260–7.

22. Brunelli A, Belardinelli R, Pompili C, et al. Minute ventilation-to-carbon dioxide output (V_E/V_{CO2}) slope is the strongest predictor of respiratory complications and death after pulmonary resection. Ann Thorac Surg 2012;93:1802–6.

23. Shafiek H, Valera JL, Togores B, et al. Risk of postoperative complications in chronic obstructive lung disease patients considered fit for lung surgery: beyond oxygen consumption. Eur J Cardiothorac Surg 2016;50:772–9.

24. Salati M, Brunelli A. Risk stratification in lung resection. Curr Surg Rep 2016;4:37.

25. Ries AL, Make BJ, Lee SM, et al. The effects of pulmonary rehabilitation in the national emphysema treatment trial. Chest 2005;128:3799–809.

26. Weinstein H, Bates AT, Spaltro BE, et al. Influence of preoperative exercise capacity on length of stay after thoracic cancer surgery. Ann Thorac Surg 2007; 84:197–202.

27. Park S, Kim JY, Lee JC, et al. Mobile phone app-based pulmonary rehabilitation for chemotherapy-treated patients with advanced lung cancer: pilot study. JMIR Mhealth Uhealth 2019;7:e11094.

28. Salati M, Brunelli A, Decaluwe H, et al, ESTS DB Committee. Report from the European Society of Thoracic Surgeons Database 2017: patterns of care and perioperative outcomes of surgery for malignant lung neoplasm. Eur J Cardiothorac Surg 2017;52(6):1041–8.

29. Brunelli A, Cicconi S, Decaluwe H, et al. Parsimonious Eurolung risk models to predict cardiopulmonary morbidity and mortality following anatomic lung resections: an updated analysis from the European Society of Thoracic Surgeons database. Eur J Cardiothorac Surg 2020;57(3):455–61.

30. Brunelli A, Rocco G, Szanto Z, et al. Morbidity and mortality of lobectomy or pneumonectomy after neoadjuvant treatment: an analysis from the ESTS database. Eur J Cardiothorac Surg 2020;57(4):740–6.

31. Yendamuri S, Groman A, Miller A, et al. Risk and benefit of neoadjuvant therapy among patients undergoing resection for non-small-cell lung cancer. Eur J Cardiothorac Surg 2018;53(3):656–63.

32. Roberts JR, Eustis C, Devore R, et al. Induction chemotherapy increases perioperative complications in patients undergoing resection for non-small cell lung carcinoma. Ann Thorac Surg 2001;72:885–8.

33. Leo F, Pelosi G, Sonzogni A, et al. Structural lung damage after chemotherapy fact or fiction? Lung Cancer 2010;67(3):306–10.

34. Cerfolio RJ, Talati A, Bryant AS. Changes in pulmonary function tests after neoadjuvant therapy predict postoperative complications. Ann Thorac Surg 2009; 88(3):930–5.

35. Leo F, Solli P, Spaggiari L, et al. Respiratory function changes after chemotherapy: an additional risk for postoperative respiratory complications? Ann Thorac Surg 2004;77(1):260–5.

36. O'Sullivan KE, Kreaden US, Hebert AE, et al. A systematic review and meta-analysis of robotic versus open and video-assisted thoracoscopic surgery approaches for lobectomy. Interact Cardiovasc Thorac Surg 2019;28(4):526–34.

37. Paul S, Altorki NK, Sheng S, et al. Thoracoscopic lobectomy is associated with lower morbidity than open lobectomy: a propensity-matched analysis from the STS database. J Thorac Cardiovasc Surg 2010;139(2):366–78.

38. Falcoz PE, Puyraveau M, Thomas PA, et al, ESTS Database Committee and ESTS Minimally Invasive Interest Group. Video-assisted thoracoscopic surgery versus open lobectomy for primary non-small-cell lung cancer: a propensity-matched analysis of outcome from the European Society of Thoracic Surgeon database. Eur J Cardiothorac Surg 2016;49(2):602–9.

39. Burt BM, Kosinski AS, Shrager JB, et al. Thoracoscopic lobectomy is associated with acceptable morbidity and mortality in patients with predicted postoperative forced expiratory volume in 1 second or diffusing capacity for carbon monoxide less than 40% of normal. J Thorac Cardiovasc Surg 2014;148(1):19–28.

40. Hurria A, Naylor M, Cohen HJ. Improving the quality of cancer care in an aging population: recommendations from an IOM report. JAMA 2013;310(17):1795–6.

41. Scott WJ, Howington J, Feigenberg S, et al. Treatment of non-small cell lung cancer stage I and stage II: ACCP evidence-based clinical practice guidelines (2nd edition). Chest 2007;132(3 Suppl):234s–42s.

42. Louie AV, van Werkhoven E, Chen H, et al. Patient reported outcomes following stereotactic ablative radiotherapy or surgery for stage IA non-small-cell lung cancer: results from the ROSEL multicenter randomized trial. Radiother Oncol 2015; 117(1):44–8.

43. Pompili C, Franks KN, Brunelli A, et al. Patient reported outcomes following video assisted thoracoscopic (VATS) resection or stereotactic ablative body radiotherapy (SABR) for treatment of non-small cell lung cancer: protocol for an observational pilot study (LiLAC). J Thorac Dis 2017;9(8):2703–13.

44. Hopmans W, Damman OC, Senan S, et al. A patient perspective on shared decision making in stage I non-small cell lung cancer: a mixed methods study. BMC Cancer 2015;15(1):959.

45. Powell HA, Jones LL, Baldwin DR, et al. Patients' attitudes to risk in lung cancer surgery: a qualitative study. Lung Cancer 2015;90(2):358–63.

46. Chow H, Edelman MJ, Giaccone G, et al. Impact of an interactive on-line tool on therapeutic decision-making for patients with advanced non-small-cell lung cancer. J Thorac Oncol 2015;10(10):1421–9.

47. Oshima Lee E, Emanuel EJ. Shared decision making to improve care and reduce costs. N Engl J Med 2013;368(1):6–8.

48. Stacey D, Paquet L, Samant R. Exploring cancer treatment decision-making by patients: a descriptive study. Curr Oncol 2010;17(4):85–93.

49. Cykert S, Kissling G, Hansen CJ. Patient preferences regarding possible outcomes of lung resection: what outcomes should preoperative evaluations target? Chest 2000;117(6):1551–9.

50. Sullivan DR, Eden KB, Dieckmann NF, et al. Understanding patients' values and preferences regarding early stage lung cancer treatment decision making. Lung Cancer 2019;131:47–57.

51. Reyna VF, Nelson WL, Han PK, et al. How numeracy influences risk comprehension and medical decision making. Psychol Bull 2009;135(6):943–73.

52. van den Bergh KA, Essink-Bot ML, van Klaveren RJ, et al. Informed decision making does not affect health-related quality of life in lung cancer screening (NELSON trial). Eur J Cancer 2010;46(18):3300–6.

53. Ashraf AA, Colakoglu S, Nguyen JT, et al. Patient involvement in the decision-making process improves satisfaction and quality of life in postmastectomy breast reconstruction. J Surg Res 2013;184(1):665–70.

Lung Cancer Screening

Humberto K. Choi, MD, FCCP*, Peter J. Mazzone, MD, MPH, FCCP

KEYWORDS

- Lung cancer • Screening • Low radiation dose chest CT scans
- Smoking cessation interventions

KEY POINTS

- Lung cancer screening with low radiation dose chest computed tomography scans decreases lung cancer mortality.
- It is important to balance the benefits of screening with the potential harms, including evaluation of false-positive results, complications from diagnostic testing, overdiagnosis, and the impact of radiation exposure.
- Integration of smoking cessation interventions may augment the benefits of lung cancer screening.
- Widespread implementation and access to high-quality lung cancer screening programs remains a challenge.

INTRODUCTION

Lung cancer is the second most common cancer diagnosed in men and women, and is the leading cause of cancer-related deaths in the United States.[1] Early detection is an important strategy to try to modify these statistics, complementing public health strategies aimed at decreasing smoking rates. Screening with a low radiation dose chest computed tomography scan (LDCT) is performed to identify lung cancer in a preclinical or asymptomatic phase. The ultimate goal is to diagnose lung cancer at an earlier stage, where curative intent treatment is more successful, resulting in a decrease in lung cancer–specific mortality.

Several professional societies have endorsed lung cancer screening based on the results of the National Lung Screening Trial (NLST).[2] It remains the strongest evidence of reduced mortality from screening with LDCT. In 2013 the US Preventive Services Task Force (USPSTF) recommended annual screening for lung cancer with LDCT for adults between 55 and 80 years old who have a 30 pack-year smoking history and who currently smoke or have quit within the last 15 years.[3] In 2015, the Centers for Medicare and Medicaid Services (CMS) issued a decision requiring Medicare coverage of lung cancer screening for its beneficiaries.[4] Several lung cancer screening programs have been implemented nationwide and many lessons have been learned since then.

Respiratory Institute, Cleveland Clinic, 9500 Euclid Avenue, Cleveland, OH 44195, USA
* Corresponding author.
E-mail address: choih@ccf.org

Surg Oncol Clin N Am 29 (2020) 509–524
https://doi.org/10.1016/j.soc.2020.06.004
1055-3207/20/© 2020 Elsevier Inc. All rights reserved.

Lung cancer screening is a complex task. A multidisciplinary team is necessary to run a screening program. Screening involves appropriate patient selection, shared decision making, balancing benefits and potential harms, and the management of screen-detected lung nodules and other findings. In this article, we discuss the evidence that supports screening and the different considerations in developing a high-quality lung cancer screening program.

EVIDENCE THAT SUPPORTS LUNG CANCER SCREENING

Early lung cancer screening trials evaluated chest radiographs (CXR) and sputum cytology as screening tests. Despite finding improved survival for those with screen detected lung cancer, the trials failed to demonstrate a reduction in lung cancer specific mortality.[5–7] Improvements in computed tomography (CT) scanning techniques, leading to increased sensitivity to detect small lung cancers, raised the interest to evaluate LDCT scans as a lung cancer screening tool.

The Early Lung Cancer Action Project and other prospective cohort studies showed that LDCT was able to identify more lung nodules and more early stage lung cancers than CXR, but this study design did not allow for a comparison of lung cancer mortality.[8]

The NLST was the first randomized controlled trial to report a significant reduction in lung cancer mortality owing to screening.[2] Between 2002 and 2009, the NLST enrolled 53,456 individuals between the ages of 55 and 74. All had a history of smoking of at least 30 pack-years and were either current smokers or former smokers who had quit within the past 15 years. The trial compared LDCT (26,723) with CXR screening (26,733) with a baseline scan followed by 2 annual LDCT or CXR rounds with 6 to 7 years of follow-up. Data from 33 medical centers in the United States showed that 3 rounds of LDCT resulted in a 16% to 20% relative reduction in the rate of death owing to lung cancer. In the LDCT arm, there were 354 deaths from lung cancer, compared with 442 in the CXR arm. Based on these results, using the NLST protocol, 320 patients would need to undergo screening to prevent 1 death owing to lung cancer. The trial also showed a 6.7% decrease in all-cause mortality with LDCT screening (1877 deaths in the LDCT arm compared with 2000 deaths in the CXR arm).

Several other randomized, controlled trials evaluating LDCT screening for lung cancer have provided valuable insight about the effectiveness of the test as a screening method, and about the natural course of the disease (**Table 1**).[9–15] The largest trial among these, the Nederlands-Leuvens Longkanker Screening Onderzoek (NELSON) trial,[9] had a smaller sample size than the NLST, but a longer follow-up (10 years), no scheduled screening in the control arm, and it included screening rounds with different intervals. Another major difference in the management of pulmonary nodules between NELSON and NLST was the use of nodule volume and volume doubling time to identify potential cases of early lung cancer. The final mortality results were recently published and they confirmed the mortality decrease with CT screening seen in the NLST.[16] The incidence of lung cancer in the screening group and no screening group was 5.58 and 4.91 cases per 1000 person-years, respectively. Lung cancer mortality was lower in the screening group by 24%. The protective effect was more pronounced in women than in men. CT screening decreased mortality by 26% in high-risk men and 33% in high-risk women over a 10-year period.[16]

POTENTIAL HARMS

An estimated 8.4 million individuals met the eligibility criteria for lung cancer screening as proposed by the USPSTF in 2013.[17] The potential eligible population was older, had a higher proportion of current smokers, and had more comorbidities than the NLST

Table 1
Trials that evaluated CT scanning for lung cancer screening

	Country	Recruitment Period	Sample Size	Screening Method	Interval	Age, Years	Smoking History	Smoking Cessation
NLST	USA	2002–2004	53,454	LDCT vs CXR	3 annual screenings	55–74	≥30 pack-years	<15 y
NELSON	Netherlands/Belgium	2003–2006	15,822	LDCT vs usual care	4 screenings with different intervals: 1 y, 2 y, and 2.5 y	50–75	≥15 cigarettes per day for ≥25 y or ≥10 cigarettes per day for ≥30 y	≤10 y
DLCST	Denmark	2004–2006	4104	LDCT vs usual care	5 annual screenings	50–70	≥20 pack-years	≤10 y
MILD	Italy	2005–2011	4099	LDCT vs usual care	Annual and biennial for 5 y	≥49	≥20 pack-years	≤10 y
UKLS	UK	2011–2014	4055	LDCT vs usual care	Single screening LDCT	50–75	Predicted risk of lung cancer ≥5%	≤10 y
LUSI	Germany	2007–2011	4052	LDCT vs usual care	Annual screening for 5 y	50–69	≥15 cigarettes per day for ≥25 y or ≥10 cigarettes per day for ≥30 y	≤10 y
ITALUNG	Italy	2004–2006	3206	LDCT vs usual care	Annual screening for 4 y	55–69	≥20 pack-years	≤10 y
DANTE	Italy	2001–2006	2450	LDCT vs clinical review	Annual screening for 4 y	60–74	>20 pack-years	≤10 y

Data from Refs.[2,9–15]

population. This finding highlights the importance of balancing the benefits and potential harms of LDCT screening in clinical practice.[18] A clear understanding of the potential harms related to LDCT screening should be considered. Some of the major concerns are the identification of many benign lung nodules, the potential for overdiagnosis of lung cancer, complications related to diagnostic evaluation, and the potential impact of radiation exposure.

In the NLST, 96% of all positive results (defined as a lung nodule ≥4 mm in diameter) in the LDCT group were not cancer.[2] Approximately 20% of all surgical resections were performed in patients with screen-detected benign nodules. The frequency of death occurring within 2 months of a diagnostic evaluation of a detected finding was 8 per 10,000 individuals screened by LDCT and 5 per 10,000 individuals screened by CXR. Overall, the frequency of major complications occurring during a diagnostic evaluation of a detected finding was 33 per 10,000 individuals screened by LDCT and 10 per 10,000 individuals screened by CXR.[2,19]

This finding illustrates the importance of every screening program having strategies for lung nodule management that minimize potential complications from their evaluation.

Overdiagnosis is an intrinsic feature of screening, because screening will detect not just aggressive tumors, but also indolent tumors that otherwise may not be clinically significant. In addition, screening individuals with comorbidities (possibly related to age and smoking history) means that a portion of those screened will die of other causes before even a typical lung cancer would have impacted their lives. These overdiagnosed cases may result in additional cost, anxiety, and morbidity associated with treatment of a screen-detected cancer that otherwise would never have needed to be detected. Patz and colleagues[20] estimated that the probability that a lung cancer detected by LDCT screening was an overdiagnosed cancer was 18.5% overall, 22.5% if the cancer detected was a non-small cell lung carcinoma, and 79% if the histology was a noninvasive adenocarcinoma in the NLST. The number of cases of overdiagnosis found among 320 participants who would need to be screened in the NLST to prevent 1 death from lung cancer was 1.38.[20]

Although there is variation in clinical practice, the effective dose of radiation of an LDCT is estimated to be 1.5 mSv per scan, which is 3 to 4 times lower than a diagnostic CT scan.[21] Estimates of the impact of cumulative radiation exposure have varied greatly. At one extreme, it was estimated that 1 in 2500 patients screened may die of radiation-related malignancy from the cumulative radiation received during screening.[19] The radiation risk may only manifest many years later and, thus, it may be less relevant for older individuals than it is for younger individuals or those with a lower risk of developing lung cancer.

IMPLEMENTATION OF SCREENING PROGRAMS

In December 2013, the USPSTF released a grade B recommendation to screen high-risk individuals, defined as those age 55 to 80 who have a minimum smoking history of 30 pack-years and who currently smoke or have quit within the past 15 years.[3] The Affordable Care Act (ACA) required that commercial insurance plans participating in the health care exchange cover screening services that receive a grade B recommendation from the USPSTF, guaranteeing coverage to insured patients younger than 65 years of age. The CMS released a decision to cover CT screening for Medicare beneficiaries who are age 55 to 77 and have the same minimum smoking history required by the USPSTF.[4] These policies minimized concern about insurance coverage becoming a barrier for screening implementation.

The adoption of lung cancer screening in the United States is growing, but remains low.[22,23] It is estimated that approximately 3.9% of 6.8 million eligible smokers were screened in 2015 according to the National Health Interview Survey.[22] It should be noted that this survey was conducted the same year as CMS approval, and current evidence suggests a substantial growth in screening program numbers and capacity. Despite this, the majority of those eligible are still not being screened. The reasons for the low adoption rate are not clear. Possible explanations include a lack of awareness, challenges related to how to best incorporate mandatory shared decision making into patient visits, uncertainty about the best approach to integrate effective treatment for tobacco dependence, and barriers related to the stigma of smoking and lung cancer itself.

Another possible reason is a lack of resources. The distribution of screening programs varies significantly across states. Kale and colleagues[23] analyzed the geographic variation of lung cancer screening facilities that are in the national registry, which is a requirement for reimbursement by CMS. They reported a cluster of states (Alabama, Arkansas, Georgia, Kentucky, Louisiana, Missouri, Mississippi, North Carolina, Oklahoma, South Carolina, Tennessee, and West Virginia) that had the highest lung cancer burden but the lowest number of screening programs. There is insufficient evidence to conclude that cost sharing or a lack of insurance coverage are causes of this disparity. However, 8 of those 12 states have not expanded Medicaid. It is not known whether the uptake of lung cancer screening in states with Medicaid expansion, as a part of the ACA implementation, is different than in nonexpansion states, but a lack of insurance coverage might contribute to the lower number of screening programs.

It is well-known that individuals of lower socioeconomic groups are less likely to receive cancer preventive services. The elimination of out-of-pocket expenses has helped to decrease this disparity, as seen in other cancer screenings, such as mammography for breast cancer.[24,25] There was a significant increase in screening mammography uptake after implementation of the ACA. The same trend was not consistently seen with colonoscopy; the uptake has been overall stagnant after ACA.[24] This difference suggests that the elimination of cost sharing is not sufficient to facilitate access to cancer prevention services. Although not sufficient, affordability is important for lung cancer screening uptake. Among respondents to the National Health Interview Survey in 2010 and 2015, more than 50% of smokers meeting criteria based on USPSTF recommendations for screening were uninsured or Medicaid insured.[22]

The implementation of a high-quality lung cancer screening program is complex. It requires the development of a broad infrastructure to meet regulatory mandates and clinical demands. Some of the aspects involved in a lung cancer screening program include patient selection, shared decision making, management of screen detected nodules, integration of smoking cessation interventions, and management of incidental findings.

Patient Selection

Several professional societies have endorsed lung cancer screening with LDCT (**Table 2**). The American College of Chest Physicians recommends screening similar to the entry criteria for the NLST: age of 55 to 77 years with at least a 30 pack-year smoking history who are current smokers or who quit within 15 years.[26] Other societies including the National Comprehensive Cancer Network and the American Association for Thoracic Surgery expanded the recommendations to include other risk factors such as environmental exposures.[27,28] For example, the American Association for Thoracic Surgery endorses LDCT screening for those ages 55 to 79 years with a 30 pack-year history of smoking; those ages 55 to 79 years with 20 a pack-year history of smoking

Table 2
USPSTF, CMS, and different profession societies recommendation regarding lung cancer screening

	Age, Years	Smoking History	Smoking Cessation	Interval	Other Recommendations
USPSTF (2013)	55–80	≥30 pack-years	<15 y	Annual	No conditions that substantially limit life expectancy
CMS (2014)	55–77	≥30 pack-years	<15 y	Annual	Shared decision making visit required.
ACCP (2018)	55–77	≥30 pack-years	<15 y	Annual	–
NCCN (2019)	55–74	≥30 pack-years	<15 y	Annual	20 pack-years, age >50, and additional risk factors
ACS (2013)	55–74	≥30 pack-years	<15 y	Annual	
AATS (2012)		≥30 pack-years		Annual	20 pack-years, age >50 y, and risk ≥5% over 5 y

Abbreviations: AATS, American Association for Thoracic Surgery; ACCP, American College of Chest Physicians; ACS, American Cancer Society; ASCO, American Society of Clinical Oncology; CMS, Center for Medicaid & Medicare Services; NCCN, National Comprehensive Cancer Network; USPSTF, United States Preventative Services Task Force.
Data from Refs.[3,4,26–28,63]

and additional comorbidities that increase the risk for lung cancer by more than 5% over 5 years; or for long-term survivors of lung cancer.[28] At the time of this writing the USPSTF has released a draft statement for public comment that would lead to an expanded pool (ages 50 to 80 years who have a 20 pack-year smoking history).

Other investigators have proposed the use of risk prediction models to select patients for screening. Two of the models that have been studied for this purpose are the Prostate, Lung, Colorectal and Ovarian Cancer Screening Trial (PLCO) 2012 model and the modified Liverpool Lung Project models (LLPv2).[15,29] Understandably, the intention of expanding the screening eligibility criteria beyond the NLST entry criteria is to find other high-risk individuals who may benefit from screening, increasing the portion of all lung cancers that could be screen detected. Patient selection using these tools have not been assessed in randomized trials. The concern with screening populations at a lower risk for lung cancer than reflected by current eligibility criteria is that we would need to screen a greater number of individuals to prevent 1 death from lung cancer, and the balance of benefits and harms may be disrupted. The concern with screening other high-risk individuals, identified through the use of a risk calculator, is that the other risk factors included in these models, such as age, the presence of emphysema or a prior cancer, modify not just the risk of developing lung cancer, but the risk of finding a lung nodule, having a complication from evaluation of a lung nodule, and the success of early lung cancer treatment. Furthermore, the implementation of risk calculator–guided screening enrollment is more complex than current eligibility criteria.

It is important for those participating in lung cancer screening to be in good enough health to be able to tolerate the evaluation and treatment of screen-detected findings for screening to be effective. In the NLST, only 2% of patients diagnosed with stage I lung cancer were treated with radiation only, which indicates that the majority of these patients were healthy enough to tolerate surgery.[2] An analysis of the screening-eligible population in the United States showed that they were older, more likely to be current smokers and to have comorbidities, and had a lower survival rate and life expectancy compared with the NLST cohort.[18] This finding suggests that the general population is more likely to have competing causes of death other than lung cancer, and comorbid conditions that could modify the benefit of screening. Unless an individual has an obvious severe, life-limiting condition, it is challenging to determine who is not well enough to participate in LDCT screening.

Shared Decision Making

The CMS has mandated a lung cancer screening counseling and shared decision-making visit before the screening examination to receive payment.[4] The purpose of the visit is to provide patients with the information and support they need to make value-based individualized decisions about whether to be screened. The shared decision-making visit is an opportunity for individuals to learn about their risk for developing lung cancer, and the benefits and potential harms of screening so that they can make informed choices that are consistent with their expectations and values.

The most effective method to conduct a shared decision-making visit has not been determined. The CMS requires that it occurs during an in-person visit with a physician, advanced practice provider, or clinical nurse specialist.[4] Regardless of the health care professionals who are conducting it, they should be well-versed and comfortable discussing the risks, benefit, and the trade-offs as they are influenced by personal risk and comorbidities. This need puts primary care providers at a disadvantage because they may not be comfortable enough, or have time, to provide a comprehensive shared decision-making visit. Decision aids and risk prediction tools are effective ways to communicate complex topics to patients. They have been shown to increase understanding and improve the comfort with decision making.[30]

At the Cleveland Clinic, we developed a centralized counseling and shared decision-making visit for our lung cancer screening program. The visit begins with a review of patient eligibility for screening. Patients then watch a 6-minute narrated video that was developed by our program. It is followed by a discussion of the individual risk of developing lung cancer with the use of an on-line decision aid (www.shouldiscreen.com/), and an opportunity for questions to be answered and additional clinical data to be collected. During the visit, the expected results are discussed (ie, a high probability of finding a lung nodule), as is the importance of compliance with annual follow-up and recommendations for evaluating screen-detected findings. We studied the impact of this visit on patient knowledge and comfort with the screening decision, and there was a significant improvement in both as measured by a previsit and postvisit questionnaire.[31]

Management of Screen-Detected Lung Nodules

Based on consensus, the American College of Radiology developed a reporting system called the Lung CT Screening Reporting and Data System (Lung-RADS), which is similar to the Breast Imaging Reporting and Data System used for mammography reporting.[32,33] Lung-RADS is a tool designed to standardize lung cancer screening CT reporting and management recommendations to facilitate results interpretation and outcome monitoring. The classification couples a category of risk of lung cancer in a detected nodule with management recommendations, largely based on the nodule size, attenuation, and change over time. **Table 3** describes the criteria for

Table 3
Examples of lung-RADS categories 2, 3 and 4 A/B

Lung-RADS	Lung Nodule Description (Average Size)	Lung-RADS Recommendation	Management Chosen	Comment
2	Right upper lobe 4.7 mm	Continue annual screening with LDCT in 12 mo	Annual screening	Nodule remained stable. Patient continued with annual screening.
3	Left upper lobe 6.4 mm	6 mo LDCT	6 mo LDCT	Nodule increased in size in 6 mo to average size of 8 mm. Upgraded to a Lung-RADS category 4B. Patient had left upper lobectomy for NSCLC.

4A	 Left upper lobe 9.7 mm	3 mo LDCT; PET/CT may be used when there is a ≥ 8 mm (≥ 268 mm^3) solid component	3 mo LDCT	Nodule remained stable in 3 mo received Lung-RADS category 2. Review of prior scans that were initially missed revealed that the nodule had remained stable for 2 y.
4 B	 Right lower lobe part solid 23 mm	Chest CT scan with or without contrast, PET/CT scan and/or tissue sampling depending on the probability of malignancy and comorbidities. PET/CT scan may be used when there is a ≥ 8 mm (≥ 268 mm^3) solid component.	Percutaneous biopsy	NSLC confirmed. Patient was treated with stereotactic ablative therapy owing to poor lung function.

Abbreviations: NSCLC, non-small cell lung cancer; PET, positron emission tomography.

defining Lung-RADS categories. It is the structured reporting system required for data entry into the only CMS-approved lung cancer screening registry.

In the NLST, the false-positive rate in the trial was 27.3%. Small nodules in the size range of 4 to 6 mm accounted for more than one-half of all positive screens across all 3 screening time points and were found to be malignant less than 1% of the time.[2] Lung-RADS increased the size threshold for a positive result from a 4-mm to a 6-mm transverse average. This effort aimed to decrease the false-positive rate at the expense of a small compromise of test sensitivity. Raising the threshold for a positive result to 6-mm would decrease the baseline NLST positive rate to approximately 13.4%.[2] In a study by Pinsky and colleagues,[34] when the authors applied Lung-RADS to the NLST group at baseline, the false-positive rate decreased from 26.6% to 12.8% and the baseline sensitivity decreased from 93.5% to 84.9%.

Small and low-risk nodules that are screen detected can be followed with an annual (category 2) or a 6-month (category 3) surveillance LDCT. The management of higher risk nodules, Lung-RADS category 4, is more challenging. Recommendations from Lung-RADS include short-term follow-up, PET scan, biopsy, or surgery.[32] Although Lung-RADS assigns a general lung cancer risk for a specific category, individual assessment of the malignancy risk is an important initial step for decision making for category 4 nodules. Malignancy risk estimation can be performed subjectively with intuition and clinical experience, or by using validated clinical prediction models. Several validated risk prediction models are available. It is important to recognize that they are most accurate when applied to individuals from populations similar to those in which they were developed. In the lung cancer screening setting, the Brock model is likely the best fit.

The Brock model was developed from the Pan-Canadian Early Detection of Lung Cancer Study (PanCan; a low-dose CT screening study), and validated on participants in cancer chemoprevention studies at the British Columbia Cancer Agency.[35] A parsimonious and a fuller model were developed from multivariable logistic regression, including known risk factors for malignant lung nodules. The variables included in the final model were age, sex, family history of lung cancer, presence of emphysema, nodule size, location of the nodule in the upper lobe, nodule attenuation on the CT scan, nodule count, and spiculated nodule border. The model showed excellent discrimination with an area under the curve of more than 0.90. Important strengths of this model are the analysis of single or multiple lung nodules and the inclusion of nodule attenuation as a variable. Although it was derived from a lung cancer screening population, it has been validated in populations with incidental nodules.[36]

Surgical lung resection is the main curative intent treatment for early stage lung cancer. Therefore, thoracic surgeons are key components of the multidisciplinary team. Lobectomy with mediastinal lymph node evaluation remains the standard in the treatment of early stage NSCLC. The minimally invasive approach with video-assisted thoracoscopy has been associated with lower morbidity, including decreased perioperative pain, less blood loss, and a shorter hospital length of stay.[37–39] Sublobar resections can be considered in patients with limited lung function or small primary tumors. The advantage of sublobar resection in high-risk patients are a lower perioperative morbidity and mortality, as well as preservation of lung function.[40,41] Segmentectomy is preferred over a wedge resection when a nodule is known to be malignant. Segmentectomy includes dissection of the bronchial tree exposing lymph nodes that are not visualized during a wedge resection, and surgical margins or more than 1 cm are more likely to be achieved.[42–44] Multiple case series have demonstrated equivalent regional recurrence rates and survival, particular in patients with tumors less than 2 cm in diameter and in elderly patients (age >75 years).[45–47] Localization techniques such as fiducial placement, labeling, and marking techniques can be used to facilitate resection of subcentimeter solid nodules deep in location, and nodules that are subsolid in attenuation that can be difficult to find by digital palpation.[48–50]

As discussed elsewhere in this article, one of the major concerns of lung cancer screening is overdiagnosis. Subsolid nodules should be managed differently than solid nodules because of their indolent behavior. A persistent subsolid nodule may be due to focal fibrosis or may represent a lesion in the spectrum of adenocarcinoma, from noninvasive atypical adenomatous hyperplasia to invasive adenocarcinoma. The prevalence of malignancy is relatively high and depends on the nodule size as well as the presence of a solid component on imaging.[51] The solid component represents the invasive foci of adenocarcinomas and it helps determine the management plan. For example, a persistent part solid nodule with solid components 8 mm or greater would be classified as Lung-RADS 4B (suspicious) and the recommendation would include consideration for a diagnostic CT scan, PET scan, or biopsy.[32] In contrast, a ground glass nodule that measures 20 mm with no solid component would be classified as Lung-RADS 2 and would be recommended to continue annual screening. Subsolid nodules typically do not require immediate resection because of their indolent behavior despite the relatively high risk of malignancy in these nodules. Supporting the conservative approach to subsolid nodules, Yankelevitz and colleagues[52] showed in a large-scale screening study that adenocarcinomas presenting as pure ground-glass nodules had an excellent prognosis with overall survival rate of 100% regardless of the time to treatment.

Integration of Smoking Cessation Interventions

Cigarette smoking is the major risk factor for lung cancer.[53] The importance of smoking cessation in the setting of lung cancer screening cannot be understated. Screening is not an alternative to smoking cessation. Rather, lung cancer screening is seen as a teachable moment for smoking cessation interventions. Every smoker should be encouraged to quit and be offered evidence-based treatment at every screening visit. It is an essential component of a screening program.[54] The integration of smoking cessation into screening programs maximizes the clinical benefit of lung cancer screening and its cost effectiveness. Tanner and colleagues[55] analyzed the effects of smoking abstinence among the individuals who participated in the NLST. The study showed that former smokers in the control arm of the NLST who were abstinent for 7 years had a 20% mortality reduction compared with active smokers, which is comparable with the benefit seen from LDCT screening. The maximum benefit was seen with the combination of smoking abstinence at 15 years and LDCT screening, which resulted in a 38% decrease in lung cancer-specific mortality.[55] Furthermore, Villanti and colleagues[56] developed a simulation model to estimate the cost-utility of annual LDCT over 15 years. The simulation showed that the addition of smoking cessation to annual screening with LDCT improved the cost effectiveness of screening between 20% and 45%. Smoking cessation resulted in increases in both the costs and quality-adjusted life years saved, reflected in cost utility rations ranging from $16,198 per quality-adjusted life years gained to $23,185 per quality-adjusted life years gained.[56]

The most effective smoking cessation intervention in the screening setting has not been determined. However, the methods applied should not be passive. Undergoing screening alone has not been shown to be enough to modify smoking behavior, but it seems that patients with abnormal findings were more likely to quit than those with normal results.[57,58] Low-intensity interventions such as providing written educational materials or brief counseling have not made a significant impact on smoking behavior.[59] A combination of counseling, behavioral, and pharmacologic treatment is most effective, but research is needed to determine if specific interventions are

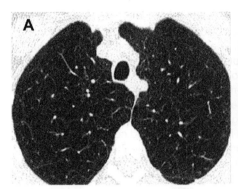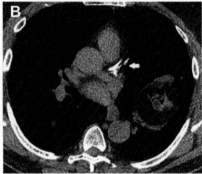

Fig. 1. Examples of pulmonary and cardiac incidental findings. (*A*) Moderate upper lobe emphysema, (*B*) Severe coronary calcification: left anterior descending (*white arrow*).

more effective for this specific group of smokers.[60] While we study the optimal timing and methods for smoking cessation interventions, it is important for screening programs to integrate their own smoking cessation resources or make referrals to established programs.

Management of Incidental Findings

Pulmonary and extrapulmonary incidental findings are common on screening LDCT.[61] In a systematic review, 14% of scans had findings that merited some form of additional evaluation.[62] The prevalence depends on how incidental findings are defined and each program's threshold to report them. We recently published our experience with incidental findings and reported every finding described by our radiologists.[61] Our study revealed that incidental findings were present in 94% of the patients screened. The most frequently reported findings were in the respiratory and cardiovascular systems (**Fig. 1**). Most findings were not felt to be actionable. Approximately 15% lead to referral to subspecialty consultants and 13% had further evaluation with testing. Serious diagnoses were found including severe coronary artery disease requiring intervention, and extrapulmonary malignancies. The evaluation of incidental findings had a significant impact on reimbursement generated by the screening program. Because incidental findings on LDCT sans are common and their impact may be significant, they should be discussed during the shared decision-making visit, and screening programs should be prepared to manage them according to their own resources.

FUTURE DIRECTIONS

Many lessons have been learned since the early stages of implementation of lung cancer screening programs. Likewise, many questions and challenges remain. The major concerns are related to how to improve patient selection for screening, how to minimize the potential harms, and how to facilitate implementation and access to screening programs. Eligibility based on age and smoking history has the advantage of its simplicity, but risk-based strategies using validated models may be able to expand screening eligibility to include other healthy high-risk individuals and assist with determining the interval between scans. Advances in molecular biomarker testing and computer-assisted image interpretation may improve the accuracy of patient selection and lung nodule management with the potential to minimize harms related to the evaluation of benign nodules. We also need to further our understanding of the reasons for the overall low uptake of lung cancer screening in the United States. Additional research and health policy evolution with a focus on access to preventive services and smoking cessation in disadvantaged populations will be necessary to optimize the impact of this life-saving tool.

REFERENCES

1. Siegel RL, Miller KD, Jemal A. Cancer statistics, 2019. CA Cancer J Clin 2019; 69:7–34.
2. National Lung Screening Trial Research Team, Aberle DR, Adams AM, et al. Reduced lung-cancer mortality with low-dose computed tomographic screening. N Engl J Med 2011;365:395–409.
3. Moyer VA, U.S. Preventive Services Task Force. Screening for lung cancer: U.S. Preventive Services Task Force recommendation statement. Ann Intern Med 2014;160:330–8.
4. Decision memo for screening for lung cancer with low dose computed tomography (LDCT). Available at: https://www.cms.gov/medicare-coverage-database/details/nca-decision-memo.aspx?NCAId=274. Accessed April 1, 2020.
5. Brett GZ. The value of lung cancer detection by six-monthly chest radiographs. Thorax 1968;23:414–20.
6. Fontana RS, Sanderson DR, Taylor WF, et al. Early lung cancer detection: results of the initial (prevalence) radiologic and cytologic screening in the Mayo Clinic study. Am Rev Respir Dis 1984;130:561–5.
7. Melamed MR, Flehinger BJ, Zaman MB, et al. Screening for early lung cancer. Results of the Memorial Sloan-Kettering study in New York. Chest 1984;86:44–53.
8. Henschke CI, McCauley DI, Yankelevitz DF, et al. Early Lung Cancer Action Project: overall design and findings from baseline screening. Lancet 1999;354: 99–105.
9. van Klaveren RJ, Oudkerk M, Prokop M, et al. Management of lung nodules detected by volume CT scanning. N Engl J Med 2009;361:2221–9.
10. Sverzellati N, Silva M, Calareso G, et al. Low-dose computed tomography for lung cancer screening: comparison of performance between annual and biennial screen. Eur Radiol 2016;26:3821–9.
11. Paci E, Puliti D, Lopes Pegna A, et al. Mortality, survival and incidence rates in the ITALUNG randomised lung cancer screening trial. Thorax 2017;72:825–31.
12. Infante M, Cavuto S, Lutman FR, et al. Long-term follow-up results of the DANTE Trial, a randomized study of lung cancer screening with spiral computed tomography. Am J Respir Crit Care Med 2015;191:1166–75.
13. Wille MM, Dirksen A, Ashraf H, et al. Results of the randomized Danish Lung Cancer Screening Trial with focus on high-risk profiling. Am J Respir Crit Care Med 2016;193:542–51.
14. Becker N, Motsch E, Gross ML, et al. Randomized Study on Early Detection of Lung Cancer with MSCT in Germany: results of the first 3 years of follow-up after randomization. J Thorac Oncol 2015;10:890–6.
15. Field JK, Duffy SW, Baldwin DR, et al. The UK Lung Cancer Screening Trial: a pilot randomised controlled trial of low-dose computed tomography screening for the early detection of lung cancer. Health Technol Assess 2016;20:1–146.
16. de Koning HJ, van der Aalst CM, de Jong PA, et al. Reduced lung-cancer mortality with volume CT screening in a randomized trial. N Engl J Med 2020;382: 503–13.

17. Ma J, Ward EM, Smith R, et al. Annual number of lung cancer deaths potentially avertable by screening in the United States. Cancer 2013;119:1381–5.
18. Howard DH, Richards TB, Bach PB, et al. Comorbidities, smoking status, and life expectancy among individuals eligible for lung cancer screening. Cancer 2015; 121:4341–7.
19. Bach PB, Mirkin JN, Oliver TK, et al. Benefits and harms of CT screening for lung cancer: a systematic review. JAMA 2012;307:2418–29.
20. Patz EF Jr, Pinsky P, Gatsonis C, et al. Overdiagnosis in low-dose computed tomography screening for lung cancer. JAMA Intern Med 2014;174:269–74.
21. Mettler FA Jr, Huda W, Yoshizumi TT, et al. Effective doses in radiology and diagnostic nuclear medicine: a catalog. Radiology 2008;248:254–63.
22. Jemal A, Fedewa SA. Lung cancer screening with low-dose computed tomography in the United States-2010 to 2015. JAMA Oncol 2017;3:1278–81.
23. Kale MS, Wisnivesky J, Taioli E, et al. The Landscape of US Lung Cancer Screening Services. Chest 2019;155:900–7.
24. Cooper GS, Kou TD, Dor A, et al. Cancer preventive services, socioeconomic status, and the Affordable Care Act. Cancer 2017;123:1585–9.
25. Trivedi AN, Leyva B, Lee Y, et al. Elimination of cost sharing for screening mammography in Medicare advantage plans. N Engl J Med 2018;378:262–9.
26. Mazzone PJ, Silvestri GA, Patel S, et al. Screening for lung cancer: CHEST guideline and expert panel report. Chest 2018;153:954–85.
27. Wood DE, Kazerooni EA, Baum SL, et al. Lung Cancer Screening, Version 3.2018, NCCN clinical practice guidelines in oncology. J Natl Compr Canc Netw 2018;16:412–41.
28. Jaklitsch MT, Jacobson FL, Austin JH, et al. The American Association for Thoracic Surgery guidelines for lung cancer screening using low-dose computed tomography scans for lung cancer survivors and other high-risk groups. J Thorac Cardiovasc Surg 2012;144:33–8.
29. Tammemagi MC, Katki HA, Hocking WG, et al. Selection criteria for lung-cancer screening. N Engl J Med 2013;368:728–36.
30. Wiener RS, Gould MK, Arenberg DA, et al. Practice AACoL-DCLCSiC. An official American Thoracic Society/American College of Chest Physicians policy statement: implementation of low-dose computed tomography lung cancer screening programs in clinical practice. Am J Respir Crit Care Med 2015;192:881–91.
31. Mazzone PJ, Tenenbaum A, Seeley M, et al. Impact of a lung cancer screening counseling and shared decision-making visit. Chest 2017;151:572–8.
32. Lung CT Screening Reporting & Data System (Lung-RADS). Available at: https://www.acr.org/Clinical-Resources/Reporting-and-Data-Systems/Lung-Rads. Accessed April 1, 2020.
33. D'Orsi CJ, Kopans DB. Mammography interpretation: the BI-RADS method. Am Fam Physician 1997;55:1548–50, 1552.
34. Pinsky PF, Gierada DS, Black W, et al. Performance of Lung-RADS in the National Lung Screening Trial: a retrospective assessment. Ann Intern Med 2015;162: 485–91.
35. McWilliams A, Tammemagi MC, Mayo JR, et al. Probability of cancer in pulmonary nodules detected on first screening CT. N Engl J Med 2013;369:910–9.
36. Choi HK, Ghobrial M, Mazzone PJ. Models to estimate the probability of malignancy in patients with pulmonary nodules. Ann Am Thorac Soc 2018;15:1117–26.
37. Cattaneo SM, Park BJ, Wilton AS, et al. Use of video-assisted thoracic surgery for lobectomy in the elderly results in fewer complications. Ann Thorac Surg 2008;85: 231–5 [discussion: 235–6].

38. Flores RM, Park BJ, Dycoco J, et al. Lobectomy by video-assisted thoracic surgery (VATS) versus thoracotomy for lung cancer. J Thorac Cardiovasc Surg 2009;138:11–8.

39. Port JL, Mirza FM, Lee PC, et al. Lobectomy in octogenarians with non-small cell lung cancer: ramifications of increasing life expectancy and the benefits of minimally invasive surgery. Ann Thorac Surg 2011;92:1951–7.

40. Jensik RJ, Faber LP, Milloy FJ, et al. Segmental resection for lung cancer. A fifteen-year experience. J Thorac Cardiovasc Surg 1973;66:563–72.

41. Keenan RJ, Landreneau RJ, Maley RH Jr, et al. Segmental resection spares pulmonary function in patients with stage I lung cancer. Ann Thorac Surg 2004;78: 228–33 [discussion: 228–33].

42. Sienel W, Dango S, Kirschbaum A, et al. Sublobar resections in stage IA non-small cell lung cancer: segmentectomies result in significantly better cancer-related survival than wedge resections. Eur J Cardiothorac Surg 2008;33:728–34.

43. El-Sherif A, Fernando HC, Santos R, et al. Margin and local recurrence after sublobar resection of non-small cell lung cancer. Ann Surg Oncol 2007;14:2400–5.

44. Kent M, Landreneau R, Mandrekar S, et al. Segmentectomy versus wedge resection for non-small cell lung cancer in high-risk operable patients. Ann Thorac Surg 2013;96:1747–54 [discussion: 1754–5].

45. Landreneau RJ, Sugarbaker DJ, Mack MJ, et al. Wedge resection versus lobectomy for stage I (T1 N0 M0) non-small-cell lung cancer. J Thorac Cardiovasc Surg 1997;113:691–8 [discussion: 698–700].

46. Koike T, Yamato Y, Yoshiya K, et al. Intentional limited pulmonary resection for peripheral T1 N0 M0 small-sized lung cancer. J Thorac Cardiovasc Surg 2003;125: 924–8.

47. Kilic A, Schuchert MJ, Pettiford BL, et al. Anatomic segmentectomy for stage I non-small cell lung cancer in the elderly. Ann Thorac Surg 2009;87:1662–6 [discussion: 1667–8].

48. Bertolaccini L, Terzi A, Spada E, et al. Not palpable? Role of radio-guided video-assisted thoracic surgery for nonpalpable solitary pulmonary nodules. Gen Thorac Cardiovasc Surg 2012;60:280–4.

49. Zaman M, Bilal H, Woo CY, et al. In patients undergoing video-assisted thoracoscopic surgery excision, what is the best way to locate a subcentimetre solitary pulmonary nodule in order to achieve successful excision? Interact Cardiovasc Thorac Surg 2012;15:266–72.

50. Sancheti MS, Lee R, Ahmed SU, et al. Percutaneous fiducial localization for thoracoscopic wedge resection of small pulmonary nodules. Ann Thorac Surg 2014; 97:1914–8 [discussion: 1919].

51. Detterbeck FC, Homer RJ. Approach to the ground-glass nodule. Clin Chest Med 2011;32:799–810.

52. Yankelevitz DF, Yip R, Smith JP, et al, International Early Lung Cancer Action Program Investigators Group. CT screening for lung cancer: nonsolid nodules in baseline and annual repeat rounds. Radiology 2015;277:555–64.

53. Malhotra J, Malvezzi M, Negri E, et al. Risk factors for lung cancer worldwide. Eur Respir J 2016;48:889–902.

54. Fucito LM, Czabafy S, Hendricks PS, et al, Association for the Treatment of Tobacco Use and Dependence/Society for Research on Nicotine and Tobacco Synergy Committee. Pairing smoking-cessation services with lung cancer screening: a clinical guideline from the Association for the Treatment of Tobacco Use and Dependence and the Society for Research on Nicotine and Tobacco. Cancer 2016;122:1150–9.

55. Tanner NT, Kanodra NM, Gebregziabher M, et al. The association between smoking abstinence and mortality in the National Lung Screening Trial. Am J Respir Crit Care Med 2016;193:534–41.

56. Villanti AC, Jiang Y, Abrams DB, et al. A cost-utility analysis of lung cancer screening and the additional benefits of incorporating smoking cessation interventions. PLoS One 2013;8:e71379.

57. Slatore CG, Baumann C, Pappas M, et al. Smoking behaviors among patients receiving computed tomography for lung cancer screening. Systematic review in support of the U.S. preventive services task force. Ann Am Thorac Soc 2014;11:619–27.

58. Tammemagi MC, Berg CD, Riley TL, et al. Impact of lung cancer screening results on smoking cessation. J Natl Cancer Inst 2014;106:dju084.

59. Iaccarino JM, Duran C, Slatore CG, et al. Combining smoking cessation interventions with LDCT lung cancer screening: a systematic review. Prev Med 2019;121: 24–32.

60. Lemmens V, Oenema A, Knut IK, et al. Effectiveness of smoking cessation interventions among adults: a systematic review of reviews. Eur J Cancer Prev 2008; 17:535–44.

61. Morgan L, Choi H, Reid M, et al. Frequency of incidental findings and subsequent evaluation in low-dose computed tomographic scans for lung cancer screening. Ann Am Thorac Soc 2017;14:1450–6.

62. Kucharczyk MJ, Menezes RJ, McGregor A, et al. Assessing the impact of incidental findings in a lung cancer screening study by using low-dose computed tomography. Can Assoc Radiol J 2011;62:141–5.

63. Wender R, Fontham ET, Barrera E Jr, et al. American Cancer Society lung cancer screening guidelines. CA Cancer J Clin 2013;63:107–17.

Intraoperative Detection and Assessment of Lung Nodules

Feredun Azari, MD[a],*,[1], Greg Kennedy, MD[a],[1], Sunil Singhal, MD[b]

KEYWORDS

- SPN • Intraoperative imaging • CT-guided biopsy • EBUS • Technetium 99 • VATS
- Indocyanine green

KEY POINTS

- R0 resection is key in lung cancer management, R1 resection patients have overall worse survival prognosis versus R0 resection.
- Preoperative nodule localization techniques include wire placement, dye marking, ultrasound examination, fluoroscopy, and intraoperative molecular imaging.
- Currently, there are limited methods of intraoperative margin assessment other than vigorous inspection using vision and palpation.
- Minimally invasive approaches can provide accurate assessment of primary tumors, mediastinal lymph node involvement, and pleural involvement.
- Folate-targeted dye detection of retained tumor cells after pulmonary adenocarcinoma is an emerging technique with the potential of transforming of intraoperative margin assessment.

INTRODUCTION

Lung cancer is the leading cause of cancer death among both men and women in the United States. It is also the leading cause of cancer death among men and the second leading cause of cancer death among women worldwide.[1] In the United States, it accounts for more cancer deaths than colon, prostate, and breast cancers combined.[2] Factors contributing to the lethality and increased mortality are grounded on asymptomatic nature of the disease leading to late detection and increased disease burden at the time of diagnosis. Although recent advances in immunotherapy and other

[a] Department of Surgery, Hospital of the University of Pennsylvania, 3400 Spruce Street, 6 White Building, Philadelphia, PA 19104, USA; [b] Department of Surgery, Division of Thoracic Surgery, University of Pennsylvania, Perelman School of Medicine, Hospital of the University of Pennsylvania, 3400 Spruce Street, 6 White Building, Philadelphia, PA 19104, USA
[1] Authors have contributed equally.
* Corresponding author.
E-mail address: Feredun.Azari@pennmedicine.upenn.edu

Surg Oncol Clin N Am 29 (2020) 525–541
https://doi.org/10.1016/j.soc.2020.06.006
1055-3207/20/© 2020 Elsevier Inc. All rights reserved.
surgonc.theclinics.com

systemic therapies have been encouraging, the 5-year survival for all comers have remained humbling at less than 20%.[2]

Given the ever-increasing prevalence and incidence of this disease, various national and international societies have implemented lung cancer screening guidelines based on current evidence. Although there have been considerable debate in the literature, these screening strategies have been beneficial in detecting early stage disease in high risk patient populations. The National Lung Screening Trial, one of the sentinel trials in this realm, demonstrated decrease in lung cancer and all-cause mortality in patients ages 55 to 74 with a 30 pack-year smoking history who underwent low-dose helical computed tomography (CT) screening.[3] This finding has shaped the US Preventative Services Task Force recommendations for lung cancer screening in high-risk patient populations.[4]

Increase in surveillance imaging as well as the ubiquitous use of cross-sectional imaging in various aspects of health care have made detection and management of solitary pulmonary nodules (SPN) an increasing clinical problem, especially in high-risk smokers. These patients have as high as 50% prevalence of SPNs.[5] Although there are institutional and societal variations in the management of these findings, there is a consensus among clinicians that high-risk patients with evidence of SPN growth on serial imaging or lesions larger than 8 mm should have tissue sampling for accurate diagnosis.[6]

CLINICAL CHALLENGES

Patients who fit the criteria for tissue sampling of concerning radiographic findings should undergo appropriate evaluation for either a transthoracic needle aspiration, transbronchial needle aspiration, or minimally invasive surgical wedge resection. Video-assisted thoracoscopic surgery (VATS) is particularly useful in cases where nonsurgical biopsy is unavailable, not practical, or nondiagnostic. VATS wedge resection provides a superior tissue sample for appropriate pathologic analysis and is therapeutic in those with early stage disease. Management of SPNs via VATS requires the thoracic surgeon to identify the lesion of interest by visual and tactile cues. This procedure can be challenging in patients with numerous, deep, and small lesions. To ameliorate the challenges posed during lesion detection, various adjuncts, including percutaneous wire placement, dye injection, intraoperative imaging, and intraoperative molecular imaging (IMI) devices, can be used.

If the patient undergoes a diagnostic or therapeutic operation, intraoperative margin assessment and attempts at R0 resection should be the paramount concern because this factor has important staging and adjuvant therapy ramifications. Specifically, patients with microscopic tumor involvement of the resection margin (R1) have a markedly worse prognosis than those with negative microscopic margins (R0).[7,8] Currently, there are limited methods of intraoperative margin assessment other than vigorous inspection using vision and palpation. Otherwise, surgeon can elect to evaluate the specimen with frozen section analysis, but this can be time consuming and often impractical. Some of the new emerging IMI techniques can alleviate these concerns and subject the patients to minimal parenchymal loss and minimize the time required for anesthesia.

NONSURGICAL BIOPSY ADJUNCTS

The recent implementation of screening guidelines and frequent use of highly accurate cross-sectional imaging techniques have increased the incidence of SPN detection. An increasing number of these patients are being evaluated by thoracic surgeons on an outpatient basis.[1] However, optimal strategies for definitive evaluation of these nodules are often heterogenous because this patient population has multiple medical comorbidities that may preclude certain operative interventions. Although VATS wedge resections can yield both therapeutic and diagnostic results, the requirement of single lung ventilation and anesthesia may not be suitable for all patients. These patients often can benefit from minimally invasive methods for SPN biopsy that use bronchoscopic and transthoracic techniques. When indicated, these procedures are generally preferred to more invasive surgery; however, they have imperfect sensitivity and lack therapeutic potential.[2,9]

With the advent of ever improving endoscopic technology and increased training available for physicians, the use of bronchoscopy in the evaluation of lung malignancies and masses are becoming more used. The bronchoscopic biopsy techniques are often undertaken under conscious sedation and involve instrumentation of airways under direct visualization. Ideal patients suitable for these interventions include those with large, visible, and central lesions. For those without the visible lesions on direct visualization, can benefit from endobronchial ultrasound-guided transbronchial needle aspiration. The addition of endobronchial ultrasound guidance to conventional bronchoscopic evaluation has been shown to substantially increase the diagnostic sensitivity.[10]

However, transbronchial tissue sampling may not appropriate for patients with more peripheral lesions. These lesions usually are best served by transthoracic needle biopsy (TTNB) or aspiration. TTNB involves percutaneously passing the needle under CT guidance through the chest wall into the lung nodule. These procedures have considerable risk of postintervention pneumothorax development, reaching as high as 19% on various literature analyses. Certain patient factors, including older age, presence of emphysematous or obstructive pulmonary disease, and active smoking, have shown to be risk factors in pneumothorax development after TTNB. Clinicians should also take into account that TTNB have false-negative rate of more than 20%, where a negative result may be discordant with imaging and provide limited value.[11,12]

The more invasive VATS provides an accurate modality for assessing primary tumors, mediastinal lymph node involvement, and pleural involvement. Although it requires general anesthesia and carries greater morbidity and mortality than minimally invasive techniques, it is often used when alternative procedures are unable to access the primary tumor or are nondiagnostic. Additionally, VATS provides an opportunity for therapeutic intervention at the time of diagnosis.

PREOPERATIVE NODULE LOCALIZATION

Localization and appropriate oncologic resection are keys for the management of any SPNs, especially for those with marginal pulmonary functions where preservation of the parenchyma is of utmost importance. Many surgeons rely on intraoperative palpation and feel, but recent literature data suggest that these techniques are suboptimal for the intraoperative localization of SPNs.[13] The difficulty of these techniques are compounded for VATS resections, which are limited by small port sizes and can require conversion to open thoracotomy in more than one-third of cases.[14] However, there are various radiologic, endoscopic, and intraoperative techniques available for the practicing thoracic surgeon for optimal localization and resection of lung nodules. These techniques are discussed elsewhere in this article.

Needle Localization

Needle localization techniques have been the mainstay of lesion localization in breast malignancies for many years with a successful track record. Thistlethwaite and associates in their institutional analysis of more than 250 patients over a decade have found that optimal characteristics of SPNs amenable for needle localization includes those greater than 2 cm from the from the pleural surface, less than 1.2 cm in size, and showing interval enlargement on serial scanning.[15] Those patients with a pulmonary artery systolic pressure of greater than 50 mm Hg, a forced expiratory volume in 1 second of less than 0.6 L, and lung nodules near vascular structures should have other techniques used for optimal patient safety.

Successful implementation of needle localization requires close collaboration between the interventional radiologists and the thoracic surgeons. Although the technical aspects of the procedure vary among the institutions, the overall steps remain the same. Common equipment used during the procedure, including the needle types, are shown in **Fig. 1**. First, patients receive light sedation and scout CT imaging is performed. After localization of the skin entry site, adequate local anesthetic is used before needle insertion. Various needles with built-in hook wires could be then inserted and advanced toward the edge of the nodule. A second needle is then inserted using a similar technique. Once appropriate positions are confirmed, the needles are removed with the wires left in place.

The success of needle localization has been well-documented in literature. Mayo and associates[16] in their analysis of 69 patients showed 97% success rate of localizing SPNs. Similar localization rates were reported by Thistlethwaite and colleagues[15] at the University of California San Diego, with 97% of 253 patients having the SPNs appropriately located preoperatively. Comparable success rates have been reproduced among international studies as well. Summary of studies investigation needle localization is presented in **Table 1**.

The success for optimal lesion detection and patient safety depends on technique and the equipment available to the operator. There are several types of guidewires available. In general, needles with established hooks, which are longer and therefore less easily displaced during repositioning or lung deflation, are preferred. Data from Miyoshi and colleagues[17] and Dendo and colleagues[18] showed a greater than 90% success rates in using established hook wires. It is thought that the hooks on these wires prevent needle dislodgement. Common complications associated with needle

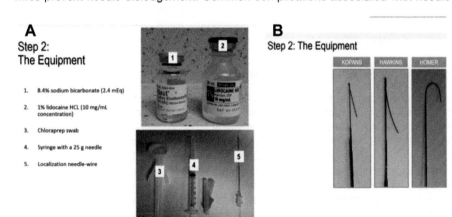

Fig. 1. Commonly used equipment for needle localization including the hook wire types available. *Part A*: demonstrates common pre-procedural equipment needed; *Part B*: demonstrates the common hookwires available for use. (*From* Kalambo M., Basak E. Dogan, Gary J. Whitman. Step by step: Planning a needle localization procedure. Clinical Imaging 2020;60(1); 100-108.)

Table 1
Studies investigating needle localization techniques reporting 70% to 90% success rate in nodule detection

Technique	First Author	Group	Year	Study Size
Microcoil	Powell	Vancouver	2004	12
Microcoil	Mayo	Vancouver	2009	69
Spiral wire	Eichfeld	Leipzig, Germany	2005	22
Hook wire	Miyoshi	Japan	2009	108
Hook wire	Dendo	Okayama, Japan	2002	150
Hook wire	Gonfiotti	Florence, Italy	2007	50

localization include pneumothorax, hemothorax, and dislodgement. These complications are readily managed by conventional postoperative care, including short-term tube thoracostomy, a without significant increase in additional surgical procedures or conversion to open thoracotomy. A literature analysis shows around a 32% risk of postprocedure pneumothorax and a 15% risk of developing a hemothorax.[11,15] The majority of study participants across studies did not require additional surgical interventions.

In summary, needle localization, where available, is a safe approach for preoperative nodule localization in those patients without significant pulmonary hypertension whose primary lesions are more than 2 cm deep and are not near major vasculature. Expertise among the operator and interventional radiologist can minimize postprocedural risks. Additionally, needles are inserted under local anesthesia while the patient is awake and can be associated with patient discomfort and uncooperativeness.

Dye, Radioisotope, and Fiducial Preoperative Localization

There are several novel and emerging techniques using dye injection, which can be used both preoperatively and intraoperatively for nodule localization. Many types of injectable dyes are used, including methylene blue, lipiodol, cyanoacrylate, India ink, and barium. These dyes are injected into or adjacent to the nodule. One should note that methylene blue, in particular, uses coaxial needle insertion into the parenchyma adjacent to the nodule of interest. Second, after the injection of methylene blue, it rapidly diffuses into the surrounding tissues, requiring a rapid transport into the operating room and swift intraoperative localization. This factor can be limiting in large hospital settings with increased operating room turnover times. To mitigate this limiting factor, McConnell and associates[19] have used an autologous blood binder, which rendered the dye useful for several hours after injection.

Conversely, to minimize adjacent dye diffusion, barium and lipiodol could be used. These agents are identified using intraoperative fluoroscopy and do not necessitate rapid patient transport into the operating room.[5] Watanabe and associates[20] described 100% success in localization of SPNs (10 ± 6 mm) using lipiodol. Similar results were reported by Fumimoto and colleagues[21] in their institutional analysis of lipiodol use for SPN detection. Although fluoroscopic guidance seems to be a feasible strategy for SPN localization before VATS resection, it is associated with an intense tissue inflammatory reaction that alters the histologic analysis. Additionally, various anaphylactoid reactions have been reported in the literature, which should be included in the preoperative informed consent. Other complications associated with lipiodol include chest wall pain (11%), hemoptysis (6%), pneumothorax (17%), and hemothorax (0.6%), and the complications and were associated with needle insertion rather than the lipiodol agent itself.[5]

Similar to gamma probe localization in breast surgery, radioisotopes can be used in comparable fashion in SPN localization. The most common radioisotope marker used for preoperative localization is technetium-99M–labeled macroaggregated albumin (traditionally used in perfusion studies). Radioisotope is coupled with noniodinated contrast and its position is confirmed with cross-sectional imaging. Subsequently, a Geiger counter is used intraoperatively during VATS to confirm the location of the nodule. The marker has a half-life of 6 to 9 hours, necessitating VATS to be performed 6 hours after injection. Various studies in literature compared technetium-99M versus needle localization techniques. Gonfiotti and associates[22] observed that both techniques were superior in locating SPNs (84% vs 96%) compared with finger palpation (26%) and there was no statistical difference in localization between them. However, as mentioned elsewhere in this article, needle localization is associated with a greater than 20% risk of developing a pneumothorax.[22] These findings were echoed by a single-institutional experience of 147 patients by Daniel and colleagues,[23] who noted greater than 95% successful localization rate with minimal complications. Similar findings were reported in various small sample case series across multiple institutions.[24]

Fiducial localization is an important adjunct for nodule localization, particularly if there is going to be a significant delay in performing definitive VATS resection. These localizers consist of 3- and 5-mm gold seeds and are placed adjacent to the nodule using a coaxial needle, similar to methylene blue injection. The advantage for the gold seeds is that they are inert and can be localized days to months after the injection. They can readily be localized intraoperatively using fluoroscopic techniques and the specimen can be confirmed with postresection back table imaging. However, these seeds can migrate and embolize into vessels and airways. Caution should be taken in deploying these seeds near critical structures.[25,26]

Three-Dimensional Navigational Printing

Increasing availability and decreased cost of operation of 3-dimensional printing have made the technology accessible for medical research. Zheng and associates[27] have published a small case series involving 16 patients where they obtained preoperative cross-sectional imaging and created a 3-dimensional digital anatomic template, which they then printed in 4 to 6 hours. The cost of each template ranged from $US80 to $US 100. This navigational template then allowed for accurate percutaneous localization based on the patient's anatomic limitations. They report a 100% success rate in nodule localization and subsequent VATS resection.[27] Although the sample size is small and the technology is in its infancy, one can expect an increased use of 3-dimensional printing in the future.

Navigational Bronchoscopy

Advances in endoscopic techniques and improvements in novel lesion detection software are improving the ability to perform minimally invasive thoracic surgery. One of these technologies that is becoming popular at large volume centers is electromagnetic navigational bronchoscopy. Electromagnetic navigational bronchoscopy combines traditional and virtual bronchoscopy for the localization of the lung nodules and allows the guidance of diagnostic as well as dye marking instruments. Furthermore, electromagnetic navigational bronchoscopy has expanded the use of bronchoscopic localization for small peripheral lesions that were previously unattainable with conventional endoscopic techniques.

The SuperDimension system (Medtronic, Minneapolis, MN) is the most commonly used electromagnetic navigational bronchoscopy system reported in the literature (**Fig. 2**). In the first phase, also known as the planning phase, the patient's CT scan is loaded into the navigational software, which allows the surgeon to identify the target lesion and pick the most appropriate bronchial pathway. A standard bronchoscopy is performed, and the landmarks are registered into the software system. The navigational system then links the images from the initial CT scan and the bronchoscopy, creating virtual images. The surgeon then navigates toward the lesion using both standard and virtual images. When the bronchoscope is wedged in the segmental bronchus and cannot advance further, the operator advances the extended working channel, which has a built-in locatable guide using the virtual image. This technique

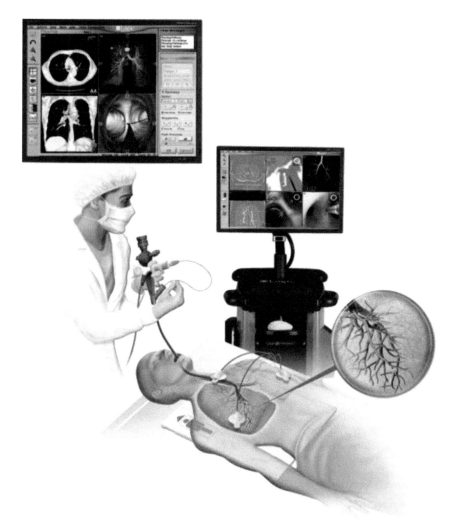

Fig. 2. The Ilogic electromagnetic navigation bronchoscopy by super dimension. (*From* Christie S., Electromagnetic Navigational Bronchoscopy and Robotic-Assisted Thoracic Surgery. AORN Journal 2007-2017; 99(6); 750-763.)

allows one to obtain cytologic brushings, place fiducials/dyes for marking, and guide stereotactic body radiation therapies.

Electromagnetic navigational bronchoscopy has been shown to effective in the diagnosis and preoperative localization of lung nodules with a lower complication profile than that of more invasive techniques. However, the diagnostic yield reported in literature ranges between 59% and 94%.[28] The reason for this large variability stems from lack of uniform selection criteria and standardized protocols. Overall, lesions larger greater than 2 cm and those that exhibit bronchus sign on the CT scan have the greatest diagnostic yield.

INTRAOPERATIVE IMAGING-GUIDED NODULE LOCALIZATION

Preoperative localization techniques are useful adjuncts that can enhance the arsenal of the thoracic surgeon, but these procedures tend to be operator dependent, have varying rates of complications, and cause discomfort to the patients. Therefore, one can use various intraoperative imaging techniques to mitigate those risks in a less costly and invasive manner. Various options for intraoperative imaging include intraoperative ultrasound examination, intraoperative CT scans or fluoroscopy, near-infrared fluorescence, and IMI.

Intraoperative Ultrasound Examination

Performing an intraoperative ultrasound examination is a real-time and alternative approach to localizing small, nonvisible, and nonpalpable pulmonary lesions without injury to lung parenchyma. It is a preferred method because it is noninvasive, nonionizing, and affordable. In fact, it is one of the earliest methods for noninvasive nodule detection, dating back to the inception of minimally invasive thoracoscopic surgery. However, using ultrasound examination to detect small nodules is heavily operator dependent because air in the lung parenchyma inhibits proper detection in conventional ultrasound probes. Nevertheless, the use of high-frequency probes has surpassed this limitation and is accurate in detecting SPNs smaller than 20 mm. Small lung lesions can be found by intraoperative ultrasound examination when they are superficial, fixed in lung parenchyma, and solid. Deeper lesions, however, require complete collapse of the lung, which can be challenging if the anesthesia team is not comfortable with single lung ventilation and/or limited by underlying patient lung mechanics, such as emphysematous disease.

Although there is no widespread use of intraoperative ultrasound examination, several small institutional studies have observed its efficacy in detecting SPNs. Hsia and colleagues[29] reported a 81.7% success rate among 153 patients over a 24-month period. Piolanti and colleagues[30] reported a 92.6% success rate in 35 patients with a mean nodule size of 13.2 mm with no reported complications. Additionally, when ultrasound examination was compared with video imaging and palpation during VATS alone in 23 patients with nodules smaller than 30 mm, ultrasound imaging was found to be 100% effective, palpation 88% effective, and imaging alone 60% effective for nodule localization ($P = .012$).[30]

Intraoperative Fluoroscopy and Computed Tomography Scans

With the advent of screening guidelines, more and more subcentimeter SPNs are detected on an annual basis. As the size of the lesion decreases, various techniques including needle and dye localization become limited in accurately detecting the lesion of interest. These challenges can be mitigated by the use of fluoroscopy intraoperatively. A common dye used for fluoroscopic detection is lipiodol, which is a lipid soluble contrast medium. Real-time CT fluoroscopy has been shown to be valuable during preoperative lipiodol marking of ground-glass opaque and deep, small, solid nodules.

Swensen and colleagues[31] reported a 97% success rate of nodule localization in 107 patients analyzed over a 17-month period. After CT-guided needle localized injection of lipiodol, they used a C-arm–shaped fluoroscopic unit to detect and resect regions of interest (**Fig. 3**). The specimen adequacy was confirmed by reimaging the resected parenchyma, looking for the presence of the lipiodol.

One of the earlier studies looking at the application of this technology was performed by Nomori and colleagues[32] with similar technical aspects to Yamashita's methods. Although a small sample size, this study showed 18 nodules in 16 patients were detected using this procedure with an average size of 7 mm. One patient had a pneumothorax that required drainage before going to the operating room. As

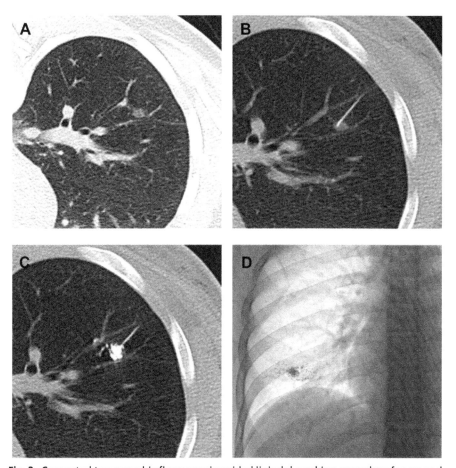

Fig. 3. Computed tomographic fluoroscopic guided lipiodol-marking procedure for ground-glass opaque (GGO) nodules. (*A*) A small GGO in the right lower lobe. (*B*) A percutaneous transhepatic cholangiography needle (23 gauge) is inserted in the center of the GGO nodule. (*C*) Lipiodol 0.3 mL is then injected into the nodule. (*D*) A radiopaque spot is clearly demonstrated on the plain chest radiograph. (*Obtained from* Thoracic Surgery Clinics. Elsevier.)

described elsewhere in this article, the use of fluoroscopic CT guidance can be enhanced by using fiducial gold seeds, but this technique requires operator expertise.

One of the limiting and inconvenient factors associated with fluoroscopic guidance is that the patient has to undergo the needle localization technique before VATS. Depending on the technique used, this process can lead to multiple trips to the health care institution, or require patient transport between procedure suites. Similar to vascular surgery, this situation has led to the development of a hybrid technique, termed image-guided VATS, by Gill and colleagues.[33] The study combines placement of fiducials using intraoperative C-arm CT guidance with standard thoracoscopic resection technique using image-guided VATS. In their phase I and II trial, they successfully resected all the specimens in 23 patients enrolled in the study with minimal complications.

Intraoperative Molecular Imaging

IMI is a novel technique aimed at localization, diagnosis and margin assessment of lung nodules. IMI involves 2 key components: fluorescent contrast agents and specialized imaging devices. A fluorescent contrast agent is given systemically and binds to tumor cells. When used in combination with a specialized imaging device, pulmonary tumors may be assessed via either thoracotomy or minimally invasive thoracoscopic techniques for fluorescence.

Currently there is only commercially available agent that has been approved by the US Food and Drug Administration, namely, indocyanine green (ICG); however, several additional contrast agents are currently being developed. Despite the limited availability of other agents, ICG has shown promise in intraoperative SPN detection. The use of electromagnetic navigational bronchoscopy using near-infrared fluorescence with ICG contrast has emerged as an accurate and efficient method for localizing pulmonary nodules. ICG is a fluorophore contrast that illuminates in the near infrared spectrum, has a high signal-to-noise ratio, is inexpensive, and is relatively nontoxic. The theory behind the use of ICG relies on the fact that malignant cells retain the dye by a nonspecific inflammatory permeability. Furthermore, infiltration of ICG into the tissues does not distort its cellular integrity, thereby allowing for accurate histopathologic analysis, including margin assessment. Since the initial 2001 study by Sakamoto and colleagues,[34] interest in ICG use for pulmonary nodule localization has increased dramatically. Early studies reported 79% to 100% success rate in nodule localization. A number of groups have since reported institutional studies regarding the accuracy of electromagnetic navigational bronchoscopy-guided near-infrared fluorescence using ICG for intraoperative localization of pulmonary lesions. Our institutional pilot study in 2015 looked at localization after administering preoperative intravenous ICG (5 mg/kg) followed by open thoracotomy within 24 hours.[9] We reported that near-infrared fluorescence detected 16 of 18 nodules (88%), which were as small as 0.2 cm in size and 1.3 cm from the pleural surface. Additionally, this approach discovered 5 subcentimeter metastatic deposits that were resected by wedge excision.

Although ICG is nontargeted and is thought to localize to the tumors through increased vasculature and dysfunctional lymphatics, other recently studied agents are targeted to tumor surface receptors. Okusanya and associates in their pilot study looking at folate-targeted dyes in tumor nodule localization demonstrated that optical fluorescent molecular imaging can be used to visually identify lung adenocarcinomas.[9,35,36] These folate targeted dyes localize to pulmonary adenocarcinomas that highly express folate receptor alpha. The folate dye used in the study was a conjugate between folate and a near-infrared dye. This conjugate forms a negatively charged fluorescent molecule that binds weakly and nonspecifically to serum proteins. In addition, in normal lung pneumocytes, folate receptor alpha is expressed on the apical (luminal) side of polarized epithelial cells; thus, it has no access to systemically administered folate.

A phase I and more recent multi-institutional phase II study have been completed and the results reported. Patients with lung nodules received the folate–near infrared tracer preoperatively. The primary goal was to determine if the tracer improved surgeons' ability to localize hard to find nodules, identify occult cancers, and discriminate close margins. Assessments were made in 3 phases: (i) lung inspection, in which the hemithorax was evaluated for other pathology, (ii) tumor resection, in which the primary tumor was resected, and (iii) the specimen check, in which the specimen was assessed on the back table for positive margins. The gold standard was pathology. One hundred ten patients were recruited; 92 were eligible for analysis. There were no drug-related serious adverse events. During the inspection phase, IMI found 10 additional cancers that were not suspected by the surgeon in 7 patients (8%). During the resection phase, IMI located 11 lesions (12%) that the surgeon could not palpate or visualize. During the specimen check phase, although the surgeon felt the margins were adequate, IMI revealed 8 positive margins (9%). The IMI learning curve was 6 cases. Benefits of IMI were most pronounced in patients undergoing sublobar pulmonary resections and those with ground-glass opacities.[37,38]

Although this finding represents an exciting avenue for intraoperative nodule localization, much work needs to be done for mainstream integration. However, early works suggest that this emerging technology is useful for real-time subcentimeter pulmonary nodule localization, margin assessment, and intraoperative diagnosis.

INTRAOPERATIVE MARGIN ASSESSMENT

Positive margins after surgery for non-small cell lung cancer occurs in approximately 5% to 15% of patients, which impacts long-term outcomes by causing local and distant disease recurrence. Numerous studies spanning multiple decades have placed importance on R0 resection as the key prognostic indicator. Therefore, every attempt should be made for sound oncologic resection of non-small cell lung cancer lesions. Despite the clinical ramifications, there are few dedicated reports that discuss intraoperative methods of margin assessment or the implications of positive margins after surgery for non-small cell lung cancer. Currently, there are limited methods whereby pulmonary tumor margins are assessed intraoperatively for both bronchial margins after pulmonary lobectomy or sublobar pulmonary resections. The ideal surgical margin for sublobar resections remains controversial. Reports suggest that for small tumors (<2 cm), the ideal surgical margin is 1.5 cm with additional resection providing no additional benefit. In larger tumors, the optimal distance from the tumor to the surgical margin is less evident, however, larger resection margin may be more favorable. Specifically, larger tumors should be resected with a margin of at least the size of the tumor in largest diameter. Most frequently, margins are assessed using gross examination either by the surgeon and/or pathologist. Additional methods of intraoperative margin assessment include frozen section, cytologic lavage analysis, intraoperative ultrasound examination, and molecular imaging.

Frozen Section

Frozen sections are one of the frequently used means for assessing margin positivity for non-small cell lung cancer. Advances in preoperative imaging and tissue sampling has led to an overall decreased use of frozen sections. However, thoracic frozen sections are still frequently used, although their indication has changed with the most common request being the characterization of margins. Margin assessment in lung sparing procedures has become a more frequently requested frozen section. With the recognition that multiple pulmonary nodules may reflect (1) synchronous primary tumors, (2) invasive cancer plus a synchronous preinvasive or minimally invasive lesion, or (3) carcinoma plus an inflammatory nodule, intraoperative sampling of ipsilateral nodules in a separate lobe or segment for lesion identification and margin assessment may be needed as part of a limited resection. Additionally, although small, there are significant false-positive and false-negative rates associated with frozen section analysis. Reasons for the false-negative rates, which are as high as 40% in some reports, include sampling error and interpretation error (misnaming malignant cells for lymphocytes, glandular tissue, metaplasia, or cautery artifact).[39,40] Furthermore, the timing required for optimal analysis by an experienced thoracic pathologist requires that the patient remain under anesthesia. This factor is particularly important, because this patient population has above average rates of significant lung and cardiovascular disease.

Data from Owen and colleagues,[40] analyzing frozen sections of bronchial margins in 270 patients, have shown that frozen section analysis rarely yields a positive result and infrequently changes intraoperative management of patients undergoing non-small cell lung cancer resection. In light of these conclusions, the National Comprehensive Cancer Network guidelines do not currently recommend frozen section analysis when performing a lobectomy or pneumonectomy.

Nevertheless, it is important to recognize that frozen section analysis is important for those undergoing sublobar resection because a positive margin can impact the exact extent of surgical resection. Despite this indication, frozen section remains costly, time consuming, and predisposes the patient to additional anesthesia. There has not been a clinical study assessing frozen section for margin assessment in this scenario.

Cytologic Lavage Analysis

Cytologic analysis of lung margins has been developed in an attempt to predict retained tumor margins at the cut end during sublobar resections. Confirmation of negative margins is thought to decrease local recurrence rates and allow for optimal oncologic resection. Miyoshi and colleagues[17] in their 2019 analysis built on techniques and findings by Higashiyama and colleagues,[41] who initially published their results on intraoperative lavage cytology dating back to 2002. In fact, they report that intraoperative lavage cytology is their primary means of assessing margin positivity for more than decade and has supplanted intraoperative frozen section analysis. The technique as described by the authors is as follows:

All autostapling cartridges used for wedge or segmental resection of pulmonary malignancies are rinsed with 50 mL saline. The washing saline is centrifuged, and the sediment is stained using Papanicolaou's method to examine for cancer cells. The result is reported to the operating room within approximately 30 minutes, and in case of a positive result, additional wedge resection is usually attempted. If there is an anatomic restriction, additional segmental resection, lobectomy, or even pneumonectomy is performed if the patient is not at high risk.

Among the 262 patients who underwent intraoperative lavage cytology, 22 (7%) had positive cytology, of whom 19 underwent additional resection. Slightly higher positive margins were detected by Higashiyama and associates (11%). During the median follow-up period of 42 months, 2% of patients with negative initial cytology developed margin recurrence.[17,41]

Intraoperative Ultrasound Examination

With the availability and cost efficacy associated with an ultrasound examination, effort has been made to use both intraoperative endoscopic and transthoracic ultrasound examinations to guide resection margins in lung tumors. Tatsumura[42] describes a technique whereby both transesophageal endoscopic ultrasound examination and intraoperative ultrasound examination were used in 71 patients with preoperatively diagnosed primary lung cancers to assess involvement of pericardium, aorta, vena cava, pulmonary vessels, left atrium, chest wall, and diaphragm. Intraoperative ultrasound examination outperformed endoscopic ultrasound examination for both the sensitivity and specificity of tumor organ involvement; however, both methods outperformed preoperative CT scan and MRI for prediction of surrounding structure involvement.[42] Although an effort has been made to use intraoperative ultrasound examination for tumor localization and assessment of surrounding structure involvement, this technique has not been described for use in determining adequate margins during sublobar resections.

Intraoperative Molecular Imaging

As detailed elsewhere in this review, intraoperative molecular imaging represents a new frontier for tumor localization and same can be said for real time intraoperative margin localization. De Jesus and colleagues[43,44] described their institutional experience using a novel folate-targeted dye (folate–fluorescein) in mice models where compared with traditional inspection (30%), IMI identified 80% of residual tumor deposits. These findings were echoed by Newton and colleagues[45] in their review of intraoperative fluorescence imaging in thoracic surgery. As these techniques and molecular tracers were identified at authors institution, there are multiple prospective trials currently underway to ascertain the efficacy of folate-based dyes in tumor localization and margin assessment.[37] There have been numerous iterations to the types of dyes used. Currently, our group is analyzing the efficacy of folate–near infrared examination, which has shown decreased autofluorescence and increased depth of penetration compared with folate-fluorescein examination, which was used in initial studies. Additionally, folate–near infrared examination had a high specificity for folate receptor alpha–expressing tumor cells lines in vitro, that folate–near infrared examination localized to murine lung cancer xenografts and spontaneous lung cancers in dogs in vivo, and that tumor margins correlated with fluorescence. With increased development of both tumor specific dyes, as well as intraoperative imaging devices, we foresee the ability of IMI to provide an accurate optical biopsy for assessment of tumor margins in the operating room in the near future.

SUMMARY

With the ever-increasing implementation of lung cancer screening programs by high-quality cross-sectional imaging, more and more SPNs are identified in this high-risk patient population. Ideally, these lesions would be managed by minimally invasive and nonsurgical techniques. However, anatomic constraints and patient comorbidities may preclude these approaches or fail in providing a diagnosis. These patients are best served by VATS surgical biopsy, which can be both diagnostic and therapeutic. For this reason, intraoperative localization of pulmonary nodules and margin assessment are challenging, although crucial, to thoracic surgeons for management of these early stage lung cancers. Several methods have been developed to improve localization and decrease time to diagnosis and rate of conversion to thoracotomy; however, none are 100% sensitive or without complications.

Depending on institutional practice patterns, equipment availability, and surgeon preference, several preoperative methods can be used. These include percutaneous CT-guided wire placement techniques, including the placement of microcoils, hook wires, and spiral wires, which can help with nodule localization during VATS and may also be used in conjunction with intraoperative fluoroscopy or ultrasound. Notably, all of these techniques require 2 procedures and have considerable complications including pneumothorax, hemothorax, and patient discomfort. Additionally, patient comorbidities such as emphysematous disease and severe pulmonary hypertension, may preclude them from these preoperative localizations.

To further enhance localization, surgeons can use preoperative dye marking Nevertheless, this again requires 2 procedures for diagnosis, which can complicate operative schedule, and remains complicated by risk of pneumothorax, dye embolism, and cases of anaphylaxis to the dye of choice. Owing to the cumbersome nature of those procedures, most thoracic surgeons still rely on finger palpation to locate nodules intraoperatively.

R0 resection is the mainstay of sound oncologic resection in non-small cell lung cancer; it has been shown that these patients have lower rates of local recurrence and better prognosis than those who do not get complete oncologic resection. With the advent of sublobar resections, which preserve lung parenchyma while performing adequate resection, margin assessment remains a cardinal step. Currently, thoracic surgeons can assess surgical margins using frozen section, cytologic analysis, and intraoperative imaging. However, currently available methods are time consuming, costly, and inaccurate. Therefore, currently, methods beyond traditional visualization and palpation are not frequently used. Although challenges for intraoperative margin assessment remain, there have been significant strides in the realm of IMI with promising early results.

REFERENCES

1. Torre LA, Siegel RL, Jemal A. Lung cancer statistics. Adv Exp Med Biol 2016; 893:1–19.
2. Hirsch FR, Scagliotti GV, Mulshine JL, et al. Lung cancer: current therapies and new targeted treatments. Lancet 2017;389(10066):299–311.
3. The National Lung Screening Trial: overview and study design1. Radiology 2011; 258(1):243–53.
4. Final Recommendation Statement: Lung Cancer: screening - US Preventive Services Task Force. Available from: https://www.uspreventiveservicestaskforce.org/Page/Document/RecommendationStatementFinal/lung-cancer-screening.   Accessed January 20, 2020.
5. Kawanaka K, Nomori H, Mori T, et al. Marking of small pulmonary nodules before thoracoscopic resection: injection of lipiodol under CT-fluoroscopic guidance. Acad Radiol 2009;16(1):39–45.
6. Sánchez M, Benegas M, Vollmer I. Management of incidental lung nodules <8 mm in diameter. J Thorac Dis 2018;10(Suppl 22):S2611–27.
7. Hofmann HS, Taege C, Lautenschläger C, et al. Microscopic (R1) and macroscopic (R2) residual disease in patients with resected non-small cell lung cancer. Eur J Cardiothorac Surg 2002;21(4):606–10.
8. Riquet M, Achour K, Foucault C, et al. Microscopic residual disease after resection for lung cancer: a multifaceted but poor factor of prognosis. Ann Thorac Surg 2010;89(3):870–5.

9. Keating J, Singhal S. Novel Methods of Intraoperative Localization and Margin Assessment of Pulmonary Nodules. Semin Thorac Cardiovasc Surg 2016;28(1): 127–36.

10. Marchand C, Medford ARL. Relationship between endobronchial ultrasound-guided (EBUS)-transbronchial needle aspiration utility and computed tomography staging, node size at EBUS, and positron emission tomography scan node standard uptake values: a retrospective analysis. Thorac Cancer 2017;8(4): 285–90.

11. Hsu H-H, Shen C-H, Tsai W-C, et al. Localization of nonpalpable pulmonary nodules using CT-guided needle puncture. World J Surg Oncol 2015;13. Available at: https://www.ncbi.nlm.nih.gov/pmc/articles/PMC4536773/. Accessed January 26, 2020.

12. Needle localization of small pulmonary nodules: lessons learned- ClinicalKey. Available at: https://www.clinicalkey.com/#!/content/journal/1-s2.0-S0022522318300552?scrollTo=%231-s2.0-S0022522318300552-fx2. Accessed January 26, 2020.

13. Mattioli S, D'Ovidio F, Daddi N, et al. Transthoracic endosonography for the intraoperative localization of lung nodules. Ann Thorac Surg 2005;79(2):443–9.

14. Suzuki K, Nagai K, Yoshida J, et al. Video-assisted thoracoscopic surgery for small indeterminate pulmonary nodules: indications for preoperative marking. Chest 1999;115(2):563–8.

15. Thistlethwaite PA, Gower JR, Hernandez M, et al. Needle localization of small pulmonary nodules: lessons learned. J Thorac Cardiovasc Surg 2018;155(5): 2140–7.

16. Mayo JR, Clifton JC, Powell TI, et al. Lung nodules: CT-guided placement of microcoils to direct video-assisted thoracoscopic surgical resection. Radiology 2009;250(2):576–85.

17. Miyoshi K, Toyooka S, Gobara H, et al. Clinical outcomes of short hook wire and suture marking system in thoracoscopic resection for pulmonary nodules. Eur J Cardiothorac Surg 2009;36(2):378–82.

18. Dendo S, Kanazawa S, Ando A, et al. Preoperative localization of small pulmonary lesions with a short hook wire and suture system: experience with 168 procedures. Radiology 2002;225(2):511–8.

19. McConnell PI, Feola GP, Meyers RL. Methylene blue-stained autologous blood for needle localization and thoracoscopic resection of deep pulmonary nodules. J Pediatr Surg 2002;37(12):1729–31.

20. Watanabe K, Nomori H, Ohtsuka T, et al. Usefulness and complications of computed tomography-guided lipiodol marking for fluoroscopy-assisted thoracoscopic resection of small pulmonary nodules: experience with 174 nodules. J Thorac Cardiovasc Surg 2006;132(2):320–4.

21. Fumimoto S, Sato K, Koyama M, et al. Combined lipiodol marking and video-assisted thoracoscopic surgery in a hybrid operating room. J Thorac Dis 2018; 10(5):2940–7.

22. Gonfiotti A, Davini F, Vaggelli L, et al. Thoracoscopic localization techniques for patients with solitary pulmonary nodule: hookwire versus radio-guided surgery. Eur J Cardiothorac Surg 2007;32(6):843–7.

23. Daniel TM, Altes TA, Rehm PK, et al. A novel technique for localization and excisional biopsy of small or ill-defined pulmonary lesions. Ann Thorac Surg 2004; 77(5):1756–62 [discussion: 1762].

24. Lin M-W, Chen J-S. Image-guided techniques for localizing pulmonary nodules in thoracoscopic surgery. J Thorac Dis 2016;8(Suppl 9):S749–55.

25. Sancheti MS, Lee R, Ahmed SU, et al. Percutaneous fiducial localization for thoracoscopic wedge resection of small pulmonary nodules. Ann Thorac Surg 2014; 97(6):1914–8 [discussion: 1919].
26. Sharma A, McDermott S, Mathisen DJ, et al. Preoperative localization of lung nodules with fiducial markers: feasibility and technical considerations. Ann Thorac Surg 2017;103(4):1114–20.
27. Zhang L, Li M, Li Z, et al. Three-dimensional printing of navigational template in localization of pulmonary nodule: a pilot study. J Thorac Cardiovasc Surg 2017; 154(6):2113–9.e7.
28. Muñoz-Largacha JA, Litle VR, Fernando HC. Navigation bronchoscopy for diagnosis and small nodule location. J Thorac Dis 2017;9(Suppl 2):S98–103.
29. Hsia DW, Jensen KW, Curran-Everett D, et al. Diagnosis of lung nodules with peripheral/radial endobronchial ultrasound-guided transbronchial biopsy. J Bronchology Interv Pulmonol 2012;19(1):5–11.
30. Piolanti M, Coppola F, Papa S, et al. Ultrasonographic localization of occult pulmonary nodules during video-assisted thoracic surgery. Eur Radiol 2003; 13(10):2358–64.
31. Swensen SJ, Yamashita K, McCollough CH, et al. Lung nodules: dual-kilovolt peak analysis with CT–multicenter study. Radiology 2000;214(1):81–5.
32. Nomori H, Horio H, Naruke T, et al. Fluoroscopy-assisted thoracoscopic resection of lung nodules marked with lipiodol. Ann Thorac Surg 2002;74(1):170–3.
33. Gill RR, Zheng Y, Barlow JS, et al. Image-guided video assisted thoracoscopic surgery (iVATS) - phase I-II clinical trial. J Surg Oncol 2015;112(1):18–25.
34. Sakamoto T, Takada Y, Endoh M, et al. Bronchoscopic dye injection for localization of small pulmonary nodules in thoracoscopic surgery. Ann Thorac Surg 2001; 72(1):296–7.
35. Okusanya OT, Deshpande C, Barbosa EM, et al. Molecular imaging to identify tumor recurrence following chemoradiation in a hostile surgical environment. Mol Imaging 2015;14(1). 7290.2014.00051.
36. Kennedy GT, Okusanya OT, Keating JJ, et al. The optical biopsy: a novel technique for rapid intraoperative diagnosis of primary pulmonary adenocarcinomas. Ann Surg 2015;262(4):602–9.
37. Predina JD, Newton AD, Keating J, et al. A phase I clinical trial of targeted intraoperative molecular imaging for pulmonary adenocarcinomas. Ann Thorac Surg 2018;105(3):901–8.
38. Predina JD, Newton AD, Keating J, et al. Intraoperative molecular imaging combined with positron emission tomography improves surgical management of peripheral malignant pulmonary nodules. Ann Surg 2017;266(3):479–88.
39. Sienko A, Allen TC, Zander DS, et al. Frozen section of lung specimens. Arch Pathol Lab Med 2005;129(12):1602–9.
40. Owen RM, Force SD, Gal AA, et al. Routine intraoperative frozen section analysis of bronchial margins is of limited utility in lung cancer resection. Ann Thorac Surg 2013;95(6):1859–65 [discussion: 1865–6].
41. Higashiyama M, Kodama K, Takami K, et al. Intraoperative lavage cytologic analysis of surgical margins in patients undergoing limited surgery for lung cancer. J Thorac Cardiovasc Surg 2003;125(1):101–7.
42. Tatsumura T. Preoperative and intraoperative ultrasonographic examination as an aid in lung cancer operations. J Thorac Cardiovasc Surg 1995;110(3):606–12.
43. De Jesus E, Keating JJ, Kularatne SA, et al. Comparison of folate receptor targeted optical contrast agents for intraoperative molecular imaging. Int J Mol

Imaging 2015;2015. Available at: https://www.ncbi.nlm.nih.gov/pmc/articles/PMC4600912/.

44. Keating JJ, Okusanya OT, De Jesus E, et al. Intraoperative molecular imaging of lung adenocarcinoma can identify residual tumor cells at the surgical margins. Mol Imaging Biol 2016;18(2):209–18.

45. Newton AD, Predina JD, Nie S, et al. Intraoperative fluorescence imaging in thoracic surgery. J Surg Oncol 2018;118(2):344–55.

.

Surgery for Locally Advanced and Oligometastatic Non–Small Cell Lung Cancer

Jenalee N. Coster, MD, Shawn S. Groth, MD, MS*

KEYWORDS

- Non–small cell lung carcinoma • Locally advanced non–small cell lung cancer
- Chest wall invasion • Superior sulcus tumors • Salvage surgery • Stage IIIA N2
- Definitive chemoradiation • Oligometastatic lung cancer

KEY POINTS

- Locally advanced non–small cell lung carcinoma is a heterogeneous, complex group of tumors that require a multidisciplinary approach.
- In the absence of N2 disease, complete surgical (R0) resection as part of a multimodal treatment strategy offers the best chance at long-term survival for select patients with locally advanced non-small cell lung carcinoma.
- Salvage lung resection after definitive chemoradiation is safe and may offer a survival advantage to select patients.
- In the absence of N2 disease, oligometastatic non–small cell lung cancer is best treated by aggressive multimodal treatment, including resection of the primary tumor and local therapy for the metastasis.

INTRODUCTION

Lung cancer, of which non–small cell lung cancer (NSCLC) is the most common type, is the leading cause of cancer-related death of men and women in the United States. Unfortunately, a majority of patients with NSCLC are diagnosed at an advanced stage. At the time of diagnosis, 24% of patients have locally advanced NSCLC, defined as tumor invasion into surrounding structures or metastasis to ipsilateral mediastinal lymph nodes.[1] Although the treatment of medically fit patients with early-stage NSCLC is well-established (i.e., surgery), the role of surgery in more advanced tumors is more controversial.[2] This complex, heterogenous group of tumors requires a thorough

Division of Thoracic Surgery, Micheal E. DeBakey Department of Surgery, Baylor College of Medicine, 7200 Cambridge St, Ste 6A. Houston, TX 77030, USA
* Corresponding author.
E-mail address: Shawn.Groth@bcm.edu

Surg Oncol Clin N Am 29 (2020) 543–554
https://doi.org/10.1016/j.soc.2020.07.001
surgonc.theclinics.com

evaluation by an experienced multidisciplinary team of medical oncologists, radiation oncologists, and thoracic surgeons. A select group of these patients derive survival benefit from surgery as part of a multimodal treatment strategy. This review discusses the evaluation, indications, and challenges of surgery for T3 (chest wall invasion) tumors, superior sulcus tumors, stage IIIA N2 disease, resectable T4 tumors, oligometastatic stage IV disease, and salvage lung resections after definitive chemoradiation.

PREOPERATIVE EVALUATION

All NSCLC patients who are potential candidates for resection must undergo a comprehensive preoperative assessment of their cardiopulmonary function to assure that the patient has sufficient cardiopulmonary reserve to undergo the operation with an acceptable risk of perioperative morbidity and mortality. This includes a thorough preoperative history and physical examination with specific attention paid to signs and symptoms of cardiopulmonary compromise. Depending on the presence and severity of clinical predictors of perioperative cardiovascular complications, such as coronary artery disease, heart failure, arrhythmias, valvular disease, diabetes mellitus, and chronic renal insufficiency, additional studies to assess cardiovascular risk may be required. Pulmonary function tests should be obtained, and the percent predicted postoperative forced expiratory volume in the first second of expiration and diffusing capacity of carbon monoxide should be determined, to further risk stratify patients.

To assure NSCLC patients are allocated to the most appropriate treatment strategy, thorough pretreatment staging is essential, including computed tomography (CT), positron emission tomography (PET), and brain magnetic resonance imaging (MRI).[2] Nodal status is one of the most important prognostic indicators[2-4] and drives preoperative decision making[2,3]; therefore, it is imperative to thoroughly assess for mediastinal nodal metastases prior to surgical intervention. Due to the potential for false-negative findings on PET and CT, the mediastinum should be pathologically evaluated with endobronchial ultrasound (EBUS) or mediastinoscopy for all patients with stage IB or higher.[2]

T3 (invasion), N0-1

According to the 8th edition of the American Joint Commission on Cancer (AJCC) Staging System for NSCLC, T3 includes local invasion into the parietal pleura, the chest wall, phrenic nerve, and pericardium.[5] Patients with chest wall invasion may present with severe pain due to pleural and chest wall involvement. Chest CT is useful for assessing the primary tumor and degree of rib involvement whereas chest MRI is useful for assessing soft tissue chest wall involvement.[4] Mediastinal staging is critical for these patients. Patients with T3N0-1M0 tumors are candidates for surgery; patients with T3N2M0 tumors are not. Patients with N2 disease are best treated with concurrent definitive chemoradiation followed by durvalumab.[2]

The location of the tumor and its extension into surrounding structures contributes have technical implications. A standard open posterolateral approach is sufficient in the majority of cases, although the safety and feasibility of a video-assisted thoracoscopic surgery (VATS) approach have been reported.[6] The chest should be entered away from the affected area and the involved chest wall should be resected en bloc with the pulmonary resection (usually a lobectomy). A mediastinal lymph node dissection or sampling should be completed. Although frozen sections of the soft tissue margins are helpful, frozen sections on the bony margin (ideally margins of 1.0 cm) are not.[4] Although some investigators have debated the benefits of skeletal resection for T3 tumors compared with an extrapleural resection,[4] Doddoli and colleagues[7] found a significant ($P = .03$) 5-year overall survival (OS) advantage with en bloc resection (60.3%) compared with extrapleural resection (39.1%) for patients with T3 tumors involving the chest wall that were resected with negative margins.

Except for defects less than 3 cm and those posterior defects above the fourth rib that otherwise would be covered by the scapula, skeletal reconstruction of the chest wall should be completed to prevent paradoxic chest wall motion. Depending on size and location of the defect and surgeon preference, polytetrafluoroethylene (PTFE), polypropylene, high-density polyethylene (HDPE) mesh, or methyl metacrylate placed between 2 pieces of HDPE mesh secured in place with nonabsorbable suture are traditional methods for reconstruction. Regardless of the chosen material, it should be secured in place with some tension to confer rigidity to the chest wall. For resectable (especially right-sided) tumors that invade the pericardium, the pericardium is reconstructed with a thin (eg, 0.1 mm), loose, fenestrated piece of PTFE mesh to prevent cardiac herniation. Diaphragm plication should be completed after resection of tumors that invade the phrenic nerve.

Given the concern for local recurrence after chest wall resection, Tandberg and colleagues[8] examined the role of adjuvant radiotherapy (RT) in those patients who underwent an R0 resection and found no significant advantage of RT with regards to local control and survival. Adjuvant chemotherapy, however, offers a survival benefit. A large retrospective study found a significant median survival benefit of 71 months versus 39 months ($P<.001$) for those patients receiving adjuvant chemotherapy.[9] Taken together these and other data support the role of adjuvant chemotherapy for T3N0 NSCLC after R0 resections. Adjuvant RT has no role after R0 resection but should be considered for R1 resections.[2]

Superior Sulcus Tumors

Superior sulcus (Pancoast) tumors (T3 invasion, N0-1 and T4 extension, N0-1) are complex due to involvement of the structures that course through the thoracic outlet (ie, branchial plexus and subclavian vessels), spine, and chest wall, which contribute technical challenges at the time of resection. These tumors may be associated with Pancoast-Tobias syndrome, which is characterized by severe and unrelenting shoulder pain with distribution down the arm and into the hand (compression of the C8-T1 nerve roots), Horner syndrome (ptosis, miosis, and anhidrosis from compression of the sympathetic chain and stellate ganglion), and atrophy of the intrinsic muscles of the hand (compression of ulnar nerve).[10,11] The presence of the Pancoast-Tobias syndrome is not a necessary condition to establish the diagnosis of a superior sulcus tumor.[10]

The pretreatment evaluation should include a dedicated chest CT. For patients who may require subclavian resection and reconstruction, CT angiogram is needed. A brachial plexus or cervical/thoracic-spine MRI is helpful for assessing nerve root and vertebral column involvement. A full-body PET and brain MRI (or CT with contrast) is needed to rule out distant metastases. Once a tumor is thought to be technically feasible for resection, invasive mediastinal nodal sampling should be completed, because nodal disease is an extremely poor prognostic indicator in superior sulcus tumors.[2,4,10,11] It is the authors' preference to stage the mediastinum with EBUS prior to neoadjuvant CRT and to restage the mediastinum with a cervical mediastinoscopy after neoadjuvant CRT.

The current recommendation for medically fit patients with resectable superior sulcus tumors is concurrent neoadjuvant chemoradiotherapy (CRT), complete surgical resection, and adjuvant chemotherapy.[2,3] Absolute contraindications for surgical resection include N2/N3 disease, involvement of the brachial plexus above the T1 nerve root, involvement of more than 50% of the vertebral bodies, and invasion into the esophagus and trachea. Involvement of the subclavian vessels and interforaminal extension of the tumor are no longer contraindications. The ipsilateral supraclavicular and scalene lymph nodes can be resected en bloc and are not a contraindication for resection.[10,11] Superior sulcus tumors often require a collaborative multispecialty surgery team of neurosurgery, vascular surgery, and thoracic surgery to aid in complete resection.

Though a posterolateral (Paulson-Shaw) thoracotomy is suitable for most tumors, an anterior (Dartevelle) thoracotomy is preferable for tumors involving the subclavian artery. Extensive vertebral body resections require posterior stabilization. Similar to early stage NSCLC, lobectomy for Pancoast tumors confers a significantly superior 5-year survival rate (60%) compared with a wedge resection (33%).[12] An in-depth description of Pancoast resection techniques is beyond the scope of this review but has been detailed elsewhere.[10,11,13]

Southwest Oncology Group Trial 9416 (Intergroup Trial 0160) was a multi-institutional prospective trial examining induction CRT prior to surgical resection for superior sulcus tumors. In this landmark trial, patients received 2 cycles of cisplatin and etoposide with concurrent 45-Gy RT and underwent subsequent resection if there was no disease progression; 61% of patients had either a pathologic complete response or minimal residual microscopic tumor with induction CRT. Pathologic complete response was a significant prognostic indicator of improved survival.[14] In a systematic review, trimodal therapy was associated with the best 5-year OS rate (35% to 84%) compared with RT alone (11% to 49%) or surgery alone (20%).[15]

Stage III (N2) NSCLC

NSCLC with N2 metastasis represents a complex group of tumors; their treatment is controversial. Randomized controlled trials have not definitively demonstrated a survival benefit of surgery for patients with N2 disease.[16] However, there may be subgroups of patients that benefit from a trimodal treatment approach. Furthermore, the presentation of N2 disease is diverse and ranges from occult, microscopic disease to bulky, infiltrative multistation nodal involvement. The management requires careful evaluation by a multidisciplinary tumor board and a multimodal treatment approach.

The heterogeneity of stage III-N2 NSCLC adds to the treatment dilemma. If occult N2 disease is discovered at time of surgery, the decision of resectability should be made by the operating surgeon. To minimize the risk of diagnosing occult N2 disease at the time of surgery, all patients with stage IB and greater should undergo pathologic mediastinal staging, independent of PET/CT findings. In the era of thoracotomies, surgeons often proceeded with resection to spare that patient another thoracotomy. In the era of VATS and robotic techniques, however, aborting surgery, giving neoadjuvant therapy, and returning for a minimally invasive resection is a reasonable alternative.[2]

For patients with known N2 disease for preoperative staging, the standard of care is neoadjuvant CRT, based on the results of a hallmark trial for N2 disease, Intergroup (INT) 0139 Trial, which compared concurrent CRT followed by resection and definitive CRT without resection. The group of patients who underwent surgery as part of their multimodal treatment strategy had a significantly better progression-free survival (PFS) (12.8 months), as compared with patients who were treated with definitive CRT (10.5 months)[hazard ratio (HR) 0.77 (95% CI, 0.62–0.96; P= .017]. However, there was no difference in OS between patients treated with CRT and surgery (23.6 months) as compared with patients treated with definitive CRT (22.2 months; HR

0.87 [0.70–1.10; P = .24]). The lack of OS benefit in the surgery group was likely driven by the high postoperative mortality (26%) after pneumonectomy, primarily caused by post-pneumonectomy acute respiratory distress syndrome (ARDS). An unplanned subgroup analysis of patients who underwent lobectomy demonstrated an improvement in 5-year OS (36% vs 18%, respectively). Though unplanned analyses should be interpreted with caution, it provides some evidence that subgroups of patients with N2 disease may benefit from surgery as part of a multimodal treatment strategy. As a result of these findings, investigators of the INT-0139 Trial recommended neoadjuvant CRT followed by lobectomy for stage IIIA-N2 disease but definitive CRT if pneumonectomy was necessary.[16]

Other retrospective studies sought to identify which subgroup of patients benefit from an aggressive trimodal therapeutic approach. Bueno and colleagues[17] determined that after induction CRT (with 40–54 Gy of RT) pathologic downstaging of mediastinal lymph nodes had a significant effect on median survival and 5-year OS (35.8% vs 9%, respectively; P = .023). In addition to nodal downstaging after neoadjuvant CRT, Stefani and colleagues[18] found 3 additional factors on multivariable analysis that had an effect on OS: clinical response to neoadjuvant chemotherapy, number of chemotherapy cycles, and histopathologic response. Furthermore, the degree of nodal burden (macroscopic vs microscopic) has also been shown to have a significant effect on OS Indeed, macroscopic disease has been shown to be associated with a 2.8-fold increased risk of death (CI 95%, 1.1%–7.3%).[19]

The benefit of nodal downstaging prior to surgery led investigators to try higher doses (50–66 Gy) of neoadjuvant RT, which were previously avoided in the neoadjuvant setting due to concerns regarding ARDS, impairments to wound healing, and development of bronchopleural fistulas, and increased mortality. Cerfolio and colleagues[20] demonstrated an 83% nodal clearance in the high-dose RT cohort, leading to a borderline significance in DFS with high dose and a trend toward significance in OS. Despite the higher dose of RT, the investigators noted that pulmonary resection could still be safely performed. Radiation Therapy Oncology Group (RTOG) 02-29 was a phase II trial, which examined the use of 50.4 Gy to the mediastinum. Primary end-points included nodal clearance and survival. Mediastinal nodal clearance was 63% after neoadjuvant CRT with significant 2-year OS advantage for those who achieved clearance of their nodal disease and underwent resection (75% for node-negative vs 52% for residual nodal involvement vs 23% for no resection; P = .0002).[21] In a meta-analysis examining neoadjuvant chemotherapy versus CRT, no increase in perioperative mortality was observed between the 2 groups. Although there was no survival benefit demonstrated with the use of RT, neoadjuvant CRT was associated with a greater tumor response, improved rate of complete surgical resection, and mediastinal downstaging.[22,23]

There is no consensus of which subset of patients with N2 disease derive benefit from resection after neoadjuvant CRT. Nonetheless, while there are no randomized clinical trials that demonstrate an unequivocal survival advantage of surgery, a CTSNet survey of thoracic surgeons found that 84% would offer neoadjuvant therapy followed by surgery for single-station microscopic N2 disease but that dropped to 62% when N2 disease became more bulky.[24] Physiologically fit patients with limited single-station disease, and who had a favorable response to neoadjuvant treatment are likely the best candidates for consideration of trimodal therapy.

Outside of clinical trials, however, there are a significant number of patients who have surgery as part of their pre-treatment plan but do not undergo resection. In a retrospective, single-institution study, Cerfolio and colleagues[24] found that only 37% of patients who completed neoadjuvant CRT underwent an operation. Patients who did not complete trimodal therapy were significantly older, lacked a response to therapy, and experienced a morbidity during neoadjuvant therapy that precluded resection.[24] Definitive CRT is the treatment of choice for patients with unresectable locally advanced NSCLC, high-risk comorbid conditions that would preclude surgical resection or patients that refuse surgery.[2]

T4 extension (mediastinum), N0-1

Similar to other locally advanced tumors, nodal disease is the most significant prognostic indicator of survival for patients with T4 tumors with mediastinal extension. As such, T4N2-3 NSCLC is unresectable.[2] For potentially resectable tumors, careful surgical planning is essential.

When considering an extended mediastinal resection and reconstruction, additional preoperative work-up may be necessary. When there is concern for left atrial involvement, ruling out coronary artery disease and valvular dysfunction is essential, and obtaining a cardiac MRI may aid in operative planning. The surgeon also may want to coordinate with anesthesia to have transesophageal echocardiography available during the operation.[25] Although only small case series are available, the data demonstrate acceptable benefit if an R0 resection can be accomplished. In 1 small case series, the 5-year OS after resection of T4 tumors with aortic invasion was 37%, atrial invasion was 25%, carinal involvement was 22%, and SVC invasion was 26%.[26]

In patients with great vessel involvement, resection can be accomplished with cardiopulmonary bypass (CPB) support. A systemic review of the literature identified 72 patients that required CPB with pulmonary resection for T4 tumors. Pneumonectomy was the most common pulmonary resection (74%) and the aorta was the most commonly resected organ (43%). The 5-year OS was 37%. The use of unplanned or emergency CPB was associated with worse survival outcomes, but perioperative 30-day and 90-day mortality rates were low, 0% and 1%, respectively.[27] CPB, when utilized in thoughtful surgical planning, is a safe option in these locally advanced tumors.

SALVAGE LUNG RESECTION

Local tumor recurrence occurs in up to 35% of patients with locally advanced NSCLC after definitive CRT and remains the dominant cause of death in these patients.[28,29] For patients with persistent or recurrent disease after definitive chemoradiation, salvage lung resection is a feasible treatment option for select patients.[28-33] Salvage resections are associated with an increased surgical risk due to post-treatment fibrosis and decreased microvascularity, which may impede healing. Nonetheless, salvage resections are indicated for progressing or persistent primary tumors, recurrent tumors, or complications after RT (eg, lung abscess, hemoptysis, empyema, and bronchial stenosis).[28-30,32]

Multiple small retrospective series have reported the feasibility of salvage resections. Kaba and colleagues[30] reported an R0 resection of 93% in a cohort of patients who primarily underwent salvage resection for progression after definitive CRT. A systematic review of 152 patients undergoing salvage lung resection noted an R0 resection rate of 85% to 100% of patients.[31] Although such resections are technically feasible, they are challenging and are associated with significant complications. Casiraghi and colleagues[32] reported a major complication rate of 25.7%, which included 2 bronchopleural fistulas and 2 bronchovascular fistulas, which led to death from massive hemoptysis (5.7% mortality). In the Swedish Cancer Institute experience, 13% of patients experienced intraoperative vascular injuries, 1 which required a conversion from a lobectomy to pneumonectomy.[33] Pneumonectomies were a large percentage of procedures performed for salvage lung resection within series under a systematic review and were associated with a 90-day mortality rate of 0% to 11.4%.[31] Salvage resections are complex but can be performed with acceptable morbidity and mortality rates and are associated with a survival benefit.

A systematic review demonstrated a mean OS rate of 9 months to 46 months and a 5-year survival rate of 20% to 75%. Distant metastases were the most common site of disease progression.[31] The indication for surgery may be important. Bauman and colleagues[28] found that persistent disease after definitive CRT (evidenced by persistently positive PET scans) was associated with superior median survival rates (43 months) compared with those patients who had recurrent disease (12 months). The extent of resection is also predictive of survival. The Swedish Cancer Institute reported their experience with salvage lung resection. Median OS was 24 months. However, they noted a significant ($P = .02$) difference in survival for patients who required nonextended resection (108.4 months) compared with an extended resection (8.9 months; $P = .02$).[33]

Salvage lung resection should be considered for persistent or recurrent disease after definitive CRT or for complications of RT requiring emergency intervention. As with all oncologic resections, R0 resections have improved survival, and patients require only a pulmonary resection (especially lobectomy) rather than an extended en bloc resection are likely to have the best outcome. Salvage lung resection may require pneumonectomy, highlighting the importance of a preoperative assessment of cardiopulmonary fitness.

STAGE IV OLIGOMETASTATIC DISEASE

Most NSCLC patients present at an advanced stage of diagnosis.[1] The heterogeneity of metastatic disease burden in NSCLC led the 8th edition of the AJCC TMN staging system to divide M1 into 3 separate subcategories: M1a is a separate tumor nodule(s) in a contralateral lobe, pleural or pericardial nodules, or malignant pleural or pericardial effusion; M1b is a single extrathoracic metastasis in a single organ; and M1c is multiple extrathoracic distant metastases in single or multiple organs.[5] This breakdown is due to the differing survival and treatment options for patients of a low burden of metastatic disease.

Oligometastatic state was first reported by Hellman and Weichselbaum[34] in 1995 to describe a state of low systemic burden of distant disease that may be amenable to aggressive local therapy. The oligometastatic state is less biologically aggressive, is limited to a single organ or a to a low-volume tumor load and often is stable over time. As a result, it is amenable to aggressive locally therapy.[35] In contrast to palliative treatment of metastatic NSCLC, which offers a limited survival benefit, long-term survival can be achieved with aggressive intervention with oligometastatic disease. It is important to recognize the nuances of this disease process to identify which patients may benefit from more aggressive treatment.

Brain

The brain is the most common site of distant metastasis in NSCLC. There are several randomized trials supporting aggressive treatment of oligometastatic brain metastases. Patchell and colleagues[36] demonstrated that patients with a single brain metastasis who underwent surgery and RT (versus RT alone) had improved survival (OS, 40 weeks vs 15 weeks, respectively), improved functional status, and decrease recurrence in the brain. Additional series reviews have demonstrated a survival benefit from aggressive management of intracranial metastases, Billing and colleagues[37] reviewed

28 patients with synchronous oligometastatic NSCLC who underwent craniectomy prior to pulmonary resection. The median time between the surgeries was 14 days. The total OS rates at 1 year, 2 years, and 5-years were 64.3%, 54.0%, and 21.5%, respectively. The degree of nodal disease had a significant negative impact on OS. No patient with positive nodal disease survived longer than 3 years.[37] Consequently, in patients with good performance status and no evidence of N2 disease, surgical resection of single brain metastases in combination with RT is recommended for these solitary intracranial metastases.[36,38,39] In particular, because of the risk of neurocognitive decline with whole brain radiation therapy (WBRT), stereotactic radiosurgery (SRS) is the preferred approach for patients whose brain metastasis is treated with RT. For patients whose brain lesion is causing mass effect, craniotomy and resection may be required.

patients with unresectable single brain metastases should be treated with definitive RT. RTOG 9508 examined patients with 1 to 3 newly diagnosed brain metastases treated with either whole-brain RT (WBRT) or WBRT with stereotactic radiosurgery (SRS), and demonstrated that WBRT with SRS had improved functional status, and in univariate analysis improved OS with a single brain metastasis.[38] The addition of WBRT with SRS was associated, however, with significant neurocognitive decline[40]; thus, SRS typically is utilized alone for single, surgically unresectable brain metastases or less than 3 brain metastases.[2]

In the absence of nodal disease, select patients with solitary brain metastasis are also candidates for aggressive local treatment of the primary tumor (resection or RT), which offers a survival advantage over chemotherapy alone.[41,42]

The data suggest that aggressive treatment of intracranial oligometastatic disease is associated with improved survival. Patients with intracranial oligometastatic disease that have good performance status, no evidence of N2 disease, limited disease in the chest, limited brain metastases may have a survival benefit from resection of the primary tumor and aggressive local therapy (surgery, or SRS) to the brain along with systemic therapy in the neoadjuvant or adjuvant setting.[36–38,40–42]

Adrenal

Isolated adrenal metastases are rare. The treatment paradigm mirrors that of isolated brain metastases—for patients with small volume disease burden in the chest, no evidence of N2 disease and a solitary oligometastatic site, aggressive local therapy to both the primary tumor and metastasis provide a survival benefit. Raz and colleagues[43] examined the surgical outcomes for patients who underwent adrenalectomy for metastatic NSCLC. The median survival was 19 months after adrenalectomy (5-year OS, 34%), compared with 6 months (5-year OS, 0%) in patients who were treated nonoperatively. In patients undergoing adrenalectomy, the median disease-free interval was 14 months. As compared with contralateral metastases, patients with ipsilateral adrenal metastases had significantly improved 5-year survival, and there was a trend of improved survival with lower lobe tumors, but it did not reach significance. No difference was found between synchronous versus metachronous adrenal metastases in this series.[43] A pooled analysis further examined the outcomes of surgical intervention on 98 patients with isolated adrenal metastases. Half of the patients had metachronous (49%) whereas half had synchronous (51%) adrenal metastases; metachronous metastases were associated with better prognosis.[39]

Summary of Oligometastatic Disease

For select patients with small volume node-negative disease in the chest and limited oligometastatic burden, numerous retrospective, single-institution studies and meta-analyses have demonstrated a survival benefit with aggressive local therapy to both the primary tumor and metastatic site in combination with systemic therapy.[35,37–44] As with all complex malignancies, a thoughtful evaluation and discussion should be undertaken by a multidisciplinary team of thoracic surgeons, medical oncologists, and radiation oncologists.

LUNG RESECTION AND IMMUNOTHERAPY

The landmark PACIFIC Trial demonstrated that durvalumab, a PD-L1 (programmed death-ligand 1) inhibitor, administered after definitive CRT for unresectable stage III NSCLC improved OS and PFS compared with placebo.[45] Based on these findings, the FDA approved durvalumab in 2017 for consolidation therapy for patients with no progression of disease after definitive CRT. Although durvalumab is approved for unresectable disease, there are trials examining immunotherapies on potentially resectable lung cancers that potentially will have an impact on how advanced, potentially resectable NSCLCs are managed in the future.

Evaluating neoadjuvant administration of nivolumab, a PD-1 (programmed cell death protein 1) inhibitor, in early stage (I–IIIA) NSCLC, investigators demonstrated that immunotherapy did not delay surgery and was associated with a 95% R0 resection; 45% had a major pathologic response (defined as no more than 10% viable tumor cells within the specimen), independent of PD-L1 status.[46] Bott and colleagues[47] reported their experience of pulmonary resection after administration of neoadjuvant nivolumab; 75% of the patients underwent lobectomy, and 54% of patients undergoing a minimally invasive approach (VATS or robotic) were converted to thoracotomy. Most of these patients required conversion to an open approach due to dense adhesions and fibrosis from immunotherapy. Importantly, neoadjuvant immunotherapy was associated with an acceptable morbidity and mortality rate. There were no reported mortalities, and the most common postoperative morbidity was atrial arrhythmia.[47] As experience with immunotherapy evolves through ongoing clinical trials, management of locally advanced and metastatic NSCLC may change.

SUMMARY

Locally advanced NSCLC is a complex, heterogeneous disease process that requires a thoughtful, multidisciplinary approach. In highly select patients with an excellent performance status and the absence of N2 disease, surgical resection of locally advanced and limited oligometastatic NSCLC offers a survival benefit when combined with a multimodal treatment strategy. With advancements in and the increasing application of immunotherapy, the multidisciplinary perspective of locally advanced NSCLC will continue to evolve.

DISCLOSURE

Dr S.S. Groth is a proctor and speaker for Intuitive Surgical Inc. (Sunnyvale, California).

REFERENCES

1. National Cancer Institute. Surveillance, epidemiology, and end results. (SEER) data. Available at: http://seer.cancer.gov/. Accessed June 15, 2020.
2. NCCN. NCCN Clinical Guidelines: non-small cell lung cancer. 2020. Available at: NCCN.org. Accessed June 15, 2020.
3. Kozower BD, Larner JM, Detterbeck FC, et al. Special Treatment Issues in Non-small cell lung cancer. Diagnosis and management of lung cancer, 3rd ed:

American College of Chest Physicians College of Chest Physicians evidence-based clinical practice guidelines. Chest 2013;143(5S):e369S–99S.

4. Riquet M, Arame A, Le Pimpec Barthes F. Non-small cell lung cancer invading the chest wall. Thorac Surg Clin 2010;20:519–27.

5. AJCC. AJCC cancer staging manual. "Lung cancer". 8th edition. New York: Springer; 2016.

6. Hennon MW, Dexter EU, Huang M, et al. Does thoracoscopic surgery decrease the morbidity of combined lung and chest wall resection? Ann Thorac Surg 2015;99:1929–35.

7. Doddoli C, D'Journo B, Le Pimpec-Barthes F, et al. Lung cancer invading the chest wall: A plea for en-bloc resection but the need for new treatment strategies. Ann Thorac Surg 2005;80:2032–40.

8. Tanberg DJ, Kelsey CR, D'Amico TA, et al. Patterns of failure after surgery for non-small cell lung cancer invading the chest wall. Clin Lung Cancer 2016; 18(4):249–65.

9. Drake JA, Sullivan JL, Weksler B. Adjuvant chemotherapy improves survival in patients with completely resected T3N0 non-small cell lung cancer invading the chest wall. J Thorac Cardiovasc Surg 2018;155:1794–802.

10. Foroulis CN, Zarogoulidis P, Darwiche K, et al. Superior sulcus (Pancoast) tumors: current evidence of diagnosis and radical treatment. J Thorac Dis 2013;5(S4): S342–58.

11. Marulli G, Battistella L, Mammana M, et al. Superior sulcus tumors (Pancoast tumors). Ann Transl Med 2016;4(12):239–52.

12. Ginsberg RJ, Martini N, Zaman M, et al. Influence of surgical resection and brachytherapy in the management of superior sulcus tumor. Ann Thorac Surg 1994;57:1440–5.

13. Ibrahim K, Walsh GL, Burt BM. Pancoast tumors. In: Sugarbaker DJ, Bueno R, Burt BM, et al, editors. Sugarbaker's adult chest surgery. 3rd edition. New York: McGraw Hill; 2020. p. 742–54.

14. Rusch VW, Giroux DJ, Kraut MJ, et al. Induction chemoradiation and surgical resection for superior sulcus non-small cell lung carcinomas: Long-term results of Southwest Oncology Group Trial 9416 (Intergroup Trial 0160). J Clin Oncol 2007;25(3):313–8.

15. Buderi SI, Shackcloth M, Woolley S. Does induction chemoradiotherapy increase survival in patients with Pancoast tumour? Interact Cardiovasc Thorac Surg 2016; 23:821–5.

16. Albain KS, Swann RS, Rusch VW, et al. Radiotherapy plus chemotherapy with or without surgical resection for Stage III non-small cell lung cancer: A phase III randomized control trial. Lancet 2009;374:379–86.

17. Bueno R, Richards WG, Swanson SJ, et al. Nodal stage after induction therapy for Stage IIIA lung cancer determines patient survival. Ann Thorac Surg 2000; 70:1826–31.

18. Stefani A, Alifano M, Bobbio A, et al. Which patients should be operated on after induction chemotherapy for N2 non-small cell lung cancer? Analysis of a 7 year experience in 175 patients. J Thorac Cardiovasc Surg 2010;140:356–63.

19. Meacci E, Cesario A, Cusumano G, et al. Surgery for patients with persistent pathological N2 IIIA stage in non-small-cell lung cancer after induction radiochemotherapy: the microscopic seed of doubt. Eur J Cardiothorac Surg 2011; 40:656–63.

20. Cerfolio RJ, Bryant AS, Spencer SA, et al. Pulmonary resection after high-dose and low-dose chest irradiation. Ann Thorac Surg 2005;80:1224–30.

21. Suntharalingam M, Paulus R, Edelman MJ, et al. Radiation Therapy Oncology Group Protocol 02-29: A Phase II trial of neoadjuvant therapy with concurrent chemotherapy and full-dose radiation therapy followed by surgical resection and consolidative therapy for locally advanced non-small cell carcinoma of the lung. Int J Radiat Oncol Biol Phys 2011;84(2):456–63.
22. Chen Y, Peng X, Zhou Y, et al. Comparing the benefits of chemoradiotherapy and chemotherapy for resectable stage IIIA/N2 non-small cell lung cancer: A meta-analysis. World J Surg Oncol 2018;16(8):1–10.
23. Veeramachaneni NK, Feins RH, Stephenson BJK, et al. Management of Stage IIIA non-small cell lung cancer by thoracic surgeons in North America. Ann Thorac Surg 2013;94:922–8.
24. Cerfolio RJ, Maniscalco L, Bryant AS. The treatment of patients with Stage IIIA non-small cell lung cancer from N2 disease: Who returns to the surgical arena and who survives. Ann Thorac Surg 2008;86:912–20.
25. Blasberg JD, Boffa DJ. Cardiopulmonary bypass for extended thoracic resections. In: Sugarbaker DJ, Bueno R, Burt BM, et al, editors. Sugarbaker's adult chest surgery. 3rd edition. New York: McGraw Hill; 2020. p. 755–61.
26. Spaggiari L, Tessitore A, Casiraghi M, et al. Survival after extended resection for mediastinal advanced lung cancer: lessons learned on 167 consecutive cases. Ann Thorac Surg 2013;95:1717–25.
27. Muralidaran A, Detterbeck FC, Boffa DJ, et al. Long-term survival after lung resection for non-small cell lung cancer with circulatory bypass: A systematic review. J Thorac Cardiovasc Surg 2011;142(5):1137–42.
28. Bauman JE, Mulligan MS, Martins RG, et al. Salvage lung resection after definitive radiation (>59 Gy) for non-small cell lung cancer: surgical and oncological outcomes. Ann Thorac Surg 2008;86:1632–9.
29. Van Breussegem A, Hendriks JM, Lauwers P, et al. Salvage surgery after high-dose radiotherapy. J Thorac Dis 2017;9(Supl3):S193–200.
30. Kaba E, Ozyurtkan MO, Ayalp K, et al. Salvage thoracic surgery in patients with lung cancer: potential indications and benefits. J Cardiothorac Surg 2018; 13(13):1–6.
31. Dickhoff C, Otten RHJ, Heymans MW, et al. Salvage surgery for recurrent or persistent tumour after radical (chemo)radiotherapy for locally advanced non-small cell lung cancer: a systematic review. Ther Adv Med Oncol 2018;10:1–12.
32. Casiraghi M, Maisonneuve P, Piperno G, et al. Salvage surgery after definitive chemotherapy for non-small cell lung cancer. Semin Thorac Surg 2017;29: 233–41.
33. Bograd AJ, Mann C, Gorden JA, et al. Salvage lung resections after definitive chemoradiotherapy: A safe and effective oncologic option. Ann Thorac Surg 2020. https://doi.org/10.1016/j.athoracsur.2020.04.035.
34. Hellman S, Weischelbaum RR. Oligometastases. J Clin Oncol 1995;13:8–10.
35. Pfannschmidt J, Dienemann H. Surgical treatment of oligometastatic non-small cell lung cancer. Lung Cancer 2010;69:251–8.
36. Patchell PA, Tibbs PA, Walsh JW, et al. A randomized trial of surgery in the treatment of single metastases to the brain. N Engl J Med 1990;322:494–500.
37. Billing PS, Miller DL, Allen MS, et al. Surgical treatment of primary lung cancer with synchronous brain metastases. J Thorac Cardiovasc Surg 2001;122:548–53.
38. Andrews DW, Scott CB, Sperduto PW, et al. Whole brain radiation therapy with or without sterotactic radiosurgery boost for patients with one to three brain metastases: phase III results of the RTOG 9508 randomised trial. Lancet 2004;363: 1665–72.

39. Gao XL, Zhang KW, Tang MB, et al. Pooled analysis for surgical treatment for isolated adrenal metastasis and non-small cell lung cancer. Interact Cardiovasc Thorac Surg 2017;24:1–7.

40. Chang EL, Wefel JS, Hess KR, et al. Neurocognition in patients with brain metastases treated with radiosurgery or radiosurgery plus whole-brain irradiation: A randomised controlled trial. Lancet Oncol 2009;10:1037–44.

41. Villareal-Garza C, de la Mata D, Zavala DG, et al. Aggressive treatment of primary tumor in patients with non-small-cell lung cancer and exclusively brain metastases. Clin Lung Cancer 2013;14(1):6–13.

42. Li D, Zhu X, Wang H, et al. Should aggressive thoracic therapy be performed in patients with synchronous oligometastatic non-small cell lung cancer? A meta-analysis. J Thorac Dis 2017;9(2):310–7.

43. Raz DJ, Lanuti M, Gaissert HC, et al. Outcomes of patients with isolated adrenal metastasis from non-small cell lung carcinoma. Ann Thorac Surg 2011;92:1788–93.

44. David EA, Clark JM, Cook DT, et al. The role of thoracic surgery in the therapeutic management of metastatic non-small cell lung cancer. J Thorac Oncol 2017;12(11):1636–45.

45. Antonia SJ, Villegas A, Daniel D, et al. Overall survival with durvalumab after chemoradiotherapy in Stage III NSCLC. N Engl J Med 2018;379:2342–50.

46. Forde PM, Chaft JE, Smith KN, et al. Neoadjuvant PD-I blockage in resectable lung cancer. N Engl J Med 2018;378:1976–86.

47. Bott MJ, Yang SC, Park BK, et al. Initial results of pulmonary resection after neoadjuvant nivolumab with resectable non-small cell lung cancer. J Thorac Cardiovasc Surg 2019l;158:269–76.

Emerging Therapies in Thoracic Malignancies— Immunotherapy, Targeted Therapy, and T-Cell Therapy in Non–Small Cell Lung Cancer

Boris Sepesi, MD[a],*, Tina Cascone, MD, PhD[b],
Stephen G. Chun, MD[c], Mehmet Altan, MD[b], Xiuning Le, MD[b]

KEYWORDS

• Immunotherapy • Targeted therapy • T cells • Adoptive therapy
• Non–small cell lung cancer

KEY POINTS

• Immunotherapy has improved survival and advanced treatment options for metastatic non–small cell lung cancer, and it is being actively studied in local and regional lung cancer settings.

• Cancer gene mutations and alterations provide a significant opportunity for the development of targeted agents, which have been very successful in cancer control and survival outcomes.

• Adoptive T-cell therapies are promising new therapeutic options for solid cancers, including lung cancer, although more research and trials are needed in this space.

INTRODUCTION

Over the past decade there have been dramatic therapeutic advances for non–small cell lung cancer (NSCLC) that have been based on an improved understanding of biomarkers, tumor immunology, driver mutations, T-cell receptors (TCRs), and adoptive immune therapies. As a result of these advances, the overall survival (OS) currently seen with immunotherapy and targeted biologic regimens is remarkably longer than with historic cytotoxic chemotherapy. These discoveries have created many new

[a] Department of Thoracic and Cardiovascular Surgery, The University of Texas MD Anderson Cancer Center, 1515 Holcombe Boulevard, Houston, TX 77030, USA; [b] Department of Thoracic/ Head and Neck Medical Oncology, The University of Texas MD Anderson Cancer Center, 1515 Holcombe Boulevard, Houston, TX 77030, USA; [c] Department of Radiation Oncology, The University of Texas MD Anderson Cancer Center, 1515 Holcombe Boulevard, Houston, TX 77030, USA
* Corresponding author. Department of Thoracic and Cardiovascular Surgery, The MD Anderson Cancer Center, 1400 Pressler Street, FCT. 196004, Unit 1489, Houston, TX 77030-4009.
E-mail address: bsepesi@mdanderson.org

Surg Oncol Clin N Am 29 (2020) 555–569
https://doi.org/10.1016/j.soc.2020.06.009
1055-3207/20/© 2020 Elsevier Inc. All rights reserved.

possible therapeutic options for lung cancer patients in both local and metastatic settings. This article reviews the current landscape of immunotherapy, targeted therapy, and adoptive therapy in NSCLC.

IMMUNOTHERAPY IN NON–SMALL CELL LUNG CANCER
Immunotherapy in Metastatic Non–Small Cell Lung Cancer

Arguably, the most important paradigm-changing innovation for NSCLC of the past decade has been the advent of anti–programmed death cell protein-1 (PD-1) and anti–programmed death ligand 1 (PD-L1) as well as cytotoxic T-lymphocyte–associated protein 4 (CTLA-4)–directed immune checkpoint blockade (ICB).[1] ICB therapy is predicated on the recognition that tumors express PD-L1 to evade the immune system by suppressing T cells by binding the PD-1 transmembrane receptor. In turn, the utilization of targeted antibodies to perturb PD-1/PD-L1 signaling has proved to have remarkable antitumor activity in NSCLC. Currently, there are 2 anti–PD-1 and 1 anti–PD-L1 agents that are approved by the Food and Drug Administration (FDA) for the treatment of metastatic NSCLC and 1 anti–PD-L1 antibody in the consolidative setting after concurrent chemoradiation for locally advanced NSCLC. Depending on the tumor PD-L1 expression level, ICBs can be utilized either as monotherapy or in combination with chemotherapy in the first-line setting for metastatic NSCLC.[2] This article reviews seminal phase III trials utilizing anti–PD-1 agents nivolumab and pembrolizumab and anti–PD-L1 agent atezolizumab in metastatic NSCLC.[2]

The initial phase III trials, which demonstrated the benefit of immunotherapy in metastatic NSCLCs, tested the anti–PD-1 antibody nivolumab in the second-line setting after recurrence or progression on cytotoxic chemotherapy. These trials included CheckMate 017[3] in squamous NSCLC and CheckMate 057[4] in nonsquamous cell lung carcinomas. Both trials demonstrated better OS with nivolumab compared with docetaxel alone and received FDA approval as the second-line therapy. Based on these encouraging results, nivolumab was added to the platinum-doublet chemotherapy in the first-line setting in the CheckMate 026[5] trial, in the hope of improving survival outcomes over standard chemotherapy. This trial did not reach the primary endpoint, however, of improved progression-free survival (PFS) or OS, suggesting that nivolumab may not enhance outcomes when combined with platinum-doublet therapy.

In the CheckMate 227[6] trial, nivolumab was combined with anti–CTLA-4 antibody ipilimumab, and compared in the first-line setting against standard chemotherapy; dual ICB therapy previously demonstrated encouraging results in metastatic melanoma.[7] The trial stratified patients based on tumor PD-L1 expression. Results in patients with PD-L1 greater than 1% demonstrated significantly longer median OS with ICB combination compared with chemotherapy.[6]

The efficacy of pembrolizumab was studied in the KEYNOTE-024,[8] KEYNOTE-042,[9] KEYNOTE-189,[10] and KEYNOTE-407[11] phase III trials and further corroborated the benefit of ICB for metastatic NSCLC. Importantly, KEYNOTE-024[8] established pembrolizumab as the first-line ICB monotherapy in wild-type epidermal growth factor receptor (EGFR) and anaplastic lymphoma kinase, metastatic NSCLC with PD-L1 expression greater than or equal to 50%. KEYNOTE-042[9] expended on pembrolizumab indications by demonstrating benefit even in patients with PD-L1 greater than 1%. KEYNOTE-189[10] and KEYNOTE-407[11] studied combination of pembrolizumab and chemotherapy in all-comers in nonsquamous and squamous cell lung carcinoma, respectively; survival outcomes were favorable with pembrolizumab in both trials.

These studies secured the indications for pembrolizumab alone or in combination with chemotherapy in the first-line metastatic NSCLC.

Atezolizumab is a monoclonal antibody directed against PD-L1 and was studied in IMpower 110 (NCT02409342), IMpower 150,[12] IMpower 130,[13] IMpower 131 (NCT02367794), and IMpower 132 (NCT02657434) trials. IMpower 110 (NCT02409342), similarly to KEYNOTE-042,[9] demonstrated survival benefit with monotherapy compared with chemotherapy in patients with PD-L1 greater than or equal to 1%. In IMpower 150[12] trial, atezolizumab, chemotherapy, and bevacizumab resulted in improved survival, even in EGFR-positive patients. IMpower 130[13] showed benefit of atezolizumab in combination with chemotherapy in the first-line metastatic nonsquamous lung cancer without EGFR or ALK mutations, whereas IMpower 131(NCT02367794), and IMpower 132 (NCT02657434) studied all-comers with metastatic squamous and nonsquamous lung cancer, respectively. Survival benefit of atezolizumab added to chemotherapy regimen was evident in both histologies; therefore, atezolizumab alone or in combination with chemotherapy is indicated in the first-line metastatic NSCLC setting.

Currently, an area of controversy and active investigation in metastatic NSCLC is the role of local consolidative therapy (LCT). Although 2 randomized phase II trials have demonstrated an improvement in PFS with LCT for oligometastatic NSCLC treated with cytotoxic chemotherapy, this paradigm has yet to be validated in patients treated with ICB.[14,15] Currently, the role of LCT for oligometastatic NSCLC treated with ICB is being tested in the context of multiple prospective clinical trials, including NRG Oncology-LU002 (NCT03137771) and the LONESTAR Trial (NCT03391869).

In summary, the advent of anti–PD-1/PD-L1 ICB has yielded major improvements in metastatic NSCLC outcomes. Current efforts to understand mechanisms of ICB resistance and the role of LCT are anticipated to further refine and improve patient care.

Immunotherapy in Locoregionally Advanced Unresectable Non–Small Cell Lung Cancer

Stage III NSCLC is a complex and heterogenous disease state, which historically has been the subject of much controversy regarding the most optimal therapeutic algorithms. Stage III generally includes either large tumors or centrally located tumors abutting or invading the mediastinum and/or cancer involved mediastinal lymph nodes, either single or multiple, or above the clavicle, which maybe bulky or nonbulky. Adding to this heterogeneity, a surgeon's judgment of what constitutes resectable and unresectable disease along with options of induction chemotherapy or chemoradiation versus definitive concomitant chemoradiation creates numerous possible treatment algorithms and sequences. For patients deemed to have unresectable disease, concurrent chemoradiation has been the standard of care for decades without significant improvements in survival since the 1990s. The PACIFIC trial changed this paradigm.[16] The PACIFIC trial enrolled surgically unresectable patients and randomized them to chemoradiation with or without 1 year of consolidative durvalumab. Initial results from this trial demonstrated improved PFS.[16] Subsequent OS analyses revealed improved OS of 83%, 74%, and 66% at 1 year, 2 years, and 3 years, respectively, all 10% to 20% better than with chemoradiation alone.[17] These results prompted FDA approval of durvalumab for stage III locally advanced NSCLC. How to further improve on these results and what to do in surgically resectable stage III NSCLC is an area of continuous study. Adjuvant durvalumab mainly improved rates of metastatic disease, including brain metastases that occurred at rates of less than 5%, which was dramatically lower than historic brain metastasis rates for stage III disease. What the rates of locoregional disease control are with this regimen is not totally clear; would trimodality therapy with concurrent chemoradiation and surgery further improve local control, and in turn survival? It also has been postulated that lower immune-priming doses of radiation might result in neoantigen activation and help prevent distant recurrence with surgical locoregional control to account for lower radiation dose. Would concomitant administration of radiation and durvalumab be even more effective? These, and many other questions remain unanswered and are tested in ongoing clinical studies.

Immunotherapy in Local and Locoregionally Advanced Resectable Non–Small Cell Lung Cancer

Currently, there are no approved immunotherapy regimens as part of the standard of care in the perioperative setting for surgically resectable NSCLCs. There are, however, numerous ongoing clinical trials testing the efficacy of mono or dual immunotherapy regimens as well as the combinations of immunotherapy and chemotherapy in the neoadjuvant setting.

Neoadjuvant Monoimmunotherapy

The first trial testing neoadjuvant ICB enrolled 21 patients with resectable stages IB–IIIA NSCLC.[18] Patients received 2 doses of neoadjuvant nivolumab followed by surgery. The aims of the trial were safety and feasibility of surgical resection within 4 weeks of the 1st dose of nivolumab, which were met. The secondary endpoint of major pathologic response (MPR) was 45% and downstaging was achieved in 40% of patients after just 2 therapeutic doses.[18] The Lung Cancer Mutation Consortium (LCMC) 3 study[19] targeted accrual has been 180 patients; preliminary results showed that 2 doses of neoadjuvant atezolizumab induced 19% MPR rate and 5% of evaluable patients achieved pathologic complete response. These results overall are similar to the MPR after 3 cycles of nivolumab in the phase 2 randomized NEOSTAR (NCT03158129) trial,[20] which demonstrated MPR of 17% in 23 treated patients. In another neoadjuvant study evaluating PD-1 inhibitor sintilimab in resectable NSCLC, 2 doses of neoadjuvant ICB induced 40.5% MPR rate,[21] which is similar to the results of phase I study MK3475-223 (NCT02938624)[22] with pembrolizumab (MPR 40%). Although there is a clear intertrial variability in terms of MPR rates after ICB monotherapy, which may be driven by several variables, including the type of immunotherapy, tumor histology, oncogenic drivers, and perhaps number of doses prior to surgery, it appears that neoadjuvant anti–PD-1/PD-L1 therapy is overall safe and feasible and its efficacy appears to be very similar or slightly better than platinum doublet chemotherapy.

Neoadjuvant Dual Immunotherapy

The combination of nivolumab and ipilimumab in the neoadjuvant setting has been studied in 2 phase II trials (NEOSTAR [NCT03158129 and NCT02259621]). Recently reported results from the NEOSTAR trial[20] investigating nivolumab given with 1 dose of ipilimumab suggested that the combination is overall well tolerated and induced 33% MPR rate. The results of NCT02259621 have not yet been presented; the trial plans to accrue 30 patients. Whether dual immunotherapy will be tested further in larger studies is currently unclear and likely depends on translational analyses from these trials, which may help identify sounds of patients responding to this therapy. Although MPR rates with dual ICB appear to be improved compared with MPR with neoadjuvant chemotherapy (15%–19%), the unprecedented MPR rates achieved after combination of immunotherapy and chemotherapy most likely will play the leading role in advancing the neoadjuvant NSCLC field forward.

Combined Neoadjuvant Immunotherapy and Chemotherapy

Several ongoing trials are investigating the paradigm of neoadjuvant combined anti–PD-1/PD-L1 inhibitors with chemotherapy for resectable NSCLC patients. The NADIM trial[23] is a single-arm phase II trial, which administered 3 doses of chemotherapy along with nivolumab prior to resection of clinically staged IIIA NSCLC. The trial enrolled 46 patients, and 89% had clinical N2 disease, majority (75%) multistation. Resectability was 89% (41/46). Importantly, the trial reported an unprecedented MPR response rates of 83% (in resected 41 patients, or 73% (34/46) if analyzed by the intention to treat). Complete pathologic response was reported in 24 patients; OS at 18-month follow-up was 91%. These results are remarkable, but require validation in currently ongoing phase III trials in order to definitively change practice paradigm for neoadjuvant therapy in NSCLC. Notable ongoing phase III trials include CheckMate 816 (NCT02998528)[24] utilizing nivolumab with chemotherapy, and randomized phase III trials: KEYNOTE-671 (NCT03425643, pembrolizumab), IMpower 030[25] (NCT03456063, atezolizumab), AEGEAN[26] (NCT03800134, durvalumab), and Check-Mate 077 (NCT04025879, nivolumab); these randomized trials will compare combined immune-chemotherapy to standard neoadjuvant chemotherapy. All are either excluding or carefully stratifying patients with targetable somatic oncogenic drivers.

Randomized phase III trials will potentially bring the combined neoadjuvant immune-chemotherapy into the realm of standard of care if they will achieve results close to the NADIM trial.

TYROSINE KINASE INHIBITORS AND TARGETED THERAPY
Targeted Therapy in Metastatic Lung Cancers

The stratification of NSCLC with molecular oncogene alterations has changed the treatment paradigm and meaningfully improved patients' survival and the quality of life.[27] A driver oncogene can be detected in two-thirds of adenocarcinomas. There are 5 oncogenes in NSCLC with FDA-approved targeted therapies for metastatic diseases, and many others are anticipated to be added to the clinical armamentarium.

The first actionable mutations in NSCLC have been EGFR mutations. In 2004, 3 groups identified tumors harboring EGFR exon19 deletion or exon21 L858R mutations that were exquisitely responsive to EGFR tyrosine kinase inhibitors (TKIs).[28–30] In metastatic setting, it was shown that the treatment with EGFR inhibitor can improve patients' PFS and quality of life compared with chemotherapy.[31–33] Although EGFR mutations are more prevalent in Asian female never-smoker patients (up to 65%), it also occurs in patients with other demographic features. Therefore, it has been recommended that all newly diagnosed metastatic NSCLC be tested for mutations in this gene. With erlotinib or gefitinib (first-generation EGFR TKIs), approximately half of the EGFR-mutant tumors acquire a new EGFR mutation T790M to displace drug binding out of the EGFR adenosine triphosphate pocket and render clinical resistance to treatment.[34] To overcome this type of resistance, newer EGFR inhibitors were designed, such as osimertinib.[35] In AURA trials, osimertinib was able to confer response in T790M tumors after progression on erlotinib or gefitinib.[36] Furthermore, in newly diagnosed metastatic patients, osimertinib was associated with better PFS[37] and OS.[38] Osimertinib currently is the preferred first-line choice for metastatic NSCLC with EGFR sensitizing mutations, with other 4 EGFR TKIs serving as alternative options.

ALK-rearranged NSCLC is another prime example of targeted therapy. It took only 3 years from discovering that ALK fusion with ELM4 is a driver fusion for NSCLC,[39] to showing that crizotinib induces response in 57% of ALK-rearranged NSCLC.[40] Similar to EGFR TKIs, newer-generation ALK TKIs, such as ceritinib,[41] alectinib,[42,43] brigatinib,[44] and lorlatinib,[45–47] demonstrated better efficacy and the ability to overcome acquired ALK mutations. Currently, the OS for patients on ALK inhibitors extends beyond 5 years (6.8 years).[48]

ROS1 is another kinase structurally very close to ALK. The fusion of ROS1 occurs in 1% to 3% of NSCLC. Not surprisingly, crizotinib,[49] certinib,[50] and lorlatinib[51] all are active in ROS1-fusion NSCLC.

BRAF V600E mutation initially was recognized in melanoma and dual inhibition of MEK and RAF was established in melanoma as an effective therapeutic strategy. In a phase II study using dabrafenib plus trametinib in BRAF V600E NSCLC patients, response rate was 68%, with almost all patients experiencing tumor reduction.[52] The FDA approved this combination based on this single-arm pivotal trial.

Most recently, NTRK inhibitors have demonstrated outstanding efficacy in tumors harboring NTRK1/2/3 fusions, regardless of the tumor type.[53] In this study, in the lung cancer subgroup, 75% patients responded well to therapy. Thus, NTRK inhibitors became the newest addition to the therapeutic options for treating lung cancers with an oncogene driver.

In addition to the FDA-approved medications for the 5 different oncogenic alterations, new targets and therapies continue to emerge and some have shown promise in their early efficacy.

RET fusion as a target for NSCLC has been recognized since 2012.[54,55] Several TKIs targeting ALK and ROS1, for example, alectinib,[56] were found to have activities for RET-fusion.

METex14 skipping was identified as a potential oncogenic driver in 2015 to 2016.[57,58] By splicing interruption with exon14, c-MET signaling is constitutively active due to the lack of degradation. Small molecule inhibitors, such as crizotinib, tepotinib, capmatinib, and savolitinib, all demonstrated efficacy in NSCLC patients with METex14 skipping mutation. Two drugs, tepotinib and capmatinib, currently are under fast-track review with regulatory agencies around the globe for approval.

Other than classic mEGFR sensitizing mutations at exon 19 and exon 21 L858R, EGFR and HER2 exon20 insertions also are known oncogenic drivers. Many novel small molecule inhibitors are under development to target this population.

In 2019, the most exciting development in targeted therapy for NSCLC has been the observation of clinical efficacies with inhibitors targeting KRAS G12C. Many agents targeting KRAS and its pathways are under clinical evaluation now.

In summary, targeted therapies with precision medicine approach have revolutionized the treatment of metastatic NSCLC. The field is moving rapidly in several different directions. Aside from the continued effort in identifying new oncogenic drivers and the development of highly potent selective therapeutics, combination therapy with other classes of medications is being explored. Combination of targeted therapy with radiation or surgical LCT consolidation (NORTHSTAR [NCT03410043] and BRIGHTSTAR [NCT03707938] trials) also have shown initial success. Combinations with chemotherapy, antiangiogenics, ICB, and immune modulation agents all are under active investigation.

Targeted Therapy in Resectable Stages I to III Non–Small Cell Lung Cancer

Building on the success in metastatic NSCLC, clinical trials are evaluating targeted therapeutics in earlier stages, as adjuvant or neoadjuvant therapies. As adjuvant therapy, several trials evaluated EGFR inhibitors as adjuvant therapy after surgical resection of stages IB–IIIA NSCLC. The initial phase III RADIANT trial showed no disease-free survival (DFS) benefit for adjuvant erlotinib in patients with EGFR amplification, but the subgroup of EGFR-mutant NSCLC favored erlotinib (median DFS, 46.4 months vs 28.5 months, respectively, with erlotinib vs without; P = .039).[59] In another randomized phase III Chinese study ADJUVANT-CTONG1104, 222 patients with N1-N2 disease (stages IIA–IIIA) were randomized to gefitinib for 2 years versus cisplatin/vinorelbine.[60] The DFS was 28.7 months for gefitinib versus 18 months for chemotherapy; hazard ratio 0.60; P = .0054). The gefitinib group had more brain recurrence than chemotherapy group.[60] In the United States, a similar adjuvant trial, Adjuvant Lung Cancer Enrichment Marker Identification and Sequencing Trial (ALCHEMIST) is a National Cancer Institute–sponsored National Clinical Trials Network initiative aiming at addressing the same question.[61] ALCHEMIST screens patients with operable lung adenocarcinoma to determine if their tumors contain EGFR or ALK. Once the presence of EGFR or ALK is confirmed, patients are randomized to monitoring versus erlotinib or crizotinib, respectively, after completion of their standard adjuvant chemotherapy. Because osimertinib has an excellent anticancer activity for brain metastases, the field has been anxiously waiting for the results of the ADUARA trial, which administered osimertinib for 3-year after lung cancer resection.[62] The data from this trial were announced via virtual 2020 American Society of Clinical Oncology meeting (due to COVID-19 pandemic). This phase III randomized trial of 682 patients was unblinded 2 years early after recommendations from an independent data monitoring committee due to 79% reduction in disease-free survival (DFS), defined as either recurrence or death, and 89% versus 53% 2-year DFS compared with placebo. This is a remarkable benefit of adjuvant osimertinib versus placebo in surgically resected patients with stages IB–IIIA EGFR positive adenocarcinoma.[63]

In the neoadjuvant setting, data on targeted therapy are sparse, partially due to the challenge of obtaining mutational status prior to surgery. A coordinated effort with multiple large academic centers through LCMC is ongoing to address the question of whether neoadjuvant targeted therapy can improve patients' outcome after surgical therapy.[63] The current study, titled, "LCMC4: Screening Patients with Suspected Early-Stage Lung Cancers for Actionable Oncogene Targets," is the fourth study conducted through the LCMC with the support of industrial and academic partners. The aim is to screen 1000 surgical patients for 10 actionable driver mutations (including EGFR, ALK, ROS1, and others). Patients with actionable mutations then will be enrolled on a mutation or alteration-specific neoadjuvant trials.

Although targeted therapy is not yet part of the standard of care in stages I–III NSCLC, the authors anticipate continued evolution of this field and incorporation of targeted therapy into future practice guidelines. The authors envision that rapid molecular testing and sequential or combination use of targeted therapy will help improve long-term outcomes in stages I–III NSCLC.

ADOPTIVE T-CELL THERAPIES, INCLUDING TUMOR-INFILTRATING LYMPHOCYTES THERAPY, CHIMERIC ANTIGEN RECEPTOR T CELLS, AND T-CELL RECEPTOR

The goal of cancer immunotherapy is to direct the immune system against tumor cells, leveraging its exquisite specificity and capacity for memory to achieve rapid and durable tumor clearance.[64] Although clinical success of ICB in cancer has embraced this concept, these therapies benefit a fraction of all patients. The major barriers to efficacy include lack of preexisting tumor-specific T-cell response and exclusion of T cells from the tumor microenvironment.[64] Adoptive T-cell therapies provide an opportunity to overcome these resistance mechanisms by infusion of large number of tumor antigen–specific cells into the host.

Tumor-Infiltrating Lymphocytes

In tumor-infiltrating lymphocytes (TILs) therapy, TILs are isolated from the tumor stroma, expanded ex vivo and reinfused peripherally after conditioning therapy.[65] Nonmyeloablative lymphodepleting preparative regimen generally is given prior to lymphocyte infusion. This preconditioning therapy consists of cyclophosphamide and fludarabine, which enables dramatic increase and persistence of transferred cells in vivo, along with enhanced TILs antitumor activity.[66,67] Lymphodepletion decreases regulatory T cells and myeloid-derived suppressor cells and provides homeostatic growth stimulus to adoptively transferred lymphocytes.[65] TILs therapy application first was used in melanoma patients[68] and induced responses in multiple melanoma studies.[66,68–70] In other solid tumors, the identification and ex vivo culturing of TILs has been difficult.[71] Although the diversity of T cells that provide broad nature of the T-cell recognition against both defined and undefined tumor antigens with this platform makes a strong argument for the utility of TIL therapies, challenges with quality and quantity of TILs remains its limitation.[72,73] Efforts on optimizing the collection, expansion and preparation for TILs are ongoing to overcome some of these challenges.[74] Number of studies in melanoma,[70,75] including in patients with advanced melanoma who progressed on multiple prior therapies, including anti–PD-1 therapy, has shown promising clinical responses with this modality and led to subsequent registration studies.[76] Experience in lung cancer with TILs therapies have been limited and currently pilot studies are ongoing to assess the utility of this approach.[77]

Chimeric Antigen Receptors

Chimeric antigen receptors (CARs) are synthetic receptors that redirect the specificity, function and metabolism of T cells.[78] CARs consist of T-cell activating domain and extracellular immunoglobulin derived heavy and light chains to direct specificity. These antibody fragments bind to specific antigens on the surface of cancer cells. Newer generations of CARs are engineered to express costimulatory receptors that can enhance proliferation and activation. CAR-based adoptive cellular therapies depend on an antibody like-mediated binding to the antigen and is independent from major histocompatibility complex (MHC) presentation.[79,80]

Advantages of CARs include the recognition of surface antigens independently from MHC restriction and antibody-like–mediated antigen recognition that allows targeting not only the cell surface proteins but also carbohydrates and glycolipids. Engineering of CAR molecules to obtain conditional activation or remote control of CAR T cells also provides additional advantages.[81,82] In hematologic cancers, these applications provided significant therapeutic success in patient subsets, which led to the FDA approval of 2 CAR-engineered T-cell (CAR-T) therapeutic medicines. Tisagenlecleucel, the anti–cluster of differentiation 19 (CD19) CAR-T therapy, has been approved for the treatment of pediatric patients and young adults with refractory or relapsed B-cell precursor acute lymphoblastic leukemia.[83] Another anti-CD19 CAR-T therapy, axicabtagene ciloleucel, was approved to treat adult patients with relapsed and refractory large B-cell lymphoma.[84]

In solid tumors, the development of CAR-T therapy has been more challenging. CARs recognize only antigens expressed on the cell surface of tumor cells. These antigens are limited due to the overall tumor heterogeneity and nonuniformity of the antigen expression. Furthermore, potential target antigens often are shared between tumors and healthy normal tissue, which makes toxicity the main limitation.[79] Few studies in thoracic malignancies showed feasibility of this platform. For example, in mesothelin-associated malignant pleural solid tumors, primarily in malignant mesothelioma, intrapleural administration of mesothelin-targeted CAR T cells in combination with anti–PD-1 therapy after a preconditioning therapy with cyclophosphamide, showed evidence of CAR T-cell antitumor activity without therapy-related major toxicity. In this study, with a minimum of 3 months' follow-up, the best overall response for a subset of 11 patients with malignant pleural mesothelioma was 72%, including 2 durable complete metabolic responses and 6 partial responses. Nine of these patients had PD-L1 less than or equal to 10%, and 6 of 8 responses were seen in PD-L1–low patients.[85] In another study, EGFR targeted CAR-T cells reported 2 partial responses and 5 stable disease for 2 months to 8 months in 11 evaluable patients.[86] CAR-T therapies have unique toxicities, such as cytokine release syndrome and neurotoxicity, which can be life threatening. Predictive algorithms have been developed for the identification of these toxicities and supportive therapies.[80]

T-Cell Receptor

The basic principle of T cell receptor gene therapy is to provide mature T lymphocytes with a high affinity TCR; both alfa and beta chains. This approach is restricted to intracellular peptides derived from tumor antigens and requires major histocompatibility complex loading and surface presentation to allow immune synapse formation. Efforts to confer durable, high-level T-cell modification largely have relied on genetic transfer of TCR genes by integrating retroviral or lentiviral vectors.[79,87,88]

The TCR-based gene therapy has certain advantages over some of the limitations that have been faced with CAR-T therapies. TCRs can recognize not only cell surface proteins but also any intracellular proteins.[64] This allows TCRs to recognize low concentrations intracellular cognate antigens. In addition, the TCR approach mimics the natural function of the T cell by recruiting the endogenous signaling molecules and adhering to correct spatial orientation between the T cell and its target.[64,79]

In this application, cancer testis antigens (CTAs) generally are selected as targets. While selecting the targets, unexpected cross-reactivity can result in potential off target effects. For example, in clinical trials evaluating the safety of engineered T cells expressing an affinity-enhanced TCR against HLA-A*01–restricted MAGE-A3 in patients with myeloma and melanoma, administration of T cells resulted in cardiogenic shock and death of the first 2 patients within a few days of T-cell infusion; these events were not predicted by preclinical studies of the high-affinity TCRs. Gross findings at autopsy revealed severe myocardial damage, and histopathologic analysis revealed T-cell infiltration. No MAGE-A3 expression was detected in heart autopsy tissues. Translational studies revealed that the recognition of an unrelated peptide derived from the striated muscle-specific protein titin by engineered TCRs caused cardiac toxicity, which led to the fatal cardiac complications.[89] Another study with MAGE-3 resulted in neurologic complications, which were attributed to reactivity to previously unrecognized expression of MAGE-A12 in the brain.[90] Subsequent studies showed safety of certain targets and currently a majority of ongoing studies in solid tumors are targeting well studied CTAs, such as NY-ESO1, LAGE 1A, MAGE-A4, and MAGE-A10. Studies in sarcoma and melanoma have been promising.[91–93] In NSCLC, although experience has been limited so far, no additional safety concerns have been raised and assessment of safety and clinical efficacy is ongoing in several studies.[94,95]

Adoptive cellular therapies are holding a great promise for the treatment of solid malignancies including lung cancer. Identification of the right patient populations and tumor subsets for these therapies, improvements in the duration of time required from the production to infusion, the optimization of conditioning regimens, genetic manipulations to overcome challenges related with T-cell trafficking, and further understanding of the tumor and tumor microenvironment are some of the ongoing efforts that provide strong hope for the future.

SUMMARY

Immunotherapy, targeted therapy, and adoptive T-cell therapy have revolutionized cancer research, added to the clinical therapeutic armamentarium, and created novel options for single, combined, or salvage modality therapies in solid organ malignancies. These tremendous advancements are most encouraging for lung cancer, which remains the leading cause of cancer related mortality. As these therapies continue to be studied and refined, it is the authors' hope that they eventually will safely enter the algorithms of standard therapeutic regimens.

DISCLOSURE

B. Sepesi receives consultant fees from Bristol-Myers Squibb and research funding from Rexanna Foundation. T. Cascone reports speaker's fees from the Society for Immunotherapy of Cancer and Bristol-Myers Squibb, consulting fees MedImmune/Astra Zeneca and Bristol-Myers Squibb, and advisory role fees from EMD Serono and Bristol-Myers Squibb. S.G. Chun is on the advisory board and receives consultant fees from Astra Zeneca. M. Altan receives advisory fees from GlaxoSmithKline and Shattuck Labs and research funding from Genentech, Nektar Therapeutics, Merck, GlaxoSmithKline, Novartis, Jounce Therapeutics, Bristol-Myers Squibb, Eli Lilly, and Adaptimmune. X. Le receives consultant and advisory fees from Eli Lilly, Astra Zeneca, and EMD Serono and research funds from Eli Lilly and Boehringer Ingelheim.

REFERENCES

1. Sharma P, Allison JP. Immune checkpoint targeting in cancer therapy: toward combination strategies with curative potential. Cell 2015;161(2):205–14.
2. Brahmer JR, Govindan R, Anders RA, et al. The Society for Immunotherapy of Cancer consensus statement on immunotherapy for the treatment of non-small cell lung cancer (NSCLC). J Immunother Cancer 2018;6(1):75.
3. Brahmer J, Reckamp KL, Baas P, et al. Nivolumab versus Docetaxel in Advanced Squamous-Cell Non-Small-Cell Lung Cancer. N Engl J Med 2015;373(2):123–35.
4. Borghaei H, Paz-Ares L, Horn L, et al. Nivolumab versus Docetaxel in Advanced Nonsquamous Non-Small-Cell Lung Cancer. N Engl J Med 2015;373(17): 1627–39.
5. Carbone DP, Reck M, Paz-Ares L, et al. First-Line Nivolumab in Stage IV or Recurrent Non-Small-Cell Lung Cancer. N Engl J Med 2017;376(25):2415–26.
6. Hellmann MD, Paz-Ares L, Bernabe Caro R, et al. Nivolumab plus Ipilimumab in Advanced Non-Small-Cell Lung Cancer. N Engl J Med 2019;381(21):2020–31.
7. Wolchok JD, Chiarion-Sileni V, Gonzalez R, et al. Overall Survival with Combined Nivolumab and Ipilimumab in Advanced Melanoma. N Engl J Med 2017;377(14): 1345–56.
8. Reck M, Rodriguez-Abreu D, Robinson AG, et al. Pembrolizumab versus Chemotherapy for PD-L1-Positive Non-Small-Cell Lung Cancer. N Engl J Med 2016; 375(19):1823–33.
9. Mok TSK, Wu YL, Kudaba I, et al. Pembrolizumab versus chemotherapy for previously untreated, PD-L1-expressing, locally advanced or metastatic non-small-cell lung cancer (KEYNOTE-042): a randomised, open-label, controlled, phase 3 trial. Lancet 2019;393(10183):1819–30.

10. Gandhi L, Rodriguez-Abreu D, Gadgeel S, et al. Pembrolizumab plus Chemo-therapy in Metastatic Non-Small-Cell Lung Cancer. N Engl J Med 2018;378(22): 2078–92.
11. Paz-Ares L, Luft A, Vicente D, et al. Pembrolizumab plus Chemotherapy for Squa-mous Non-Small-Cell Lung Cancer. N Engl J Med 2018;379(21):2040–51.
12. Reck M, Shankar G, Lee A, et al. Atezolizumab in combination with bevacizumab, paclitaxel and carboplatin for the first-line treatment of patients with metastatic non-squamous non-small cell lung cancer, including patients with EGFR muta-tions. Expert Rev Respir Med 2020;14(2):125–36.
13. West H, McCleod M, Hussein M, et al. Atezolizumab in combination with carbo-platin plus nab-paclitaxel chemotherapy compared with chemotherapy alone as first-line treatment for metastatic non-squamous non-small-cell lung cancer (IM-power130): a multicentre, randomised, open-label, phase 3 trial. Lancet Oncol 2019;20(7):924–37.
14. Gomez DR, Blumenschein GR Jr, Lee JJ, et al. Local consolidative therapy versus maintenance therapy or observation for patients with oligometastatic non-small-cell lung cancer without progression after first-line systemic therapy: a multicentre, randomised, controlled, phase 2 study. Lancet Oncol 2016; 17(12):1672–82.
15. Iyengar P, Wardak Z, Gerber DE, et al. Consolidative Radiotherapy for Limited Metastatic Non-Small-Cell Lung Cancer: A Phase 2 Randomized Clinical Trial. JAMA Oncol 2018;4(1):e173501.
16. Antonia SJ, Villegas A, Daniel D, et al. Durvalumab after Chemoradiotherapy in Stage III Non-Small-Cell Lung Cancer. N Engl J Med 2017;377(20):1919–29.
17. Antonia SJ, Villegas A, Daniel D, et al. Overall Survival with Durvalumab after Chemoradiotherapy in Stage III NSCLC. N Engl J Med 2018;379(24):2342–50.
18. Forde PM, Chaft JE, Pardoll DM. Neoadjuvant PD-1 Blockade in Resectable Lung Cancer. N Engl J Med 2018;379(9):e14.
19. Kwiatkowski DJ, Rusch VW, Chaft JE, et al. Neoadjuvant atezolizumab in resect-able non-small cell lung cancer (NSCLC): Interim analysis and biomarker data from a multicenter study (LCMC3). J Clin Oncol 2019;37(15_suppl):8503.
20. Cascone T, William WN, Weissferdt A, et al. Neoadjuvant nivolumab (N) or nivo-lumab plus ipilimumab (NI) for resectable non-small cell lung cancer (NSCLC): Clinical and correlative results from the NEOSTAR study. J Clin Oncol 2019; 37(15_suppl):8504.
21. Gao S, Li N, Gao S, et al. Neoadjuvant PD-1 inhibitor (Sintilimab) in NSCLC. J Thorac Oncol 2020;15(5):816–26.
22. Bar J, Urban D, Ofek E, et al. Neoadjuvant pembrolizumab (Pembro) for early stage non-small cell lung cancer (NSCLC): Updated report of a phase I study, MK3475-223. J Clin Oncol 2019;37(15_suppl):8534.
23. Provencio M, Nadal E, Insa A, et al. OA13.05 NADIM Study: Updated Clinical Research and Outcomes. J Thorac Oncol 2019;14(10):S241.
24. Felip E, Brahmer J, Broderick S, et al. P2.16-03 CheckMate 816: A Phase 3 Trial of Neoadjuvant Nivolumab Plus Ipilimumab or Chemotherapy vs Chemotherapy in Early-Stage NSCLC. J Thorac Oncol 2018;13(10):S831–2.
25. Rizvi N, Gandara D, Solomon B, et al. P2.17-27 IMpower030: Phase III Study Evaluating Neoadjuvant Treatment of Resectable Stage II-IIIB NSCLC with Atezo-lizumab + Chemotherapy. J Thorac Oncol 2018;13(10):S863.
26. Heymach J, Taube J, Mitsudomi T, et al. P1.18-02 The AEGEAN Phase 3 Trial of Neoadjuvant/Adjuvant Durvalumab in Patients with Resectable Stage II/III NSCLC. J Thorac Oncol 2019;14(10):S625–6.

27. Halliday PR, Blakely CM, Bivona TG. Emerging Targeted Therapies for the Treatment of Non-small Cell Lung Cancer. Curr Oncol Rep 2019;21(3):21.
28. Paez JG, Janne PA, Lee JC, et al. EGFR mutations in lung cancer: correlation with clinical response to gefitinib therapy. Science 2004;304(5676):1497–500.
29. Pao W, Miller V, Zakowski M, et al. EGF receptor gene mutations are common in lung cancers from "never smokers" and are associated with sensitivity of tumors to gefitinib and erlotinib. Proc Natl Acad Sci U S A 2004;101(36):13306–11.
30. Lynch TJ, Bell DW, Sordella R, et al. Activating mutations in the epidermal growth factor receptor underlying responsiveness of non-small-cell lung cancer to gefitinib. N Engl J Med 2004;350(21):2129–39.
31. Mok TS, Wu YL, Thongprasert S, et al. Gefitinib or carboplatin-paclitaxel in pulmonary adenocarcinoma. N Engl J Med 2009;361(10):947–57.
32. Rosell R, Carcereny E, Gervais R, et al. Erlotinib versus standard chemotherapy as first-line treatment for European patients with advanced EGFR mutation-positive non-small-cell lung cancer (EURTAC): a multicentre, open-label, randomised phase 3 trial. Lancet Oncol 2012;13(3):239–46.
33. Sequist LV, Yang JC, Yamamoto N, et al. Phase III study of afatinib or cisplatin plus pemetrexed in patients with metastatic lung adenocarcinoma with EGFR mutations. J Clin Oncol 2013;31(27):3327–34.
34. Kobayashi S, Ji H, Yuza Y, et al. An alternative inhibitor overcomes resistance caused by a mutation of the epidermal growth factor receptor. Cancer Res 2005;65(16):7096–101.
35. Cross DA, Ashton SE, Ghiorghiu S, et al. AZD9291, an irreversible EGFR TKI, overcomes T790M-mediated resistance to EGFR inhibitors in lung cancer. Cancer Discov 2014;4(9):1046–61.
36. Janne PA, Yang JC, Kim DW, et al. AZD9291 in EGFR inhibitor-resistant non-small-cell lung cancer. N Engl J Med 2015;372(18):1689–99.
37. Soria JC, Ohe Y, Vansteenkiste J, et al. Osimertinib in untreated EGFR-mutated advanced non-small-cell lung cancer. N Engl J Med 2018;378(2):113–25.
38. Ramalingam SS, Vansteenkiste J, Planchard D, et al. Overall survival with osimertinib in untreated, EGFR-mutated advanced NSCLC. N Engl J Med 2020;382(1):41–50.
39. Soda M, Choi YL, Enomoto M, et al. Identification of the transforming EML4-ALK fusion gene in non-small-cell lung cancer. Nature 2007;448(7153):561–6.
40. Butrynski JE, D'Adamo DR, Hornick JL, et al. Crizotinib in ALK-rearranged inflammatory myofibroblastic tumor. N Engl J Med 2010;363(18):1727–33.
41. Shaw AT, Engelman JA. Ceritinib in ALK-rearranged non-small-cell lung cancer. N Engl J Med 2014;370(26):2537–9.
42. Shaw AT, Gandhi L, Gadgeel S, et al. Alectinib in ALK-positive, crizotinib-resistant, non-small-cell lung cancer: a single-group, multicentre, phase 2 trial. Lancet Oncol 2016;17(2):234–42.
43. Gainor JF, Shaw AT. J-ALEX: alectinib versus crizotinib in ALK-positive lung cancer. Lancet 2017;390(10089):3–4.
44. Lin JJ, Zhu VW, Schoenfeld AJ, et al. Brigatinib in Patients With Alectinib-Refractory ALK-Positive NSCLC. J Thorac Oncol 2018;13(10):1530–8.
45. Shaw AT, Felip E, Bauer TM, et al. Lorlatinib in non-small-cell lung cancer with ALK or ROS1 rearrangement: an international, multicentre, open-label, single-arm first-in-man phase 1 trial. Lancet Oncol 2017;18(12):1590–9.
46. Shaw AT, Friboulet L, Leshchiner I, et al. Resensitization to Crizotinib by the Lorlatinib ALK Resistance Mutation L1198F. N Engl J Med 2016;374(1):54–61.

47. Shaw AT, Solomon BJ, Besse B, et al. ALK resistance mutations and efficacy of lorlatinib in advanced anaplastic lymphoma kinase-positive non-small-cell lung cancer. J Clin Oncol 2019;37(16):1370–9.
48. Pacheco JM, Gao D, Smith D, et al. Natural history and factors associated with overall survival in stage IV ALK-rearranged non-small cell lung cancer. J Thorac Oncol 2019;14(4):691–700.
49. Shaw AT, Riely GJ, Bang YJ, et al. Crizotinib in ROS1-rearranged advanced non-small-cell lung cancer (NSCLC): updated results, including overall survival, from PROFILE 1001. Ann Oncol 2019;30(7):1121–6.
50. Lim SM, Kim HR, Lee JS, et al. Open-label, multicenter, phase II study of Ceritinib in patients with non-small-cell lung cancer harboring ROS1 rearrangement. J Clin Oncol 2017;35(23):2613–8.
51. Shaw AT, Solomon BJ, Chiari R, et al. Lorlatinib in advanced ROS1-positive non-small-cell lung cancer: a multicentre, open-label, single-arm, phase 1-2 trial. Lancet Oncol 2019;20(12):1691–701.
52. Planchard D, Besse B, Groen HJM, et al. Dabrafenib plus trametinib in patients with previously treated BRAF(V600E)-mutant metastatic non-small cell lung cancer: an open-label, multicentre phase 2 trial. Lancet Oncol 2016;17(7):984–93.
53. Drilon A, Laetsch TW, Kummar S, et al. Efficacy of Larotrectinib in TRK fusion-positive cancers in adults and children. N Engl J Med 2018;378(8):731–9.
54. Lipson D, Capelletti M, Yelensky R, et al. Identification of new ALK and RET gene fusions from colorectal and lung cancer biopsies. Nat Med 2012;18(3):382–4.
55. Ju YS, Lee WC, Shin JY, et al. A transforming KIF5B and RET gene fusion in lung adenocarcinoma revealed from whole-genome and transcriptome sequencing. Genome Res 2012;22(3):436–45.
56. Lin JJ, Kennedy E, Sequist LV, et al. Clinical activity of Alectinib in advanced RET-rearranged non-small cell lung cancer. J Thorac Oncol 2016;11(11):2027–32.
57. Awad MM, Oxnard GR, Jackman DM, et al. MET Exon 14 mutations in non-small-cell lung cancer are associated with advanced age and stage-dependent MET genomic amplification and c-Met Overexpression. J Clin Oncol 2016;34(7): 721–30.
58. Paik PK, Drilon A, Fan PD, et al. Response to MET inhibitors in patients with stage IV lung adenocarcinomas harboring MET mutations causing exon 14 skipping. Cancer Discov 2015;5(8):842–9.
59. Kelly K, Altorki NK, Eberhardt WE, et al. Adjuvant Erlotinib versus placebo in patients with stage IB-IIIA non-small-cell lung cancer (RADIANT): a randomized, double-blind, phase III trial. J Clin Oncol 2015;33(34):4007–14.
60. Zhong WZ, Wang Q, Mao WM, et al. Gefitinib versus vinorelbine plus cisplatin as adjuvant treatment for stage II-IIIA (N1-N2) EGFR-mutant NSCLC (ADJUVANT/ CTONG1104): a randomised, open-label, phase 3 study. Lancet Oncol 2018; 19(1):139–48.
61. Govindan R, Mandrekar SJ, Gerber DE, et al. ALCHEMIST trials: a golden opportunity to transform outcomes in early-stage non-small cell lung cancer. Clin Cancer Res 2015;21(24):5439–44.
62. Wu YL, Herbst RS, Mann H, et al. ADAURA: Phase III, double-blind, randomized study of osimertinib versus placebo in EGFR mutation-positive early-stage NSCLC after complete surgical resection. Clin Lung Cancer 2018;19(4):e533–6.
63. Herbst RS, Tsuboi M, John T, et al. Osimertinib as adjuvant therapy in patients with stage IB-IIIA EGFR mutation positive NSCLC after complete tumor resection: ADAURA. ASCO20 Virtual Scientific Program. Abstract LBA5. Presented in pre-meeting press briefing on May 26, 2020.

64. LCMC4. Available at: https://www.lungcancerresearchfoundation.org/research/applications-2/. Accessed May 1, 2020.

65. Anandappa AJ, Wu CJ, Ott PA. Directing traffic: how to effectively drive T cells into tumors. Cancer Discov 2020;10(2):185–97.

66. Rosenberg SA. Cell transfer immunotherapy for metastatic solid cancer–what clinicians need to know. Nat Rev Clin Oncol 2011;8(10):577–85.

67. Dudley ME, Wunderlich JR, Robbins PF, et al. Cancer regression and autoimmunity in patients after clonal repopulation with antitumor lymphocytes. Science 2002;298(5594):850–4.

68. Dudley ME, Yang JC, Sherry R, et al. Adoptive cell therapy for patients with metastatic melanoma: evaluation of intensive myeloablative chemoradiation preparative regimens. J Clin Oncol 2008;26(32):5233–9.

69. Rosenberg SA, Packard BS, Aebersold PM, et al. Use of tumor-infiltrating lymphocytes and interleukin-2 in the immunotherapy of patients with metastatic melanoma. A preliminary report. N Engl J Med 1988;319(25):1676–80.

70. Besser MJ, Shapira-Frommer R, Itzhaki O, et al. Adoptive transfer of tumor-infiltrating lymphocytes in patients with metastatic melanoma: intent-to-treat analysis and efficacy after failure to prior immunotherapies. Clin Cancer Res 2013; 19(17):4792–800.

71. Rosenberg SA, Yang JC, Sherry RM, et al. Durable complete responses in heavily pretreated patients with metastatic melanoma using T-cell transfer immunotherapy. Clin Cancer Res 2011;17(13):4550–7.

72. Antonia SJ, Vansteenkiste JF, Moon E. Immunotherapy: beyond Anti-PD-1 and Anti-PD-L1 therapies. Am Soc Clin Oncol Educ Book 2016;35:e450–8.

73. Wu R, Forget MA, Chacon J, et al. Adoptive T-cell therapy using autologous tumor-infiltrating lymphocytes for metastatic melanoma: current status and future outlook. Cancer J 2012;18(2):160–75.

74. Geukes Foppen MH, Donia M, Svane IM, et al. Tumor-infiltrating lymphocytes for the treatment of metastatic cancer. Mol Oncol 2015;9(10):1918–35.

75. Sarnaik A, Kluger HM, Chesney JA, et al. Efficacy of single administration of tumor-infiltrating lymphocytes (TIL) in heavily pretreated patients with metastatic melanoma following checkpoint therapy. J Clin Oncol 2017;35(15_suppl):3045.

76. Goff SL, Dudley ME, Citrin DE, et al. Randomized, prospective evaluation comparing intensity of lymphodepletion before adoptive transfer of tumor-infiltrating lymphocytes for patients with metastatic melanoma. J Clin Oncol 2016;34(20):2389–97.

77. Sarnaik A, Khushalani NI, Chesney JA, et al. Safety and efficacy of cryopreserved autologous tumor infiltrating lymphocyte therapy (LN-144, lifileucel) in advanced metastatic melanoma patients who progressed on multiple prior therapies including anti-PD-1. J Clin Oncol 2019;37(15_suppl):2518.

78. Chesney JA, Lutzky J, Thomas SS, et al. A phase II study of autologous tumor infiltrating lymphocytes (TIL, LN-144/LN-145) in patients with solid tumors. J Clin Oncol 2019;37(15_suppl):TPS2648.

79. June CH, Sadelain M. Chimeric antigen receptor therapy. N Engl J Med 2018; 379(1):64–73.

80. Ott PA, Dotti G, Yee C, et al. An update on adoptive T-cell therapy and neoantigen vaccines. Am Soc Clin Oncol Educ Book 2019;39:e70–8.

81. Salter AI, Pont MJ, Riddell SR. Chimeric antigen receptor-modified T cells: CD19 and the road beyond. Blood 2018;131(24):2621–9.

82. Wu CY, Roybal KT, Puchner EM, et al. Remote control of therapeutic T cells through a small molecule-gated chimeric receptor. Science 2015;350(6258): aab4077.
83. Kloss CC, Condomines M, Cartellieri M, et al. Combinatorial antigen recognition with balanced signaling promotes selective tumor eradication by engineered T cells. Nat Biotechnol 2013;31(1):71–5.
84. Maude SL, Laetsch TW, Buechner J, et al. Tisagenlecleucel in children and young adults with B-cell lymphoblastic leukemia. N Engl J Med 2018;378(5):439–48.
85. Neelapu SS, Locke FL, Bartlett NL, et al. Axicabtagene Ciloleucel CAR T-cell therapy in refractory large B-cell lymphoma. N Engl J Med 2017;377(26):2531–44.
86. Adusumilli PS, Zauderer MG, Rusch VW, et al. A phase I clinical trial of malignant pleural disease treated with regionally delivered autologous mesothelin-targeted CAR T cells: Safety and efficacy AACR Annual Meeting, March 29-April 3, 2019:Atlanta, Georgia Abstract CT036.
87. Feng K, Guo Y, Dai H, et al. Chimeric antigen receptor-modified T cells for the immunotherapy of patients with EGFR-expressing advanced relapsed/refractory non-small cell lung cancer. Sci China Life Sci 2016;59(5):468–79.
88. He Q, Jiang X, Zhou X, et al. Targeting cancers through TCR-peptide/MHC interactions. J Hematol Oncol 2019;12(1):139.
89. Zhao L, Cao YJ. Engineered T cell therapy for cancer in the Clinic. Front Immunol 2019;10:2250.
90. Linette GP, Stadtmauer EA, Maus MV, et al. Cardiovascular toxicity and titin cross-reactivity of affinity-enhanced T cells in myeloma and melanoma. Blood 2013; 122(6):863–71.
91. Morgan RA, Chinnasamy N, Abate-Daga D, et al. Cancer regression and neurological toxicity following anti-MAGE-A3 TCR gene therapy. J Immunother 2013; 36(2):133–51.
92. Ramachandran I, Lowther DE, Dryer-Minnerly R, et al. Systemic and local immunity following adoptive transfer of NY-ESO-1 SPEAR T cells in synovial sarcoma. J Immunother Cancer 2019;7(1):276.
93. Robbins PF, Morgan RA, Feldman SA, et al. Tumor regression in patients with metastatic synovial cell sarcoma and melanoma using genetically engineered lymphocytes reactive With NY-ESO-1. J Clin Oncol 2011;29(7):917–24.
94. Robbins PF, Kassim SH, Tran TLN, et al. A pilot trial using lymphocytes genetically engineered with an NY-ESO-1–reactive T-cell receptor: long-term follow-up and correlates with response. Clin Cancer Res 2015;21(5):1019–27.
95. Lam VK, Hong DS, Heymach J, et al. Initial safety assessment of MAGE-A10c796TCR T-cells in two clinical trials. J Clin Oncol 2018;36. suppl; abstr 3056.

Mediastinal Germ Cell Tumors
Updates in Diagnosis and Management

Amanda R. Stram, MD, PhD[a,b], Kenneth A. Kesler, MD[c,d],*

KEYWORDS

- Germ cell tumors • Mediastinal tumors • Nonseminomatous germ cell cancer
- Thoracic surgery • Chemotherapy

KEY POINTS

- Primary mediastinal nonseminomatous germ cell tumors represent a rare but important malignancy that occurs in otherwise young and healthy patients.
- Treatment is challenging and involves cisplatin-based chemotherapy followed by surgery to remove residual disease.
- Avoiding bleomycin-containing chemotherapy in the treatment of primary mediastinal nonseminomatous germ cell tumors is important.
- Prechemotherapy and postchemotherapy pathology as well as postoperative serum tumor markers are independent predictors of long-term survival.

INTRODUCTION

The mediastinum is the most common site of extragonadal origin of germ cell tumors, with 5% to 10% of germ cell tumors arising primarily within the anterior mediastinum and accounting for 15% to 20% of all anterior mediastinal tumors.[1,2] Mediastinal germ cell tumors comprise 3 distinct histologic types: teratoma (mature and immature subtypes), seminoma, and nonseminomatous germ cell tumors (NSGCTs). Mature teratomas comprise 60% to 70% of mediastinal germ cell tumors and are considered benign, and surgical resection is curative. Immature teratomas behave more aggressively and have poor outcomes compared with their mature counterparts. Primary mediastinal seminomas represent about 40% of malignant mediastinal germ cell tumors. Seminomas are sensitive to chemotherapy and have excellent cure rates with

a Department of Surgery, Division of Cardiothoracic Surgery, Indiana University Melvin and Bren Simon Cancer Center, 545 Barnhill Drive, Indianapolis, IN 46202, USA; b Department of Surgery, Thoracic Surgery Division, Indiana University, 545 Barnhill Drive, Indianapolis, IN 46202, USA; c Department of Surgery, Division of Cardiothoracic Surgery, Indiana University Melvin and Bren Simon Cancer Center, 545 Barnhill Drive EM #212, Indianapolis, IN 46202, USA; d Department of Surgery, Thoracic Surgery Division, Indiana University, 545 Barnhill Drive EM #212, Indianapolis, IN 46202, USA
* Corresponding author. 545 Barnhill Drive EM #212, Indianapolis, IN 46202.
E-mail address: kkesler@iupui.edu

Surg Oncol Clin N Am 29 (2020) 571–579
https://doi.org/10.1016/j.soc.2020.06.005
surgonc.theclinics.com

cisplatin-based treatment. Primary mediastinal NSGCTs (PMNSGCTs) represent most malignant mediastinal germ cell tumors. These tumors are typically aggressive with a poor-risk profile, and overall 5-year survival is approximately 45%.[3–5] Treatment of PMNSGCTs consists of cisplatin-based chemotherapy followed by surgical resection of residual tumor mass. The diagnosis and contemporary multimodality strategy for the treatment of PMNSGCT are discussed here.

Pathogenesis

PMNSGCTs represent a rare but important malignancy, accounting for 1% of all mediastinal tumors and most of the malignant germ cell tumors of the mediastinum. These tumors occur almost exclusively in young adult men, most commonly between the ages of 20 and 40 years.

On histology, these neoplasms are typically mixed, and contain at least 1 nonseminomatous germ cell cancer subtype (yolk sac tumor, embryonal carcinoma, choriocarcinoma) as well as some form of teratomatous disorder, ranging from mature teratoma to teratoma with immature or atypical elements. Occasionally, frank malignant transformation of teratoma into so-called non–germ cell cancers (sarcomas and epithelial carcinomas) is found. The tumor admixture can contain variable proportions of these nonseminomatous histologies, as well as malignant seminoma.

DIAGNOSIS

Patients with PMNSGCTs are usually symptomatic on presentation. Clinical findings are consistent with a growing mediastinal mass, such as cough, shortness of breath, chest pain, or superior vena cava syndrome. Computed tomography (CT) imaging usually reveals a large heterogeneous mass in the anterior mediastinum (**Fig. 1**). These masses are aggressive tumors and local invasion into surrounding structures is a common finding at presentation. Metastatic disease was present at diagnosis in 32% of 244 patients in our recent institutional series, with lung being the most common site, followed by mediastinal and extrathoracic lymph nodes, liver, and central nervous system (CNS).[6] Chest and abdominal CT scans are standard imaging tests for staging, with other radiologic studies, including PET scan and MRI, acquired on a case-by-case basis.

Obtaining serum tumor markers (STMs) on a young man presenting with an anterior mediastinal mass is essential to establish a diagnosis of PMNSGCT. Any increase in alpha fetoprotein (AFP) level or significant increase in β-human chorionic gonadotropin (βHCG) greater than 100 unit/L is diagnostic of PMNSGCT. In patients with diagnostic increase in STM level, prompt cytologic confirmation can be obtained with CT-guided biopsy, if desired. Biopsy, either CT guided or surgical when CT-guided is not feasible, is obtained in cases where AFP level is normal and βHCG level marginally increased, potentially indicating seminoma.

TREATMENT
Chemotherapy

The treatment strategy for PMNSGCT is multimodal therapy with cisplatin-based chemotherapy as initial treatment followed by surgical resection of residual tumor. There is no role for radiation therapy in the treatment of PMNSGCT. Development of cisplatin-based combination chemotherapy for NSGCT has been responsible for vastly improved long-term survival rates compared with outcomes in the precisplatin era. Four courses of bleomycin, etoposide, and cisplatin chemotherapy have traditionally been considered the standard of care for patients with poor-risk NSGCT, including

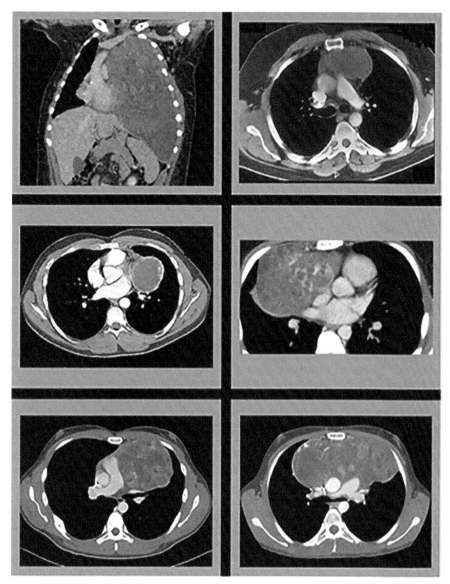

Fig. 1. Illustrative chest CT images of patients presenting with PMNSGCT, showing heterogeneous tumors arising from the anterior mediastinum.

PMNSGCT. However, postchemotherapy surgery for PMNSGCT is usually extensive and carries significant risk of pulmonary-related morbidity, including development of acute respiratory distress syndrome (ARDS). Pulmonary toxicity is a well-known consequence of bleomycin. In order to avoid the compounding effect of bleomycin on the postoperative pulmonary risk associated with mediastinal and intrathoracic resection, over the past 15 years, our institution has been using an etoposide, ifosfamide, and cisplatin (VIP) regimen as the chemotherapy of choice for PMNSGCT. The authors have experienced a relative reduction in postoperative respiratory failure rate in patients with PMNSGCT with use of non–bleomycin-containing regimens, despite similar extent of surgery, including pulmonary resections.[7,8] We recently updated our institutional experience and showed a 14.8% rate of postoperative pulmonary failure, which carried 40.7% mortality in these otherwise young and healthy patients, after receiving bleomycin-containing regimens, compared with an incidence of 2.6% in patients who received VIP.[6] Postoperative pulmonary complications and ARDS carry significant associated morbidity. Therefore, following chemotherapy strategies that minimize the risks of ARDS remains important.

Surgery

Ideally, STM levels normalize after chemotherapy, or at least significantly decrease, and tumor dimension shrinks. However, there always remains a residual mediastinal mass, most of which contain residual disease for which surgical resection is indicated. Most residual tumor masses contain teratoma, persistent nonseminomatous germ cell cancer, and non–germ cell cancer cells, and complete tumor necrosis is found in only a minority of cases.[9] Surgery to remove residual disease is typically planned 4 to 6 weeks following chemotherapy to allow for patient recovery. The standard of care for patients with testicular NSGCT who relapse serologically shortly after first-line chemotherapy involves second-line chemotherapy, before considering surgery. However, response rates of standard cisplatin-based salvage chemotherapy for PMNSGCT are notoriously poor.[10] Moreover, although increased STM levels are diagnostic of PMNSGCT, postchemotherapy STM levels lack high sensitivity or specificity for residual NSGCT. In addition, the propensity of PMNSGCT to transform into non–germ cell cancers, which are typically STM negative as well as refractory to chemotherapy, further questions the role of second-line chemotherapy before surgery. Therefore, the authors subscribe to a policy of removing residual disease if deemed operable, regardless of STM status, because the overall results of surgical salvage in patients with residual malignancy after first-line chemotherapy seem to be superior to the response rates of second-line chemotherapy.[11,12]

Patients are rarely considered to be inoperable; however, extensive great vessel or middle mediastinal involvement may preclude safe resection. For patients with persistent metastatic disease after first-line chemotherapy, the authors use an individualized approach. In patients with normal STM levels after first-line chemotherapy, nonpulmonary and pulmonary metastases are resected when feasible, particularly if suspicious for teratoma. Extrathoracic metastases are typically removed as a staged procedure before or after mediastinal surgery. Surgery is undertaken for select patients with increased STM levels and limited areas of pulmonary metastases deemed resectable at the time of surgery to remove the residual mediastinal mass. For patients with increased STM levels after first-line chemotherapy and systemic or extensive pulmonary metastases, second-line chemotherapy, more recently in the form of high-dose chemotherapy with peripheral stem cell transplant, should be given before proceeding with surgery.[13] Patients with increased STM levels after first-line chemotherapy caused by an isolated CNS metastasis can be treated with stereotactic radiation and/or surgery with CNS disease control before removal of mediastinal disease. Rare patients show a so-called growing teratoma syndrome, defined by a rapidly growing symptomatic mediastinal mass with decreasing STM level before completion of 4 chemotherapy cycles.[14] In these cases, chemotherapy is discontinued and urgent surgery undertaken.

Surgery can be challenging, because chemotherapy results in fibrosis of mediastinal tissues surrounding residual disease. Our technique to remove residual mediastinal tumor has been described.[15] We start by selecting an approach (median sternotomy, clamshell with transverse sternotomy, anterolateral thoracotomy, or sternotomy combined with separate thoracotomy) to optimize exposure of technically difficult areas anticipated during surgery. Surgical removal involves en bloc dissection of the residual mass and surrounding involved structure with an ultimate goal of obtaining an R0 resection (**Table 1**). A balanced surgical approach is used to spare critical structures such as phrenic nerves, main pulmonary arteries, great veins, and cardiac chambers where the residual mass abuts but does not grossly invade, using intraoperative frozen section for margin control. In cases where phrenic nerves are removed en bloc, prophylactic diaphragm plication can be performed on an individual basis. With respect to the great veins, reconstruction is done in all cases where en bloc superior vena cava resection is required. If 1 innominate vein is involved, ligation can be performed without reconstruction. A single vein reconstruction technique is used for cases that

Table 1
Anatomic structures removed en bloc with the residual mass after chemotherapy in 244 operative survivors with primary mediastinal nonseminomatous germ cell tumors

Variable (Total n = 244)	Number (%)
Organs removed, any	228 (93.4)
1	37 (15.2)
>1	191 (78.3)
Pericardium	195 (79.9)
Phrenic nerve	74 (30.3)
Right phrenic nerve	19 (7.8)
Left phrenic nerve	51 (20.9)
Diaphragm plication	15 (6.1)
Great vein, any	64 (26.2)
Right innominate	12 (4.9)
Left innominate	54 (22.1)
Superior vena cava	25 (10.2)
Inferior vena cava	1 (0.4)
Cardiac chamber	9 (3.9)
Right atrium	5 (2.2)
Left atrium	2 (0.9)
Left ventricle	2 (0.9)
Chest wall	9 (3.9)
Diaphragm	8 (3.5)
Pulmonary resection	165 (72.3)
Segment or wedge	77 (33.8)
Lobectomy	55 (24.1)
1	35 (15.4)
>1	20 (8.8)
Pneumonectomy	12 (5.3)

Data from Outcomes Following Surgery for Primary Mediastinal Nonseminomatous Germ Cell Tumors in the Cisplatin Era. Kesler, Kenneth A. et al. The Journal of Thoracic and Cardiovascular Surgery, Published online April 22, 2020

require bilateral innominate vein removal, preferably the right innominate to superior vena cava with ligation of the left innominate vein. Our conduit preference for great vein reconstruction is cryopreserved descending thoracic aortic allografts. Cardiopulmonary bypass capabilities should be made available for select patients with great vessel or cardiac involvement. Perioperative fluid and oxygen administration should be kept to a minimum, particularly in patients who may have received bleomycin before surgery.

Follow-up

Patients who present to surgery with increased STM levels should have the levels measured before hospital discharge and at 1 month postoperatively. Patients with pathologic evidence of viable NSGCT and normal postoperative STM levels should be given 2 additional cycles of etoposide/cisplatin. Current practice includes consideration of high-dose chemotherapy for patients with persistently increased postoperative STM levels and recurrent PMNSGCT.[13] Routine long-term follow-up includes chest radiographs and STM levels every 2 months for the first year, every 4 months for the second year, every 6 months in years 3 through 5, then annually. For patients who pathologically show a component of teratoma, CT imaging is also recommended during follow-up. Patients with recurrent disease are treated on an individual basis, with surgery favored for teratoma and limited areas of malignancy.

Outcomes

STMs seem to remain important from a prognosis standpoint. By univariate analysis, our recent study showed that preoperative increased AFP level, increased STM levels in general, and increasing STM levels were predictive of poor survival, whereas normal STM level was protective. Even though increased postchemotherapy STM levels did not remain statistically significant in the multivariate model, persistent increase of STM levels after surgery, likely indicating residual microscopic NSGCT, was predictive of adverse survival.[6] Our institutional approach now uses high-dose chemotherapy in patients with increasing postoperative STM levels with an expectation of low but improving cure rates.[13] A multicenter review of patients with extragonadal NSGCT, including 341 with PMNSGCT, identified pretreatment increased βHCG level and non-pulmonary visceral metastases as adverse risk factors for survival.[5] Of note, less than half of the patients with PMNSGCT in this study underwent postchemotherapy surgery. Although prechemotherapy tumor histology was not provided, it is plausible that increased βHCG level was a surrogate for the presence of choriocarcinoma, which was independently predictive in our recent series. In contrast, pure mediastinal seminomas have extremely high cure rates with cisplatin-based chemotherapy alone.[3,4] Although all patients in our recent series had serologic or pathologic evidence of NSGCT, it is perhaps not surprising that the subset of cases with tumors containing a malignant seminoma component had significantly improved survival.

Although overall 5-year survival averages 45%, individual survival after surgery for PMNSGCT has been reported to range widely, with rates reported between 30% and 90%. Similar to prechemotherapy pathology, features identified in resected mediastinal masses can be variable and mixed, potentially containing elements of tumor necrosis, teratoma, and malignancy. Current and previous studies from our institution as well as a report from Memorial Sloan Kettering Cancer Center continue to show that the pathology features identified in the residual mass following chemotherapy is independently predictive of long-term survival and largely responsible for variable survival rates (**Fig. 2**).[6,7,16] Patients who show complete tumor necrosis have excellent long-term prognosis. Patients with pathologic evidence of teratoma, with or without tumor

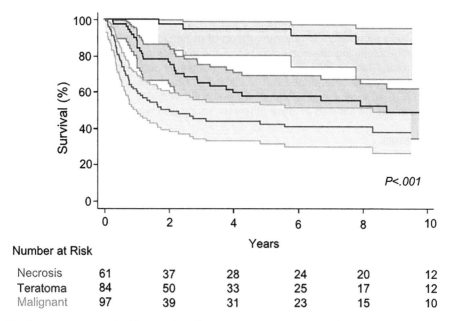

Fig. 2. Long-term survival in a series of 244 operative survivors with primary mediastinal nonseminomatous germ cell tumors based on the worst pathologic diagnosis microscopically identified in the residual mass (necrosis, teratoma, or malignant). (*Data from* Outcomes Following Surgery for Primary Mediastinal Nonseminomatous Germ Cell Tumors in the Cisplatin Era. Kesler, Kenneth A. et al. The Journal of Thoracic and Cardiovascular Surgery, Published online April 22, 2020.)

necrosis, show intermediate survival. The poorer prognosis of PMNSGCT compared with testicular NSGCT is caused not only by a relative resistance to cisplatin-based chemotherapy but also by a higher propensity of teratoma in PMNSGCT to undergo malignant transformation into nongerm cancers.[17,18] Teratoma with stromal atypia arguably represents the precursor to non–germ cell cancer. Although sarcomas predominate, the spectrum of non–germ cell disorders in residual mass lesions is a testimony to the pluripotent nature of these tumors. Interestingly, the subset of patients who pathologically show teratoma with stromal atypia have long-term survival similar to patients with residual malignancy, which diminishes overall survival in the teratoma category. We speculate that pathologic sampling error in large residual masses where small areas of frank non–germ cell cancer are missed, or perhaps observer variability (severe atypia vs frank non–germ cell cancer), could be contributing factors to this finding.

Surgery has the ability to salvage patients with pathologic evidence of malignancy in the form of either viable NSGCT and/or non–germ cell cancers with poor but possible long-term survival. Impressively, patients with less than 50% of the residual mass containing viable malignancy have been shown to have long-term survival equivalent to the overall survival of patients whose worst disorder was teratoma. However, survival significantly diminishes when 50% or more of the residual mass contains viable malignancy.[6,7]

SUMMARY

PMNSGCTs represent a challenging group of malignant germ cell tumors. Avoiding bleomycin-containing chemotherapy before these major thoracic surgical procedures is important. Prechemotherapy and postchemotherapy pathology, as well as postoperative STM levels, are independent predictors of long-term survival. Although overall PMNSGCT survival remains inferior to testicular NSGCT, an aggressive surgical approach can be justified in these otherwise young and healthy patients.

DISCLOSURE

The authors declare no conflict of interest. There was no external funding source.

REFERENCES

1. Takeda S, Miyoshi S, Ohta M, et al. Primary germ cell tumors in the mediastinum: a 50-year experience at a single Japanese institution. Cancer 2003;97(2):367–76.
2. Sellke FW, Del Nido PJ, Swanson SJ. Sabiston & Spencer surgery of the chest. Philadelphia: Elsevier; 2016. Available at: https://RX8KL6YF4X.search.serialssolutions.com/ejp/?libHash=RX8KL6YF4X#/search/?searchControl=title&searchType=title_code&criteria=TC0001573183.
3. Bokemeyer C, Nichols CR, Droz JP, et al. Extragonadal germ cell tumors of the mediastinum and retroperitoneum: results from an international analysis. J Clin Oncol 2002;20(7):1864–73.
4. Kesler KA, Rieger KM, Ganjoo KN, et al. Primary mediastinal nonseminomatous germ cell tumors: the influence of postchemotherapy pathology on long-term survival after surgery. J Thorac Cardiovasc Surg 1999;118(4):692–700.
5. Hartmann JT, Nichols CR, Droz JP, et al. Prognostic variables for response and outcome in patients with extragonadal germ-cell tumors. Ann Oncol 2002;13(7):1017–28.
6. Kesler KA, Stram AR, Timsina LR, et al. Outcomes following surgery for primary mediastinal nonseminomatous germ cell tumors in the cisplatin era. J Thorac Cardiovasc Surg 2020. https://doi.org/10.1016/j.jtcvs.2020.01.118.
7. Kesler KA, Rieger KM, Hammoud ZT, et al. A 25-year single institution experience with surgery for primary mediastinal nonseminomatous germ cell tumors. Ann Thorac Surg 2008;85(2):371–8.
8. Ranganath P, Kesler KA, Einhorn LH. Perioperative morbidity and mortality associated with bleomycin in primary mediastinal nonseminomatous germ cell tumor. J Clin Oncol 2016;34(36):4445–6.
9. Vuky J, Bains M, Bacik J, et al. Role of postchemotherapy adjunctive surgery in the management of patients with nonseminoma arising from the mediastinum. J Clin Oncol 2001;19(3):682–8.
10. Hartmann JT, Einhorn L, Nichols CR, et al. Second-line chemotherapy in patients with relapsed extragonadal nonseminomatous germ cell tumors: results of an international multicenter analysis. J Clin Oncol 2001;19(6):1641–8.
11. Schneider BP, Kesler KA, Brooks JA, et al. Outcome of patients with residual germ cell or non-germ cell malignancy after resection of primary mediastinal nonseminomatous germ cell cancer. J Clin Oncol 2004;22(7):1195–200.
12. Radaideh SM, Cook VC, Kesler KA, et al. Outcome following resection for patients with primary mediastinal nonseminomatous germ-cell tumors and rising serum tumor markers post-chemotherapy. Ann Oncol 2010;21(4):804–7.

13. Adra N, Abonour R, Althouse SK, et al. High-dose chemotherapy and autologous peripheral-blood stem-cell transplantation for relapsed metastatic germ cell tumors: the indiana university experience. J Clin Oncol 2017;35(10):1096–102.
14. Kesler KA, Patel JB, Kruter LE, et al. The "growing teratoma syndrome" in primary mediastinal nonseminomatous germ cell tumors: criteria based on current practice. J Thorac Cardiovasc Surg 2012;144(2):438–43.
15. Kesler KA. Technique of mediastinal germ cell tumor resection. Oper Tech Thorac Cardiovasc Surg 2009;14(1):55–65.
16. Sarkaria IS, Bains MS, Sood S, et al. Resection of primary mediastinal nonseminomatous germ cell tumors: a 28-year experience at memorial sloan-kettering cancer center. J Thorac Oncol 2011;6(7):1236–41.
17. Malagon HD, Valdez AM, Moran CA, et al. Germ cell tumors with sarcomatous components: a clinicopathologic and immunohistochemical study of 46 cases. Am J Surg Pathol 2007;31(9):1356–62.
18. Contreras AL, Punar M, Tamboli P, et al. Mediastinal germ cell tumors with an angiosarcomatous component: a report of 12 cases. Hum Pathol 2010;41(6):832–7.

Thymic Malignancy—Updates in Staging and Management

Jesse M.P. Rappaport, MD[a], James Huang, MD, MPH[b],
Usman Ahmad, MD[a,c,d],*

KEYWORDS

- Thymoma • Thymic carcinoma • Multimodal therapy • Neoadjuvant
- Chemotherapy • Chemoradiation

KEY POINTS

- Complete resection is the therapy of choice for early-stage thymic malignancies.
- Patients with advanced-stage disease (without extrathoracic involvement) should be considered for multimodal treatment, including surgery.
- Neoadjuvant therapy may improve resectability and should be considered in locally advanced tumors.
- Limited pleural disease in stage IVA and locoregional recurrence should be considered for trimodality treatment.
- Thymic carcinoma histology portends worse disease-free survival and overall survival.

INTRODUCTION

Thymic malignancies, although rare compared with lung or esophageal cancer, are the most common tumors of the anterior mediastinum. True incidence is unknown but is estimated to be approximately 2.2 to 2.6 per million per year for thymomas and 0.3 to 0.6 per million per year for thymic carcinomas.[1] Thymomas typically are indolent and present with localized disease but have the potential for intrathoracic and extrathoracic metastasis. Thymic carcinoma, compared to thymoma, represents a worse histology and disease course with much higher rates of nodal and systemic involvement.[2]

[a] Department of Cardiothoracic Surgery, Heart, Vascular and Thoracic Institute, Cleveland Clinic, Cleveland, OH, USA; [b] Thoracic Service, Department of Surgery, Memorial Sloan Kettering Cancer Center, 1275 York Avenue, New York, NY 10065, USA; [c] Taussig Cancer Center, Cleveland Clinic, Cleveland, OH, USA; [d] Transplant Institute, Cleveland Clinic, Cleveland, OH, USA
* Corresponding author. Department of Cardiothoracic Surgery, Heart, Vascular and Thoracic Institute, Cleveland Clinic, 9500 Euclid Avenue, Desk J4, Cleveland, OH 44195, USA.
E-mail address: AHMADU@ccf.org

Surg Oncol Clin N Am 29 (2020) 581–601
https://doi.org/10.1016/j.soc.2020.06.010
1055-3207/20/© 2020 Elsevier Inc. All rights reserved.

surgonc.theclinics.com

Thymomas commonly are associated with myriad paraneoplastic disorders, most common being myasthenia gravis. It is less common to find a concomitant paraneoplastic syndrome in thymic carcinoma or neuroendocrine tumors.[3] Histology plays an important role in disease biology, and worse differentiation is associated with shorter disease-free survival and overall survival (OS).

In general, early-stage tumors (without invasion into surrounding vascular structures or lung parenchyma) are treated with upfront resection. Excellent long-term OS is noted in completely resected thymomas and ranges from 80% to 90% at 10 years. Completely resected early-stage thymic carcinoma has a 5-year OS of approximately 70%.[2]

Locally advanced disease with invasion into surrounding resectable structures or with oligometastatic pleural or pericardial implants typically is managed with multimodal therapy. Resection is attempted after some form of neoadjuvant therapy (either chemotherapy alone or chemotherapy with radiation). Unresectable disease can be treated with definitive chemoradiation.

This review addresses the recent updates and advances in staging and treatment paradigms for thymic tumors. Also highlighted is the importance of multidisciplinary and multi-institutional collaborations in moving the field forward. At the present time, the International Thymic Malignancy Interest Group (ITMIG) offers a virtual tumor board where any physician can upload the case data and get input from an international multidisciplinary panel.[4,5]

GENERAL APPROACH AND PRINCIPLES

Because complete resection clearly is associated with improved OS for all histologic subtypes, work-up and treatment planning centers around optimizing R0 (complete microscopic) resection. For early-stage tumors with no radiographic evidence of vascular, pulmonary, or great vessel involvement and no evidence of intrathoracic or extrathoracic metastases, upfront resection is the standard of care. Based on tumor size and surgeon experience, this can be performed through sternotomy or thoracotomy or using a minimally invasive technique. Lately robotic thymectomy through unilateral or bilateral pleural approach has gained popularity. Although tissue diagnosis is not necessary for small tumors that appear amenable to complete resection, it should be considered if the possibility of an alternate diagnosis (lymphoma or germ cell tumor) exists. Tissue diagnosis is necessary if neoadjuvant therapy is needed.[6]

The general approach to patients with locally advanced thymic tumors includes multidisciplinary evaluation typically by a cardiothoracic surgeon, medical oncologist, radiation oncologist, radiologist, pathologist, and neurologist (for patients with concomitant paraneoplastic syndromes). Multidisciplinary evaluation and discussion can greatly facilitate the management of these challenging cases.

Radiographic evaluation should include high-resolution computed tomogram (CT) scan with intravenous contrast (preferentially given through the left or right upper extremity to opacify the innominate vein or right brachiocephalic vein or CT venogram protocol if there is concern for invasion of these structures) is essential for delineating the anatomic relationships of the tumor and adjacent organs.[7] The value of positron emission tomography in assessing local invasion is unclear but is important in staging and ruling out metastatic disease, particularly in more aggressive histologies, such as thymic carcinoma.[8]

UPDATES IN STAGING

Thymic tumor staging has gone through several iterations, and proposals based on TNM, local invasion, and histology have been made over several decades. Historically, the Masaoka-Koga[9,10] system had been the most widely adapted system for the past decade and recently has been replaced by an updated TNM system that was part of the 8th edition of the American Joint Committee on Cancer stage classification.[11] Previous staging systems were based on studies with a small number of patients. For example, the Masaoka classification was based on a retrospective series of 96 cases.[9] To overcome this issue, an international collaboration resulted in a robust retrospective database of approximately 10,000 cases from all over the world. This became the substrate for the latest TNM staging system and categorization.[8] Both staging systems are shown in **Tables 1–3** and **Fig. 1**. Both staging systems now are used widely[6] as the adoption of and transition to TNM system evolves.

The most important prognostic factors still remain tumor stage and achieving an R0 resection, leading to a 10-year OS rate of 80% to 90% for surgically resected localized tumors (Masaoka-Koga stage I and II).[12,13] The general treatment paradigm, therefore, puts radical R0 resection at the center of multimodal therapy. In addition to thymectomy, with the introduction of TNM 8th edition, there is now growing support for including regional lymphadenectomy/sampling (**Fig. 2**); however, the survival benefit of lymph node staging has not yet been demonstrated.[14]

Comparisons of the TNM staging with Masaoka-Koga staging showed a shift in proportion of stages in 3 studies. Fukui and colleagues[15] assessed 154 patients who underwent complete resection and found the TNM staging correlated with recurrence-free survival, but they did not find an apt correlation with OS. Conversely, Ried and colleagues[16] found good correlation between Masaoka-Koga stage and TNM stage in respect to both OS and disease-free survival with their series of 76 surgical patients. In another series of 181 patients, the Masaoka-Koga staging system was able to statistically predict time to recurrence, but not OS. Neither time to recurrence nor OS was statistically correlated with TNM staging.[17] Given the indolent nature of the disease, recurrence-free survival is an important parameter when studying disease course and treatment outcomes.

INDUCTION CHEMOTHERAPY

Several chemotherapy regimens have been tried with varying outcomes.[12] Cooperative group studies examined cisplatin, doxorubicin, and cyclophosphamide (CAP) regimen led by Eastern Cooperative Oncology Group[18] and etoposide-cisplatin led by the European Organisation for Research and Treatment of Cancer[19] in patients

Table 1 Masaoka-Koga staging	
Category	**Definition**
Stage I	Grossly and microscopically encapsulated
Stage II	
A	Microscopic transcapsular invasion
B	Macroscopic capsular invasion
Stage III	Macroscopic invasion of neighboring organs, including pericardium, lung, or the main blood vessels
Stage IV	
A	Pleural or pericardial dissemination
B	Hematogenous or lymphatic dissemination

Table 2
International Association for the Study of Lung Cancer/International Thymic Malignancy Interest Group TNM staging

Category	Definition (Involvement of)[a,b]
T1	
a	Encapsulated or unencapsulated, with or without extension into mediastinal fat
b	Extension into mediastinal pleura
T2	Pericardium
T3	Lung, brachiocephalic vein, superior vena cava, chest wall, phrenic nerve, hilar (extrapericardial) pulmonary vessels
T4	Aorta, arch vessels, main pulmonary artery, myocardium, trachea, or esophagus
N0	No nodal involvement
N1	Anterior (perithymic) nodes
N2	Deep intrathoracic or cervical nodes
M0	No metastatic pleural, pericardial, or distant sites
M1	
a	Separate pleural or pericardial nodule(s)
b	Pulmonary intraparenchymal nodule or distant organ metastasis

[a] Involvement must be pathologically proved in pathologic staging.
[b] A tumor is classified according to the highest T level of involvement that is, present with or without any invasion of structures of lower T levels.

with metastatic or unresectable disease. Reasonable response and toxicity profiles were noted.[18,19] Other smaller retrospective series have shown reasonable clinical response (62%–100%) and R0 resection rates of 22% to 92% (**Table 4**).

A few notable prospective studies include a single-arm prospective trial of CAP regimen, which was used as induction therapy in 22 patients with unresectable thymoma[20]; 6 of 16 patients had greater than 80% tumor necrosis on pathologic evaluation. At 5 years, disease-free survival was 77% and OS was 95%.

Table 3
International Association for the Study of Lung Cancer (IASLC) / International Thymic Malignancies Interest Group (ITMIG) staging groups

T/M	Subcategory	N0	N1	N2
T1	1a	I	IVa	IVb
	1b			
T2		II	IVa	IVb
T3		IIIa	IVa	IVb
T4		IIIb	IVa	IVb
M1	a	IVa	IVa	IVb
	b	IVb	IVb	IVb

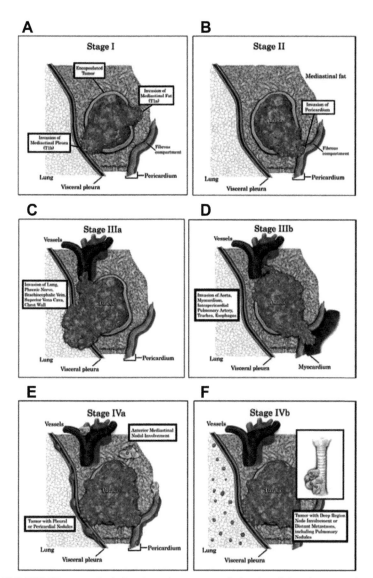

Fig. 1. IASLC/ITMIG stage depiction based on anatomic landmark involvement. (*From* Detterbeck F C, Stratton K, Giroux D, et al. The IASLC/ITMIG Thymic Epithelial Tumors Staging Project: Proposal for an Evidence-Based Stage Classification System for the Forthcoming (8th) Edition of the TNM Classification of Malignant Tumors. J Thorac Oncol. 2014;9: S65–S72.)

A phase II Japan Clinical Oncology Group study reported results with either chemotherapy (cisplatin, vincristine, doxorubicin, and etoposide) or radiation followed by resection. In the chemotherapy group, 62% of patients had radiographic response and 14% had complete pathologic response.[21] An Italian[22] prospective analysis of 30 stages III and IVA thymoma patients treated with neoadjuvant cisplatin, epirubicin, and etoposide reported 73% response rate and 77% complete resection rate.

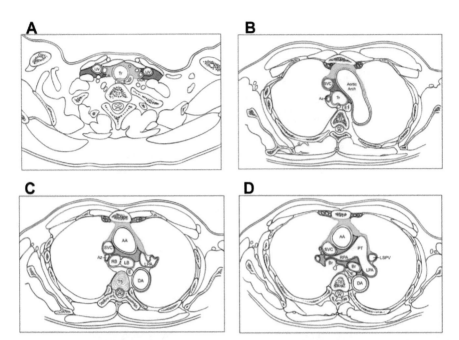

Fig. 2. ITMIG/IASLC lymph node map. Anterior and deep node regions as depicted on axial images. Anterior region (*blue*); deep region (*purple*). (*A*) Thoracic inlet; (*B*) para-aortic level; (*C*) at AP window level; and (*D*) at carina. (*From* Bhora F Y, Chen D J, Detterbeck F C, et al. The ITMIG/IASLC Thymic Epithelial Tumors Staging Project: A Proposed Lymph Node Map for Thymic Epithelial Tumors in the Forthcoming 8th Edition of the TNM Classification of Malignant Tumors. J Thorac Oncol. 2014;9: S88–S96.)

A series from the Japanese Association for Research of the Thymus (JART) database reported on 441 patients with clinical stage III thymoma, of whom 113 had induction treatment. Treatment response was 52%; however, induction was associated with worse prognosis. The investigators attributed this to selection bias to more patients with advanced disease receiving induction treatment.[23] Another study, using a database of 1486 patients from the Korean Association for Research on the Thymus, found no difference in complete resection rate, OS, or disease-free survival when comparing a matched cohort of patients who received upfront surgery with induction therapy plus surgery. The chemotherapy regimens were heterogeneous, but the majority included cisplatin in combination with a second agent.[24]

A European Society of Thoracic Surgeons database[25] review of treated patients showed higher use of neoadjuvant treatment in unresectable patients. Chemotherapy regimens included cisplatin, doxorubicin, cyclophosphamide, and vincristine and were administered in 25% of the patients. No association between induction treatment and cancer-specific or recurrence-free survival was noted in advanced-stage or unresectable patients, making the results rather inconclusive.

A series from the Réseau Tumeurs Thymiques et Cancer (RYTHMIC) network in France reviewed 236 patients (119 thymoma and 117 thymic carcinoma) and found that 91 patients underwent induction therapy, with a majority (70%) receiving cyclophosphamide, doxorubicin, and cisplatin.[26] They found an objective response rate of 83% for thymoma, and, of the 57 patients who underwent operative treatment, 70% achieved complete resection.

Table 4
Results of multimodality treatment in thymoma using induction chemotherapy

Author	y	N	Stage	Chemotherapy	Response Rate (%)	Complete Resection Rate (%)	Postoperative Radiotherapy	Disease-Free Survival	Overall Survival
Prospective									
Macchiarini et al,[78] 1991	1988–1990	7	III	Cisplatin, epirubicin, etoposide	100	57	45 Gy (R0)	—	—
Rea et al,[79] 1993	1985–1991	16	III, IIVA	Doxorubicin, cisplatin, vincristine, cyclophosphamide	100	69	11 cases	—	70%—3 y
Berruti et al,[80] 1993	1990–1992	6	III, IVA	Doxorubicin, cisplatin, vincristine, cyclophosphamide	83	83	—	—	—
Venuta et al,[81] 1997	1989-onwards	15	III	Cisplatin, epirubicin, etoposide	67	91	40 Gy (R0)	—	—
Kim et al,[20] 2004	1990–2000	22	III, IVA	Cisplatin, doxorubicin, cyclophosphamide, prednisone	77	76	50 Gy (R0)	77%—5 y	95%—5 y
Yokoi et al,[82] 2007	1988–2003	14	III, IVA	Cisplatin, doxorubicin, methylprednisolone	93	22	50 Gy	—	89%—5 y and 10 y
Lucchi et al,[22] 2006	1989–2004	30	III, IVA	Cisplatin, epirubicin, etoposide	73	77	45 Gy (R0)	—	82%—10 y
Kunitoh et al,[21] 2010	1997–2005	21	III	Cisplatin, vincristine, doxorubicin, etoposide	62	43	48 Gy (R0)	32%—8 y	69%—8 y
Retrospective									
Bretti et al,[83] 2004	1990–1992	25	III, IVA	Doxorubicin, cisplatin, vincristine, cyclophosphamide (18 cases) Cisplatin, etoposide (7 cases)	72	44	45 Gy (R0)	—	—
Yamada et al,[23] 2015	1991–2010	113	III	Not specified	52	—	—	—	—
Leuzzi et al,[25] 2016	1990–2010	88	III	Cisplatin, doxorubicin, cyclophosphamide, vincristine	—	65	—	—	—
Nakamura et al,[51] 2019	2003–2007	19	IVA	Cisplatin, doxorubicin, methylprednisolone	79	—	—	46%—10 y	77%—10 y

(continued on next page)

Table 4
(continued)

Author	y	N	Stage	Chemotherapy	Response Rate (%)	Complete Resection Rate (%)	Postoperative Radiotherapy	Disease-Free Survival	Overall Survival
Ma et al,[84] 2019	2005–2013	15	III, IV	Platinum-based	—	—	45–54 Gy	32%—5 y	89%— 5y
Kanzaki et al,[85] 2019	1997–2018	26	III, IV	Cisplatin-based (20 cases), Carboplatin-based (9 cases)	38	83	5 cases	50%—10 y	87%—10 y

Data from Refs.[20–23,25,51,78–85]

Overall, the favorable outcomes from the prospective and larger retrospective experience support the use of neoadjuvant chemotherapy. Most regimens are well tolerated with an acceptable toxicity profile and results in reasonable response rates in locally advanced tumors.

INDUCTION CHEMORADIATION

Similar to locally advanced lung and esophageal tumors,[27,28] the benefit of neoadjuvant radiation in improving local disease control and improving resectability has been explored. In a prospective intergroup trial,[29] patients with localized unresectable thymoma and thymic carcinoma underwent 4 cycles of CAP followed by 54 Gy of radiation as definitive therapy. Among the 23 assessable patients, the overall response rate to initial chemotherapy was 69.6%. After radiation, 1 patient with partial response had complete response; 4 patients who previously had minimal response now showed complete or partial response (5-year OS 53%).

Some of the initial experience came from Wright and colleagues,[30] who reported a series of 10 patients with stage III or stage IVA thymic tumors utilizing concurrent chemoradiation (cisplatin and etoposide with 40–45 Gy): 4 patients had partial response; 8 patients had complete and 2 had incomplete resection; and 4 patients had a pathologic complete response.

A multi-institutional phase II study of induction treatment with cisplatin, etoposide, and 45 Gy of radiation[31] included 22 patients with stage III disease (>5 cm tumors with suspicion of local invasion). In 7 thymic carcinoma and 14 thymoma patients; 21 completed induction treatment and a partial radiographic response was noted in 10 (47%) patients. Grade 3 or grade 4 toxicity was noted in 9 cases (41%). During surgery, 17 had an R0 resection, 3 had R1 resection, and 1 had R2 resection. There were no complete responses and 5 cases had less than 10% viable tumor. Postoperative complications were noted in 8 (36%) patients. This study was notable for high treatment toxicity with as well as perioperative mortality with 2 in-hospital deaths. Overall, 5-year survival was 71% and freedom from progression was 83%.

Findings from chemoradiation experience are summarized in **Table 5**. Higher toxicity with chemoradiation may be related to large radiation fields over the mediastinum and both lungs, especially with larger tumors.[30–32] In addition to higher acute toxicity and perioperative morbidity, long-term effects, including coronary and valvular disease, cannot be discounted.[31]

INDUCTION RADIATION

Most institutions now favor the use of chemotherapy in the induction setting. In a multi-institutional study from European Society of Thoracic Surgeons database, only 12 of 2030 (1%) of patients underwent induction radiation alone.[33] A review of the ITMIG database showed that for thymic carcinomas, 48 of 1042 (6%) of the cases had induction radiation only.[2]

In a historical series of 34 stage III thymoma patients, 8 received preoperative radiation with cobalt 60 whereas 26 did not. Patients who underwent a complete resection had improved survival; however, there was no difference in OS between patients who did or did not receive preoperative radiation.[34] More modern radiation treatments have since been reported by others. Ribet and colleagues[35] reported a series of 113 patients, where 19 patients had preoperative radiation. In this group, complete resection was achieved in 10 of 19 patients, with 5-year OS of 44%. Akaogi and colleagues[36] reported a series of 12 patients with thymic tumor invading the great vessels (vena cava, pulmonary artery, and aorta). Patients were treated with preoperative

Table 5
Results of multimodality treatment in thymoma using induction chemoradiation therapy

Author	y	N	Stage	Chemotherapy	Radiation	Response Rate (%)	Complete Resection (%)	Disease-Free Survival	Overall Survival
Prospective									
Loehrer et al,[29] 1997[a]	1983–1995	23	III, IV	Cisplatin, cyclophosphamide, doxorubicin	45 Gy	70	No resection	—	53%—5 y
Korst et al,[31] 2014	2007–2012	21	I, II, III	Cisplatin, etoposide	45 Gy	47	77	83%—5 y (freedom from progression	71%—5 y
Retrospective									
Wright et al,[30] 2008	1997–2006	10	III, IVA	Cisplatin, etoposide	40–45 Gy	40	80	—	69%—5 y

[a] Chemoradiation as definitive therapy only. No surgery.
Data from Refs.[29-31]

radiation (12–21 Gy). The rate of complete resection was 75%. Ten patients also received adjuvant radiation (mean, 42.3 Gy). The OS was 72% at 5 years and 48% at 10 years. Selection bias, changes in radiation technology, and improvement in surgical management likely make some of these results inapplicable to contemporary practice.

UPDATES IN SURGICAL RESECTION

Surgical resection remains the definitive local therapy of choice for thymic tumors. Regardless of the approach or tumor stage, the goal of surgery is complete resection with en bloc removal of the entire thymus gland and perithymic fat without violation of the tumor capsule.

For early-stage disease, minimally invasive techniques are increasingly utilized with acceptable oncologic outcomes. A study utilizing the National Cancer Database focused on 943 stage I and II thymoma patients found an increase utilization of minimal invasively resection from 2010 and 2014 of approximately 20% with comparable R0 rate to open resection.[37] Large database studies, including those from ITMIG database, show acceptable R0 resection rates with the use of minimally invasive approaches.[38,39] A more recent systematic review of open, video-assisted thoracoscopic surgery, and robotic thymectomy concluded that the minimally invasive approaches offer significant morbidity advantages over open surgery and should be considered when feasible to obtain an R0 resection in early-stage disease.[40]

Regardless of approach, there is growing evidence to suggest the importance of systematic lymph node sampling even in early-stage tumors. In a multicenter observational study of 275 patients, The Chinese Alliance for Research in Thymomas found lymph node metastases in 2.1% of thymoma cases, 25% of thymic carcinoma cases, and 50% of neuroendocrine tumors. They also noted an increase in lymph node positivity with increasing T stage.[41] Appropriate nodal staging should be kept in perspective when choosing the surgical approach.

In locally advanced disease, the surgical team should be prepared to asses and resect tumors invading surrounding viscera. Although innominate vein, superior vena cava, pleura, pericardium, and nonanatomic lung resections do not add significant morbidity, greater resections, including lobectomy or pneumonectomy and great vessel reconstruction, can be technically and physiologically challenging. Patients with locally advanced disease should be assessed on a case-by-case basis in a multidisciplinary fashion. In well-selected cases, the authors have been able to resect and reconstruct ascending aorta, coronary bypass grafts, and pulmonary arterial trunk; however, these surgeries require significant preparation and carry significant morbidity. If such extensive resection is expected, consideration should be given to limiting neoadjuvant regimen to chemotherapy only and use radiation in the adjuvant setting to treat residual disease or high-risk tumor bed.

Even in clinical stage IVA tumors with pleural or pericardial implants, resection has been undertaken with reasonable results.[42] Obtaining en bloc R0 oncologic resection in these patients, however, requires careful selection of patients with the use of detailed preoperative assessment and the use of neoadjuvant treatments.

POSTOPERATIVE RADIATION THERAPY

There are no randomized trials focused on post-operative radiation; however, reasonable-sized institutional and database studies favor the use of postoperative radiation treatment (PORT) in appropriately selected patients. PORT has been shown to be a significant factor in improving OS. Specifically, in an analysis of the National Cancer

Database, 49% (n = 2001) of patients who underwent resection for thymoma or thymic carcinoma received PORT. Patients who received PORT had a survival benefit across advanced stages (IIB–IV), positive resection margins, and histologic subtypes.[43]

In early-stage, completely resected thymoma, studies show mixed results on the potential benefit of PORT. In a meta-analysis of 14 studies looking at completely resected thymoma, Zhou and colleagues[44] found no benefit to PORT in stage I disease but some benefit in stage II and stage III. This is echoed by the ITMIG analysis of PORT versus surgery alone in 1263 stages II–III thymoma patients who underwent R0 resection, showing 5-year and 10-year survival benefits of 95% and 86%, respectively, compared with 90% and 79%, respectively.[45] A study utilizing the JART database, however, which included patients with incomplete resection (R1/2), found no recurrence-free or OS benefit of PORT in thymoma and only a benefit in recurrence-free survival in thymic carcinoma.[46]

For stages III to IV, PORT seems much more widely accepted for resected tumors. Studies have shown that aggressive treatment with induction chemotherapy, surgical resection, and PORT can lead to improved survival in later stages.[47] A review of 146 patients with stages III–IVA thymoma demonstrated an increased OS and freedom from recurrence with the use of trimodality treatment in the stage III group but not yet shown in the stage IVA group.[48] This again is highlighted by a study of the Surveillance, Epidemiology, and End Results (SEER) database, which demonstrated at least improvement in disease-specific survival.[49] Patients with thymic carcinoma appear to benefit from adjuvant radiation therapy more consistently, especially those with locally advanced disease and incomplete resection.[2]

SPECIAL CONSIDERATIONS
Stage IVA Disease

In extensive pleural disease, extrapleural pneumonectomy (EPP) potentially can achieve a macroscopic complete resection, also allowing for hemithoracic radiation without the risk of pneumonitis. In patients with limited pleural disease, partial pleurectomy is considered adequate resection. In both scenarios, induction chemotherapy is strongly considered. The role of radiation is limited by the large size of the required treatment field.

The few data on pleural lavage show feasibility, particularly in recurrent disease, but true added benefit is unclear. In a notable series of 35 stage IVA patients with thymoma (17), thymic carcinoma (4), and recurrent thymoma (14), induction chemotherapy was administered to all thymic carcinoma and 13 thymoma patients. Along with EPP or local resection, the pleural space was intraoperatively perfused with cisplatin and doxorubicin at 45°C for 60 minutes; 90-day mortality was 2.5%. After median follow-up of 62 months, the 5-year and 10-year progression-free survival rates were 61% and 43%, respectively, for primary thymomas, and 48% and 18%, respectively, for recurrent thymomas.[50] Local control was not achieved in thymic carcinoma patients and all died within 4 years. Heated povidone was used in a series of 6 thymoma patients with pleural disease; induction chemotherapy was administered followed by complete pleurectomy. Povidone-iodine solution (diluted in a 1:10 ratio in sterile water and heated to 40°C–41°C) was instilled in the pleural space for at least 15 minutes. After median follow-up of 18 months, 1 patient had died of unrelated reasons and 1 patient underwent re-resection for recurrence, whereas the remaining 4 patients were free of disease.

Choe and colleagues[42] analyzed 72 primary stage IVA patients with thymoma (57) and thymic carcinoma (15) and found that 48 patients underwent thymectomy with pleurectomy, 7 received EP, 10 underwent thymectomy alone, and 7 were unresectable. In 73%, a macroscopic complete resection was achieved with a 5-year, 10-year, and 15-year OS rates of 73%, 51%, and 18%, respectively; 83% had received induction chemotherapy and 64% received postoperative treatment (31 radiation, 2 brachytherapy, 8 chemotherapy, and 5 chemoradiation). Progression/recurrence was common (64%) with median time to progression of 2.2 years and a median of 3 episodes of progression per patient. Re-resection was common in this population with at least 1 additional operation in 21 patients (46% of those with progression).

In a study of 19 stage IVA patients (13 primary and 6 recurrent pleural disease), 78.9% had partial response with induction chemotherapy (cisplatin, doxorubicin, and methylprednisolone). Ten patients underwent EPP and 9 underwent resection of pleural dissemination. Between these 2 groups, they demonstrated similar OS, but progression-free survival in the EPP group was higher; however, no statistical comparison was made.[51] A series from the European Society of Thoracic Surgeons Thymic Working Group included 152 patients (70.4% primary dissemination and 29.6% recurrent pleural disease) who underwent EP (n = 40), total pleurectomy (n = 23), local pleurectomy (n = 88) without significant difference in freedom from recurrence or OS between the groups.[52]

These treatment protocols may have utility in the treatment of extensive pleural disease where pleural metastases limit the ability to achieve complete resection. To date, however, there are no validated prospective data that demonstrate efficacy in these difficult cases.

Thymic Carcinoma

Although thymoma represents a majority of data accumulated, the severity of thymic carcinoma by comparison remains apparent with a 5-year OS rates of 80%, 63%, 42%, and 30% for stages I/II, III, IVA, and IVB, respectively, according to the largest series by ITMIG, with a total of 1042 cases.[2] Recurrence rates at 5 years and 10 years in this cohort ranged, respectively, from 15% for stages I and II, to 35% and 38% for stage III, and to 45% and 52% for stages IVA/B.

In review of treatment patterns, the authors have previously shown that trimodality therapy improved OS.[2] On multivariable analysis, complete surgical resection (R0) and radiation treatment improved OS, but only radiation treatment and male gender were associated with recurrence-free survival. The authors were not able to differentiate between the benefits of adjuvant versus neoadjuvant treatment in this cohort of patients. In another study of 306 thymic carcinoma patients, perioperative therapy did not afford the same benefit to OS; however, tumor size and PORT were associated with better recurrence-free survival after an R0 resection.[53] PORT again was found e beneficial, specifically for locally advanced tumors, in a review of the SEER database looking at thymic carcinoma cases between 2004 and 2013.[54] Hamaji and colleagues[55] also found similar results in their meta-analysis looking at a total of 973 cases of thymic carcinoma demonstrating a benefit of PORT for both OS and progression-free survival (hazard ratios of 0.66 and 0.54, respectively).

General principles of management of thymic carcinoma are similar to thymoma, except that local invasion is more common and the index of suspicion of invasion should be higher. Utilization of neoadjuvant and adjuvant therapies show significant improvement in survival.

MANAGEMENT OF RECURRENT DISEASE

Standard definition of recurrence as recommended by ITMIG include all cases of disease presence after an R0 resection. They can be classified as local (site of original tumor), regional (intrathoracic not contiguous with original tumor or thymus), and distant (intraparenchymal and extrathoracic). A majority of recurrences are locoregional (>90%) for thymoma and more likely to be distant in thymic carcinoma.[56] Recurrences should be managed based on location, prior treatment responses, and ability for re-resection.

Due to thymoma's primarily locoregional recurrence, re-resection may be viable through EPP or pleurectomy with or without lung resection. The addition of intrathoracic hyperthermic chemotherapy perfusion has been attempted for disease control. In a series of 13 patients with recurrent pleural thymoma who underwent re-resection and hyperthermic intrathoracic perfusion chemotherapy, there were no perioperative toxicities and the mean survival was 58 months with a 5-year survival of 92%.[57] Maury and colleagues[58] published on 19 consecutive cases of patients who underwent either pleurectomy (4), pleurectomy and wedge resection (14), or pleuropneumonectomy with concurrent intrathoracic chemohyperthermia for thymoma pleural recurrence. They had no perioperative deaths, a median disease-free survival of 42 months, and 5-year survival of 86%.

At this time, however, experience is limited and heterogenous. Multimodal therapy appears to impart reasonable local control with unclear survival benefit. In localized unresectable disease, radiotherapy typically is employed, whereas unresectable regional/distant disease requires systemic treatments.

TARGETED THERAPIES AND IMMUNOTHERAPIES

Despite thymic tumors harboring a variety of targetable mutations,[59,60] there has been limited success with targeted therapies (**Table 6**).

Due to the activation of the PI3K/AKT pathway in thymic tumors,[61] the mammalian target of rapamycin (mTOR) inhibitor everolimus has been studied in phase II trial showing median progression-free survival of 10.1 months and OS of 25.7 months in advanced, treatment refractory thymoma and thymic carcinoma.[62]

Despite high rates of overexpression of epidermal growth factor receptor, activating mutations rarely are seen.[59] Two phase II studies using gefitinib and erlotinib showed poor response rates in chemorefractory patients.[63,64] A phase II study of CAP plus cetuximab as induction therapy followed by surgery in locally advanced chemotherapy-naive patients was designed and currently is ongoing at the Memorial Sloan Kettering Cancer Center (NCT01025089). Patients receive 4 cycles of CAP concurrently with cetuximab on a weekly basis, followed by surgical resection. Similarly, KIT overexpression has reported in thymic carcinomas; however, fewer than 10% of the tumors harbor a KIT mutation and to date no response has been reported with the use of imatinib.[65]

Insulinlike growth factor receptor overexpression has been shown in thymic tumors[66] and a phase II study enrolled 49 patients (37 thymoma and 12 thymic carcinoma) with refractory or recurrent disease: 5 thymoma patients had partial response to cixutumumab, 28 had stable disease, and 4 progressed. Of the 12 thymic carcinoma patients treated, none responded, 5 had stable disease, and 7 had progressive disease.[67]

Vascular endothelial growth factors (VEGFs) and VEGF receptors have been found as possible targets in high-risk thymomas and thymic carcinomas,[68] and thus antiangiogenic factors, such as sunitinib, pose possibilities. In an open-label phase II study of chemorefractory tumors, sunitinib demonstrated partial response in 6 thymic carcinoma cases and stable disease in 15 of 23 thymic carcinoma cases. One of 16 thymoma patients had a partial response while 12 had stable disease.[69] In a

Table 6
Results of targeted therapies and immunotherapies

Author	y	N	Agent	Response Rate (%)	Disease Control (%)	Progression-Free Survival, Median	Overall Survival, Median
Targeted therapy							
Zucali et al,[62] 2018	2011–2013	51	Everolimus	12	88	10 m	26 m
Rajan et al,[67] 2014	2009–2012	49	Cixutumumab	10	78	8 m	16 m
Thomas et al,[69] 2015	2012–2013	40	Sunitinib	18	85	8 m	17 m
Remon et al,[70] 2016	2012–2015	28	Sunitinib	22	63	4 m	15 m
Immunotherapy							
Giaccone et al,[74] 2018	2015–2016	40	Pembrolizumab	23	75	4 m	25 m
Cho et al,[75] 2019	2016	33	Pembrolizumab	21	79	6 m	15 m
Rajan et al,[77] 2019	2013–2019	8	Avelumab	57	38	—	—

Data from Refs.[62,67,69,70,74,75,77]

retrospective review of off-label use, the RYTHMIC cohort of 28 patients (20 thymic carcinoma and 8 thymoma) demonstrated a response rate of 22% and a disease control rate of 63%, with median progression-free survival of 3.7 months and median OS of 14.5 months.[70]

The recent developments with immunotherapy have increased the potential for opportunities to investigate novel combined therapy approaches in these tumors. Both thymoma and thymic carcinoma have shown expression of programmed cell death protein 1 (PD-1) and programmed death-ligand 1 (PD-L1),[71–73] leading to the evaluation of pembrolizumab in chemorefractory tumors. In a study of 40 patients with thymic carcinoma, 1 patient had complete response, 8 had partial response, and 21 had stable disease. Median progression-free survival was 4.2 months and median OS was 24.9 months.[74] Another phase II trial by Cho and colleagues[75] demonstrated response in 5 of 26 refractory thymic carcinoma cases and 2 of 7 refractory thymoma cases with a median progression-free survival of 6.1 months. Both studies showed high incidence of treatment related autoimmunity and recommend close monitoring.

Similarly, other PD-L1 antibodies have been studied. In a phase II trial of 15 cases of unresectable or recurrent thymic carcinoma treated with nivolumab demonstrated 11 patients with stable disease, but no patients had treatment response. The median progression-free survival was 3.8 months and OS was 12.7 months.[76] A second multicenter nivolumab phase II trial is ongoing in Europe (NCT03134118). Rajan and colleagues[77] evaluated the effect of avelumab in a phase I trial for advanced thymoma and thymic carcinoma and found of 7 thymoma patients, 2 with partial response, 2 with unconfirmed partial response, and 2 with stable disease. The 1 thymic carcinoma patient had stable disease. Again, immune-related adverse events were common occurring in all responders.

Although promising responses have been noted, these therapies have yet to be completely evaluated and adverse autoimmune effects appear common in this patient population.

CONFLICTS OF INTEREST

Supported in part by the Daniel and Karen Lee Endowed Chair in Thoracic Surgery and the Drs Sidney and Becca Fleischer Heart and Vascular Education Chair.

REFERENCES

1. de Jong WK, Blaauwgeers JLG, Schaapveld M, et al. Thymic epithelial tumours: A population-based study of the incidence, diagnostic procedures and therapy. Eur J Cancer 2008;44(1):123–30.
2. Ahmad U, Yao X, Detterbeck F, et al. Thymic carcinoma outcomes and prognosis: Results of an international analysis. J Thorac Cardiovasc Surg 2015;149(1): 95–101.e2.
3. Padda SK, Yao X, Antonicelli A, et al. Paraneoplastic Syndromes and Thymic Malignancies: An Examination of the International Thymic Malignancy Interest Group Retrospective Database. J Thorac Oncol 2018;13(3):436–46.
4. Sigurdson SS, Roden AC, Marom EM, et al. Case presentation and recommendations from the April 2018 ITMIG tumor board: an international multidisciplinary team. Mediastinum 2019;3:4.
5. Sigurdson S, Roden AC, Marom EM, et al. Case presentation and recommendations from the April 2019 ITMIG tumor board: an international multidisciplinary team. Mediastinum 2019;3:41.
6. Ruffini E, Fang W, Guerrera F, et al. The International Association for the Study of Lung Cancer Thymic Tumors Staging Project: The Impact of the Eighth Edition of the Union for International Cancer Control and American Joint Committee on Cancer TNM Stage Classification of Thymic Tumors. J Thorac Oncol 2020. https://doi.org/10.1016/j.jtho.2019.11.013.
7. Marom EM, Rosado-De-Christenson ML, Bruzzi JF, et al. Standard report terms for chest computed tomography reports of anterior mediastinal masses suspicious for thymoma. J Thorac Oncol 2011;6(7 SUPPL. 3). https://doi.org/10.1097/JTO.0b013e31821e8cd6.
8. Detterbeck FC, Stratton K, Giroux D, et al. The IASLC/ITMIG thymic epithelial tumors staging project: Proposal for an evidence-based stage classification system for the forthcoming (8th) edition of the TNM classification of malignant tumors. J Thorac Oncol 2014;9(9):S65–72.
9. Masaoka A, Monden Y, Nakahara K, et al. Follow-up study of thymomas with special reference to their clinical stages. Cancer 1981;48(11):2485–92.
10. Koga K, Matsuno Y, Noguchi M, et al. A review of 79 thymomas: Modification of staging system and reappraisal of conventional division into invasive and non-invasive thymoma. Pathol Int 1994;44(5):359–67.
11. Brierley JD, Gospodarowicz MK, Wittekind C. TNM classification of malignant tumours. 8. Hoboken: Wiley-Blackwell; 2016.

12. Detterbeck FC, Parsons AM. Thymic tumors. Ann Thorac Surg 2004;77(5): 1860–9.

13. Detterbeck FC, Parsons AM. Management of Stage I and II Thymoma. Thorac Surg Clin 2011;21(1):59–67.

14. Hwang Y, Park IK, Park S, et al. Lymph node dissection in thymic malignancies: Implication of the itmig lymph node map, TNM stage classification, and recommendations. J Thorac Oncol 2016;11(1):108–14.

15. Fukui T, Fukumoto K, Okasaka T, et al. Clinical evaluation of a new tumour-node-metastasis staging system for thymic malignancies proposed by the International Association for the Study of Lung Cancer Staging and Prognostic Factors Committee and the International Thymic Malignancy Interest Group. Eur J Cardiothorac Surg 2016;49(2):574–9.

16. Ried M, Eicher MM, Neu R, et al. Evaluation of the new TNM-staging system for thymic malignancies: Impact on indication and survival. World J Surg Oncol 2017;15(1). https://doi.org/10.1186/s12957-017-1283-4.

17. Meurgey A, Girard N, Merveilleux du Vignaux C, et al. Assessment of the ITMIG Statement on the WHO Histological Classification and of the Eighth TNM Staging of Thymic Epithelial Tumors of a Series of 188 Thymic Epithelial Tumors. J Thorac Oncol 2017;12(10):1571–81.

18. Loehrer PJ, Kim K, Aisner SC, et al. Cisplatin plus doxorubicin plus cyclophosphamide in metastatic or recurrent thymoma: final results of an intergroup trial. The Eastern Cooperative Oncology Group, Southwest Oncology Group, and Southeastern Cancer Study Group. J Clin Oncol 1994;12(6):1164–8.

19. Giaccone G, Ardizzoni A, Kirkpatrick A, et al. Cisplatin and etoposide combination chemotherapy for locally advanced or metastatic thymoma. A phase II study of the European Organization for Research and Treatment of Cancer Lung Cancer Cooperative Group. J Clin Oncol 1996;14(3):814–20.

20. Kim ES, Putnam JB, Komaki R, et al. Phase II study of a multidisciplinary approach with induction chemotherapy, followed by surgical resection, radiation therapy, and consolidation chemotherapy for unresectable malignant thymomas: Final report. Lung Cancer 2004;44(3):369–79.

21. Kunitoh H, Tamura T, Shibata T, et al. A phase II trial of dose-dense chemotherapy, followed by surgical resection and/or thoracic radiotherapy, in locally advanced thymoma: Report of a Japan Clinical Oncology Group trial (JCOG 9606). Br J Cancer 2010;103(1):6–11.

22. Lucchi M, Melfi F, Dini P, et al. Neoadjuvant chemotherapy for stage III and IVA thymomas: a single-institution experience with a long follow-up. J Thorac Oncol 2006;1(4):308–13. Available at: http://www.ncbi.nlm.nih.gov/pubmed/17409875. Accessed January 15, 2020.

23. Yamada Y, Yoshino I, Nakajima J, et al. Surgical outcomes of patients with stage III thymoma in the Japanese nationwide database. Ann Thorac Surg 2015;100(3): 961–7.

24. Park S, Park IK, Kim YT, et al. Comparison of Neoadjuvant Chemotherapy Followed by Surgery to Upfront Surgery for Thymic Malignancy. Ann Thorac Surg 2019;107(2):355–62.

25. Leuzzi G, Rocco G, Ruffini E, et al. Multimodality therapy for locally advanced thymomas: A propensity score-matched cohort study from the European Society of Thoracic Surgeons Database. J Thorac Cardiovasc Surg 2016;151:47–57.e1. Mosby Inc.

26. Merveilleux du Vignaux C, Dansin E, Mhanna L, et al. Systemic Therapy in Advanced Thymic Epithelial Tumors: Insights from the RYTHMIC Prospective Cohort. J Thorac Oncol 2018;13(11):1762–70.

27. Rusch VW, Giroux DJ, Kraut MJ, et al. Induction chemoradiation and surgical resection for superior sulcus non-small-cell lung carcinomas: Long-term results of Southwest Oncology Group trial 9416 (Intergroup trial 0160). J Clin Oncol 2007;25(3):313–8.

28. Van Hagen P, Hulshof MCCM, Van Lanschot JJB, et al. Preoperative chemoradiotherapy for esophageal or junctional cancer. N Engl J Med 2012;366(22): 2074–84.

29. Loehrer PJ, Chen M, Kim KM, et al. Cisplatin, doxorubicin, and cyclophosphamide plus thoracic radiation therapy for limited-stage unresectable thymoma: An intergroup trial. J Clin Oncol 1997;15(9):3093–9.

30. Wright CD, Choi NC, Wain JC, et al. Induction Chemoradiotherapy Followed by Resection for Locally Advanced Masaoka Stage III and IVA Thymic Tumors. Ann Thorac Surg 2008;85(2):385–9.

31. Korst RJ, Bezjak A, Blackmon S, et al. Neoadjuvant chemoradiotherapy for locally advanced thymic tumors: A phase II, multi-institutional clinical trial. J Thorac Cardiovasc Surg 2014;147(1). https://doi.org/10.1016/j.jtcvs.2013.08.061.

32. Huang J, Riely GJ, Rosenzweig KE, et al. Multimodality Therapy for Locally Advanced Thymomas: State of the Art or Investigational Therapy? Ann Thorac Surg 2008;85(2):365–7.

33. Ruffini E, Detterbeck F, van raemdonck D, et al. Tumours of the thymus: A cohort study of prognostic factors from the European Society of Thoracic Surgeons database. Eur J Cardiothorac Surg 2014;46(3):361–8.

34. Yagi K, Hirata T, Fukuse T, et al. Surgical treatment for invasive thymoma, especially when the superior vena cava is invaded. Ann Thorac Surg 1996;61(2): 521–4.

35. Ribet M, Voisin C, Gosselin B, et al. Lympho-epithelial thymoma. Anatomo-clinical and therapeutic study of 113 cases. Rev Mal Respir 1988;5(1):53–60. Available at: http://www.ncbi.nlm.nih.gov/pubmed/3368635. Accessed January 15, 2020.

36. Akaogi E, Ohara K, Mitsui K, et al. Preoperative radiotherapy and surgery for advanced thymoma with invasion to the great vessels. J Surg Oncol 1996; 63(1):17–22.

37. Burt BM, Nguyen D, Groth SS, et al. Utilization of Minimally Invasive Thymectomy and Margin-Negative Resection for Early-Stage Thymoma. Ann Thorac Surg 2019;108(2):405–11.

38. Burt BM, Yao X, Shrager J, et al. Determinants of Complete Resection of Thymoma by Minimally Invasive and Open Thymectomy: Analysis of an International Registry. J Thorac Oncol 2017;12(1):129–36.

39. Friedant AJ, Handorf EA, Su S, et al. Minimally invasive versus open thymectomy for thymic malignancies: Systematic review and meta-analysis. J Thorac Oncol 2016;11(1):30–8.

40. O'Sullivan KE, Kreaden US, Hebert AE, et al. A systematic review of robotic versus open and video assisted thoracoscopic surgery (VATS) approaches for thymectomy. Ann Cardiothorac Surg 2019;8(2):174–93.

41. Fang W, Wang Y, Pang L, et al. Lymph node metastasis in thymic malignancies: A Chinese multicenter prospective observational study. J Thorac Cardiovasc Surg 2018;156(2):824–33.e1.

42. Choe G, Ghanie A, Riely G, et al. Long-term, disease-specific outcomes of thymic malignancies presenting with de novo pleural metastasis. J Thorac Cardiovasc Surg 2020;159:705–14.e1. Mosby Inc.

43. Jackson MW, Palma DA, Camidge DR, et al. The Impact of Postoperative Radiotherapy for Thymoma and Thymic Carcinoma. J Thorac Oncol 2017;12(4): 734–44.

44. Zhou D, Deng XF, Liu QX, et al. The effectiveness of postoperative radiotherapy in patients with completely resected thymoma: A meta-analysis. Ann Thorac Surg 2016;101(1):305–10.

45. Rimner A, Yao X, Huang J, et al. Postoperative radiation therapy is associated with longer overall survival in completely resected stage II and III thymoma-an analysis of the international thymic malignancies interest group retrospective database. J Thorac Oncol 2016;11(10):1785–92.

46. Omasa M, Date H, Sozu T, et al. Postoperative radiotherapy is effective for thymic carcinoma but not for thymoma in stage II and III thymic epithelial tumors: The Japanese Association for Research on the Thymus Database Study. Cancer 2015;121(7):1008–16.

47. Willmann J, Rimner A. The expanding role of radiation therapy for thymic malignancies. J Thorac Dis 2018;10:S2555–64.

48. Modh A, Rimner A, Allen PK, et al. Treatment modalities and outcomes in patients with advanced invasive thymoma or thymic Carcinoma a retrospective multi-center study. Am J Clin Oncol 2016;39(2):120–5.

49. Weksler B, Shende M, Nason KS, et al. The role of adjuvant radiation therapy for resected stage III thymoma: A population-based study. Ann Thorac Surg 2012; 93(6):1822–9.

50. Yellin A, Simansky DA, Ben-Avi R, et al. Resection and heated pleural chemoperfusion in patients with thymic epithelial malignant disease and pleural spread: A single-institution experience. J Thorac Cardiovasc Surg 2013;145:83–9.

51. Nakamura S, Kawaguchi K, Fukui T, et al. Multimodality therapy for thymoma patients with pleural dissemination. Gen Thorac Cardiovasc Surg 2019;67(6):524–9.

52. Moser B, Fadel E, Fabre D, et al. Surgical therapy of thymic tumours with pleural involvement: an ESTS Thymic Working Group Project. Eur J Cardiothorac Surg 2017;52(2):346–55.

53. Hishida T, Nomura S, Yano M, et al. Long-term outcome and prognostic factors of surgically treated thymic carcinoma: results of 306 cases from a Japanese Nationwide Database Study. Eur J Cardiothorac Surg 2016;49(3):835–41.

54. Lim YJ, Song C, Kim JS. Improved survival with postoperative radiotherapy in thymic carcinoma: A propensity-matched analysis of Surveillance, Epidemiology, and End Results (SEER) database. Lung Cancer 2017;108:161–7.

55. Hamaji M, Shah RM, Ali SO, et al. A Meta-Analysis of Postoperative Radiotherapy for Thymic Carcinoma. Ann Thorac Surg 2017;103(5):1668–75.

56. Huang J, Rizk NP, Travis WD, et al. Comparison of patterns of relapse in thymic carcinoma and thymoma. J Thorac Cardiovasc Surg 2009;138(1):26–31.

57. Ambrogi MC, Korasidis S, Lucchi M, et al. Pleural recurrence of thymoma: surgical resection followed by hyperthermic intrathoracic perfusion chemotherapy†. Eur J Cardiothorac Surg 2015. https://doi.org/10.1093/ejcts/ezv039.

58. Maury JM, Girard N, Tabutin M, et al. Intra-Thoracic Chemo-Hyperthermia for pleural recurrence of thymoma. Lung Cancer 2017;108:1–6.

59. Henley J, Koukoulis G, Loehrer P. Epidermal growth factor receptor expression in invasive thymoma. J Cancer Res Clin Oncol 2002;128(3):167–70.

60. Girard N, Shen R, Guo T, et al. Comprehensive genomic analysis reveals clinically relevant molecular distinctions between thymic carcinomas and thymomas. Clin Cancer Res 2009;15(22):6790–9.

61. Alberobello AT, Wang Y, Beerkens FJ, et al. PI3K as a potential therapeutic target in thymic epithelial tumors. J Thorac Oncol 2016;11(8):1345–56.

62. Zucali PA, De Pas T, Palmieri G, et al. Phase II study of everolimus in patients with thymoma and thymic carcinoma previously treated with cisplatin-based chemotherapy. J Clin Oncol 2018;36:342–9. American Society of Clinical Oncology.

63. Kurup A, Burns M, Dropcho S, et al. Phase II study of gefitinib treatment in advanced thymic malignancies. J Clin Oncol 2005;23(16_suppl):7068.

64. Bedano PM, Perkins S, Burns M, et al. A phase II trial of erlotinib plus bevacizumab in patients with recurrent thymoma or thymic carcinoma. J Clin Oncol 2008; 26(15_suppl):19087.

65. Giaccone G, Rajan A, Ruijter R, et al. Imatinib mesylate in patients with WHO B3 thymomas and thymic carcinomas. J Thorac Oncol 2009;4(10):1270–3.

66. Girard N, Teruya-Feldstein J, Payabyab EC, et al. Insulin-like growth factor-1 receptor expression in thymic malignancies. J Thorac Oncol 2010;5(9):1439–46.

67. Rajan A, Carter CA, Berman A, et al. Cixutumumab for patients with recurrent or refractory advanced thymic epithelial tumours: A multicentre, open-label, phase 2 trial. Lancet Oncol 2014;15(2):191–200.

68. Lattanzio R, La Sorda R, Facciolo F, et al. Thymic epithelial tumors express vascular endothelial growth factors and their receptors as potential targets of antiangiogenic therapy: A tissue micro array-based multicenter study. Lung Cancer 2014;85(2):191–6.

69. Thomas A, Rajan A, Berman A, et al. Sunitinib in patients with chemotherapy-refractory thymoma and thymic carcinoma: An open-label phase 2 trial. Lancet Oncol 2015;16(2):177–86.

70. Remon J, Girard N, Mazieres J, et al. Sunitinib in patients with advanced thymic malignancies: Cohort from the French RYTHMIC network. Lung Cancer 2016;97: 99–104.

71. Arbour KC, Naidoo J, Steele KE, et al. Expression of PD-L1 and other immunotherapeutic targets in thymic epithelial tumors. In: Ahmad A, editor. PLoS One 2017;12(8):e0182665.

72. Weissferdt A, Fujimoto J, Kalhor N, et al. Expression of PD-1 and PD-L1 in thymic epithelial neoplasms. Mod Pathol 2017;30(6):826–33.

73. Katsuya Y, Horinouchi H, Asao T, et al. Expression of programmed death 1 (PD-1) and its ligand (PD-L1) in thymic epithelial tumors: Impact on treatment efficacy and alteration in expression after chemotherapy. Lung Cancer 2016;99:4–10.

74. Giaccone G, Kim C, Thompson J, et al. Pembrolizumab in patients with thymic carcinoma: a single-arm, single-centre, phase 2 study. Lancet Oncol 2018; 19(3):347–55.

75. Cho J, Kim HS, Ku BM, et al. Pembrolizumab for patients with refractory or relapsed thymic epithelial tumor: An open-label phase II trial. J Clin Oncol 2019;37(24):2162–70.

76. Katsuya Y, Horinouchi H, Seto T, et al. Single-arm, multicentre, phase II trial of nivolumab for unresectable or recurrent thymic carcinoma: PRIMER study. Eur J Cancer 2019;113:78–86.

77. Rajan A, Heery CR, Thomas A, et al. Efficacy and tolerability of anti-programmed death-ligand 1 (PD-L1) antibody (Avelumab) treatment in advanced thymoma. J Immunother Cancer 2019;7(1):269.

78. Macchiarini P, Chella A, Ducci F, et al. Neoadjuvant chemotherapy, surgery, and postoperative radiation therapy for invasive thymoma. Cancer 1991;68(4): 706–13.
79. Rea F, Sartori F, Loy M, et al. Chemotherapy and operation for invasive thymoma. J Thorac Cardiovasc Surg 1993;106(3):543–9. Available at: http://www.ncbi.nlm. nih.gov/pubmed/8361199. Accessed January 15, 2020.
80. Berruti A, Borasio P, Roncari A, et al. Neoadjuvant chemotherapy with adriamycin, cisplatin, vincristine and cyclophosphamide (ADOC) in invasive thymomas: Results in six patients. Ann Oncol 1993;4(5):429–31.
81. Venuta F, Rendina EA, Pescarmona EO, et al. Multimodality treatment of thymoma: a prospective study. Ann Thorac Surg 1997;64(6):1585–91 [discussion: 1591–2].
82. Yokoi K, Matsuguma H, Nakahara R, et al. Multidisciplinary treatment for advanced invasive thymoma with cisplatin, doxorubicin, and methylprednisolone. J Thorac Oncol 2007;2(1):73–8.
83. Bretti S, Berruti A, Loddo C, et al. Multimodal management of stages III-IVa malignant thymoma. Lung Cancer 2004;44(1):69–77.
84. Ma WL, Lin CC, Hsu FM, et al. Clinical Outcomes of Up-front Surgery Versus Surgery After Induction Chemotherapy for Thymoma and Thymic Carcinoma: A Retrospective Study. Clin Lung Cancer 2019;20(6):e609–18.
85. Kanzaki R, Kanou T, Ose N, et al. Long-term outcomes of advanced thymoma in patients undergoing preoperative chemotherapy or chemoradiotherapy followed by surgery: A 20-year experience. Interact Cardiovasc Thorac Surg 2019;28(3): 360–7.

Updates in Staging and Management of Malignant Pleural Mesothelioma

Andrea S. Wolf, MD, MPH*, Raja M. Flores, MD

KEYWORDS

- Surgery for malignant pleural mesothelioma • Extrapleural pneumonectomy
- Pleurectomy/decortication • Perioperative mortality • Quality of life

KEY POINTS

- While without treatment, malignant pleural mesothelioma (MPM) confers poor survival, cancer-directed surgery as part of multimodality treatment has been associated with a 15% 5-year survival.
- Extrapleural pneumonectomy (EPP) and radical or extended pleurectomy/decortication (P/D) are the 2 types of resection performed in this context. Preoperative staging is critical to patient selection for surgery and, generally, P/D is recommended over EPP in most cases.
- Adjuvant therapy with intraoperative platforms, traditional chemotherapy, hemithoracic radiotherapy before or after resection, and new immunotherapy agents are instrumental in achieving durable long-term results for MPM patients. This article outlines the latest understanding of the staging of this disease and describes the current state of literature and practice for MPM.

INTRODUCTION

Malignant pleural mesothelioma (MPM) is a primary malignancy of the pleura best known for its association with asbestos exposure. A locally aggressive disease, MPM is difficult to eradicate, with progression and/or recurrence so frequent they are considered the rule, not the exception. Left untreated, the median overall survival of for MPM is 7 months.[1] Resection, chemotherapy, radiotherapy, and immunotherapy have been used in various combinations, and in the context of multimodality therapy, curative-intent surgery has been associated with improved survival.[2–5]

Surgery for MPM includes both diagnostic and therapeutic procedures to stage and treat this disease. Surgical biopsy via pleuroscopy or video-assisted thoracoscopic surgery distinguishes MPM from metastatic disease of other primaries, such as

Department of Thoracic Surgery, The Icahn School of Medicine at Mount Sinai, 1190 Fifth Avenue, Box 1023, New York, NY 10029, USA
* Corresponding author.
E-mail address: andrea.wolf@mountsinai.org

Surg Oncol Clin N Am 29 (2020) 603–612
https://doi.org/10.1016/j.soc.2020.06.002
1055-3207/20/© 2020 Elsevier Inc. All rights reserved.

lung, colorectal, and breast cancers. Moreover, surgical biopsy most accurately predicts tumor histology (epithelial, sarcomatoid, biphasic, and so forth).[6] While the therapeutic benefit of surgery is the subject of ongoing discussion, cancer-directed surgery for MPM has been associated with a 5-year survival of 15%, not dissimilar to other aggressive solid cancers such as locally advanced esophageal or pancreatic carcinoma.[7–10]

STAGING IN MALIGNANT PLEURAL MESOTHELIOMA

As with any solid malignancy, patients who present with MPM require staging to determine prognosis and guide therapy. An ideal staging system stratifies patients into discrete groups (with sufficient numbers in each group) based on prognosis in which analysis results in survival curves with clear separation and reduced survival with each advancement in stage. Multiple staging systems have been developed and described for MPM, generally limited by the rarity and relative poor survival for most patients with this disease.[11]

Published staging systems that have been based on retrospective data from mostly surgical studies. Butchart and colleagues[12] described the first staging system for MPM based on their single-institution study of 29 patients undergoing extrapleural pneumonectomy (EPP) for MPM, in which 9 (31%) died in the hospital and 3 (10.3%) survived 2 or more years. The Brigham and Women's Hospital published the first iteration of the Brigham staging system based on a series of 52 patients undergoing EPP, chemotherapy, and radiotherapy.[13] This group published revised editions of this system based on updates in the original dataset.[14] Analysis of a large cohort of mostly new cases was used to derive proposed adjustments for the staging of patients with epithelial disease in 2010.[15]

Additional staging systems have incorporated clinical variables available before surgical resection (or, if none is performed, factors available as part clinical staging) as datasets became available that included large enough cohorts of patients treated operatively.[16] The International Union Against Cancer (UICC) and American Joint Committee on Cancer (AJCC) first proposed tumor, node, and metastasis criteria for MPM in the 4th edition of the UICC/AJCC staging system in 1992.[17,18] Modifications were proposed by the International Mesothelioma Interest Group in 1994, which have subsequently been adopted as the international standard.[19] In the 25 years since, the International Association for the Study of Lung Cancer staging committee has subsequently assembled an international database combining retrospective datasets from participating institutions with an ongoing prospective registry with continued efforts to standardize documentation of clinical, demographic, pathologic, and treatment variables.[20–22]

Clinical Staging of Malignant Pleural Mesothelioma for Preoperative Evaluation

All MPM patients are staged with PET-computed tomography to evaluate for nodal and/or distant metastases. High PET-avidity in the pleural tumor is associated with worse survival.[23] Mediastinal nodal evaluation with endobronchial ultrasound or mediastinoscopy should be considered, and certainly if there are enlarged or PET-avid mediastinal lymph nodes. Some clinicians advocate routine pathologic mediastinal staging, but the variable nodal drainage of the pleura and unpredictable patterns of nodal metastatic spread from MPM have resulted in poor sensitivity of cervical mediastinoscopy for detecting extrapleural nodal spread of disease.[24,25] Diffuse chest wall, subdiaphragmatic, and mediastinal invasion are assessed with chest MRI.[26] Laparoscopic staging to rule out intra-abdominal spread of MPM should be performed if imaging suggests subdiaphragmatic extension of tumor and/or ascites, although some surgeons perform this in all patients. In general, cancer-directed surgical resection is not offered to patients with intra-abdominal invasion of disease.

SURGICAL RESECTION FOR MALIGNANT PLEURAL MESOTHELIOMA

Although few MPM patients undergo resection in the general population, up to 40% are offered surgery at tertiary referral centers.[27] In a study of 5937 MPM patients in the Surveillance, Epidemiology, and End Results (SEER) dataset diagnosed between 1990 and 2004, Flores and colleagues[27] found that 22% of patients underwent cancer-directed surgery. Updated, more comprehensive datasets were analyzed in more recent studies and also found that cancer-directed surgery was predictive of longer survival.[7,28] In 1 study exploring racial disparities, surgery was an independent predictor of reduced mortality (hazard ratio [HR] = 0.68; 95% CI, 0.63–0.74) and surgery was associated with a median overall survival of 11 months (compared with 7 months without, $P<.0001$), but fewer black patients were treated with resection.[28]

In MPM, surgical resection includes either EPP or radical or extended pleurectomy/decortication (P/D). EPP is the en bloc removal of the lung, parietal and visceral pleurae, diaphragm, and pericardium. Radical or extended P/D includes resection of the parietal and visceral pleurae, with or without removal of the diaphragm and/or pericardium if involved with tumor, but always preserving the underlying lung. While individual surgeon, patient, and tumor-specific factors determine which procedure is performed, most experts recommend radical or extended P/D as the procedure of choice, and all clinicians and investigators agree that surgery should be performed in the context of multimodality therapy whenever possible. Preoperative, intraoperative, and/or postoperative adjuvant treatment includes chemotherapy, intracavitary chemotherapy or photodynamic therapy, preoperative or postoperative external beam radiotherapy, and immunotherapy.[29–35]

Selecting Patients for Surgery

Historically, it was believed that resection should be considered for patients with more disease characteristics such that the possible benefit of surgery would offset its risk. Criteria for patient selection for surgery are therefore based on identifying patients with favorable clinical and demographic characteristics. Positive prognostic factors for MPM are epithelial histology, female gender, and earlier stage. In a retrospective study of 945 patients, epithelial histology, female gender, early stage, absence of tobacco or asbestos exposure, and left-sided tumors were associated with longer survival.[36–38] In a SEER analysis of 14,229 MPM patients diagnosed between 1973 and 2009, female gender was a significant predictor of longer survival, independent of age, stage, race, and treatment (adjusted HR = 0.78; 95% CI, 0.75–0.82).[4] Another study of the impact of gender on survival found that the association with positive effect on survival was only present for young women with epithelial tumors.[5] In this series evaluating patients who survived at least 3 years after EPP, women under the age of 56 years with epithelial MPM had a median survival longer than 7 years, compared with less than 4.5 years for older women.[5] For men and women, higher stage and nonepithelial histology are associated with lower survival.[2,36]

Outcomes of Extrapleural Pneumonectomy

Because EPP is generally performed in the context of multimodality therapy, studies evaluating results for EPP reflect effects of EPP and adjuvant treatment, such as chemotherapy, radiotherapy, and/or immunotherapy. In an early series of 183 patients who underwent EPP with adjuvant chemotherapy and radiotherapy, perioperative mortality was 3.8% and morbidity was 50%.[14] Median survival for those who survived surgery was 19 months. Patients with epithelial disease, negative margins, and normal extrapleural (mediastinal) nodes had a median long-term survival of 51 months.

Heated intraoperative chemotherapy (HIOC) has been used successfully as an adjunct to surgery for MPM. In a phase I study of EPP with HIOC, a median survival of 26 moths was seen in patients who received cisplatin doses of 175 to 200 mg/m^2.[39] Median survival was 39 months for stage I/II epithelial patients, compared with 15 months for those with stage III epithelial disease. The same investigators published a larger phase II study of 121 patients, reporting an overall median survival of 12.8 months, and for patients with early-stage tumors, 21 months.[40] In a trial evaluating EPP and adjuvant chemotherapy in 302 patients in Scotland, those with stage I/II MPM had a median survival of 35 months.[41] Those who underwent EPP alone had a survival of 13 months. Batirel and colleagues[42] in Turkey analyzed results for 20 patients undergoing EPP and adjuvant radiotherapy and platinum-based chemotherapy, reporting a median survival of 17 months in this cohort. Yan and colleagues[8] reported a retrospective series of 70 patients undergoing EPP followed by chemotherapy and/or radiotherapy, resulting in a median survival of 20 months. Adjuvant radiotherapy and pemetrexed were independent predictors of longer survival.

In 1 trial of 19 patients undergoing induction chemotherapy, EPP, followed by adjuvant radiotherapy, Weder and colleagues[30] found an overall median survival of 23 months, with 13 patients completing the full regimen. In a large, multicenter prospective study of 61 patients, the same investigators reported that 58 (95%) completed induction chemotherapy, 45 (74%) underwent EPP, and 36 (59%) received at least part of planned adjuvant radiotherapy.[43] Overall median survival was 19.8 months, with 23 months for patients who underwent EPP after completing chemotherapy.

In a phase II trial of neoadjuvant chemotherapy, EPP, and hemithoracic radiotherapy, Flores and colleagues[29] reported an overall median survival of 19 months. For 8 patients who completed cisplatin-gemcitabine chemotherapy and EPP, median survival was 35 months. In a phase II multicenter trial of 77 patients, the same group treated 77 patients with cisplatin-pemetrexed, EPP, and radiotherapy, with 40 (52%) patients completing the full regimen and surviving a median of 29 months.[44] Perioperative mortality was 3.7% and local recurrence occurred in 14% of patients. The overall median survival was 16.8 months. de Perrot and colleagues[45] found similarly promising results in a retrospective analysis of 60 patients treated with cisplatin-based chemotherapy followed by EPP and adjuvant radiotherapy. Median overall survival was 14 months, but for 30 (50%) patients who completed the full regimen, those with no nodal disease on final pathologic analysis had a median survival of 59 months. The same investigators enrolled 25 patients in a phase I/II trial of induction radiotherapy with 25 Gy intensity-modulated radiotherapy 1 week before EPP, with patients with positive nodes on final pathologic analysis receiving adjuvant chemotherapy.[46] There was 1 (4%) postoperative death. With a median follow-up of 23 months, 3-year survival was 84% for patients with epithelial disease and 13% for those with biphasic disease.

Recurrence After Extrapleural Pneumonectomy

While metastasis in MPM is less common than that seen with other solid malignancies, local recurrence is the rule, rather than the exception, and represents the most common cause of death in most patients after EPP. Whereas hematoge-nous spread occurs rarely, recurrence is more commonly locoregional (to the ipsi-lateral chest and abdomen). Baldini and colleagues[47] described a series of all patients undergoing EPP-based multimodality therapy, excluding 11 patients who died perioperatively or lacked information regarding location of recurrence. In 54 patients (72% of all recurrences), recurrence first occurred in the ipsilateral hemi-thorax or mediastinum. The remaining recurrences occurred in the abdomen (53%), contralateral chest (38%), and distant sites (7%), with many patients recur-ring in multiple concurrent sites. The authors concluded that treatment failure most commonly occurred in the ipsilateral chest. Flores and colleagues[48,49] pub-lished a retrospective study of 663 patients treated with various surgery-based multimodality protocols. Of 385 patients undergoing EPP, 57% recurred, with 33% of first recurrences occurring in the ipsilateral chest or pericardium. Other sites were abdomen (31%), contralateral chest (22%), abdomen and chest (8%), and bone (3%).

Outcomes of Pleurectomy/Decortication

Over the decades, increasing evidence and experience has suggested that the high mortality and morbidity of EPP was not met with obvious benefit in long-term mortal-ity.[50] Most clinicians now agree that P/D, the lung-sparing resection for MPM, is rec-ommended for cancer-directed surgery in this disease.[51]

As in EPP, patients undergoing P/D are treated with adjuvant therapy in an effort to decrease the likelihood of local recurrence. In 1 prospective phase I/II trial, 44 patients underwent P/D with HIOC, with a median survival of 14 months seen in patients who were resectable. The subset of patients who received high-dose intraoperative cisplatin ($175–450$ mg/m^2) had a median survival of 18 months.[31] Postoperative hemi-thoracic radiotherapy has been used successfully as adjuvant therapy, but the pres-ence of the remaining underlying lung parenchyma makes this a complex and highly specialized technique. In the largest retrospective series, 123 patients treated with a median of 42.5 Gy hemithoracic radiotherapy after P/D experienced a local control rate of 42% and median survival of 13.5 months.[52,53] The same investigators used 46.8 Gy intensity-modulated radiotherapy in another series and found 1- and 2-year survival of 75% and 53%, respectively, with grade 3/4 pneumonitis occurring in 20% of patients.

Recurrence After Pleurectomy/Decortication

Despite best attempts at intraoperative and postoperative adjunctive therapy, most patients who undergo P/D recur, with the most common site of treatment failure in the ipsilateral chest. The ipsilateral hemithorax and/or mediastinum were the site(s) of more frequent first recurrence in 95% of 59 patients undergoing P/D in 1 large series evaluating this issue.[54] Flores's series comparing EPP to P/D had similar findings, with 65% of first relapse presenting as local recurrence.[48]

DATA COMPARING EXTRAPLEURAL PNEUMONECTOMY WITH PLEURECTOMY/DECORTICATION

As P/D became the procedure of choice for most surgeons treating MPM, many studies evaluated outcomes for the 2 operations. P/D is associated with better periop-erative morbidity and mortality. One Society of Thoracic Surgeons Database study found higher rates of acute respiratory distress syndrome, reintubation, unexpected reoperation, sepsis, and mortality after EPP compared with P/D.[55]

In the largest retrospective study comparing EPP to P/D, Flores and colleagues[48] found higher cumulative survival for curative-intent P/D than EPP for patients with early-stage disease. For patients with later-stage disease, EPP was associated with better survival. One meta-analysis of a small portion of the literature comparing the 2 operations found significantly lower mortality and a trend toward higher cumulative survival with P/D.[56] Another meta-analysis of 24 independent datasets from all English-language observational studies published from 1990 to 2014 compared 1391 patients who underwent EPP with 1512 patients who underwent P/D.[57,58] The proportion of patients with epithelial histology varied widely among the studies. There was significantly higher 30-day mortality associated with EPP (4.5% versus 1.7%, $P<.05$) with little heterogeneity between studies. For the 17 studies including data on median survival, 53% demonstrated higher median survival with EPP (and 47% with P/D). Of 7 studies reporting at least 2-year survival, there was no significant survival difference, but there was significant heterogeneity among studies.[57]

Given an association with higher risk and lack of clear survival benefit over P/D, EPP has been the subject of controversy, with some practitioners advocating against it.[59] The Mesothelioma and Radical Surgery (MARS) trial, which failed to complete successful randomization, was an attempt to compare EPP with no surgery for MPM. Post-hoc analyses explored long-term outcomes, but these studies lacked adequate power to draw meaningful conclusions. A phase III randomized control trial of P/D versus no surgery for patients undergoing platinum-pemetrexed chemotherapy for MPM, MARS2 (NCT02040272), is currently ongoing.[60]

IMMUNOTHERAPY IN MALIGNANT PLEURAL MESOTHELIOMA

The observation of longer-than-expected survival for MPM patients with chronic inflammatory states from smoldering postoperative infection combined with successful use of checkpoint inhibitors in other solid thoracic malignancies[61] has led to optimism that the tumor microenvironment in MPM may be modulated to promote antitumor response. In fact, although sarcomatoid histology and high tumor-infiltrating lymphocyte are considered poor prognosticators,[62] patients with these features have demonstrated clinical responsiveness in small trials of programmed cell death protein-1 (PD-1) blockade.[63] Immunotherapy alone has been tested as second- and third-line treatment options for MPM, with response rates of 20% to 30%.[64] Success with the additive and/or synergistic impact of chemotherapy combined with PD-1 blockade in non-small cell lung cancer[65,66] has led many investigators to recruit for trials of chemo-immunotherapy in MPM and also led many clinicians to use these combinations off-label in practice. Novel therapeutics in the form of oncolytic viruses, vaccines, chimeric antigen receptor T cell, checkpoint inhibition, and antibody-drug conjugates are the subject of ongoing investigation as components of multimodality therapy for MPM.[35]

SUMMARY

Despite its reputation as an aggressive and fatal disease, MPM has multiple treatment options, specifically in the context of surgery-based multimodality therapy, which is associated with a 15% 5-year survival. Staging patients preoperatively and selecting the appropriate type of resection for the appropriate patient is critical. Generally, P/D is better tolerated and evidence suggests that survival is not worse than that associated with EPP. Locoregional recurrence is common after both procedures but patients who have undergone P/D have avoided the morbidity of EPP and are generally better positioned to tolerate adjuvant therapy and treatment of recurrent disease. Traditional adjuvant therapy before or after surgery with chemotherapy and/or radiotherapy is currently part of the standard protocols, although there are no data to support one or-der of treatment over another. Combination with immunotherapy represents the new-est horizon with initial studies suggesting we may be able to harness individual patients' immune systems to fight this challenging disease.

CONFLICTS OF INTEREST

No conflicts of interest to disclose.

REFERENCES

1. Sugarbaker DJ, Jaklitsch MT, Bueno R, et al. Prevention, early detection, and management of complications after 328 consecutive extrapleural pneumonecto-mies. J Thorac Cardiovasc Surg 2004;128:138–46.
2. Wolf AS, Richards WG, Tilleman TR, et al. Characteristics of malignant pleural mesothelioma in women. Ann Thorac Surg 2010;90:949–56 [discussion: 56].
3. Sugarbaker DJ, Wolf AS. Surgery for malignant pleural mesothelioma. Expert Rev Respir Med 2010;4:363–72.
4. Taioli E, Wolf AS, Camacho-Rivera M, et al. Women with malignant pleural meso-thelioma have a threefold better survival rate than men. Ann Thorac Surg 2014; 98:1020–4.
5. Sugarbaker DJ, Wolf AS, Chirieac LR, et al. Clinical and pathological features of three-year survivors of malignant pleural mesothelioma following extrapleural pneumonectomy. Eur J Cardiothorac Surg 2011;40:298–303.
6. Chirieac LR, Hung YP, Foo WC, et al. Diagnostic value of biopsy sampling in pre-dicting histology in patients with diffuse malignant pleural mesothelioma. Cancer 2019;125:4164–71.
7. Taioli E, Wolf AS, Camacho-Rivera M, et al. Determinants of survival in malignant pleural mesothelioma: a surveillance, epidemiology, and end results (SEER) study of 14,228 patients. PLoS One 2015;10:e0145039.
8. Yan TD, Boyer M, Tin MM, et al. Extrapleural pneumonectomy for malignant pleural mesothelioma: outcomes of treatment and prognostic factors. J Thorac Cardiovasc Surg 2009;138:619–24.
9. Taioli E, Wolf AS, Camacho-Rivera M, et al. Racial disparities in esophageal can-cer survival after surgery. J Surg Oncol 2016;113:659–64.
10. Mayo SC, Nathan H, Cameron JL, et al. Conditional survival in patients with pancreatic ductal adenocarcinoma resected with curative intent. Cancer 2012; 118:2674–81.
11. Richards WG. Recent advances in mesothelioma staging. Semin Thorac Cardio-vasc Surg 2009;21:105–10.
12. Butchart EG, Ashcroft T, Barnsley WC, et al. Pleuropneumonectomy in the man-agement of diffuse malignant mesothelioma of the pleura. Experience with 29 pa-tients. Thorax 1976;31:15–24.
13. Sugarbaker DJ, Strauss GM, Lynch TJ, et al. Node status has prognostic signif-icance in the multimodality therapy of diffuse, malignant mesothelioma. J Clin On-col 1993;11:1172–8.
14. Sugarbaker DJ, Flores RM, Jaklitsch MT, et al. Resection margins, extrapleural nodal status, and cell type determine postoperative long-term survival in trimo-dality therapy of malignant pleural mesothelioma: results in 183 patients. J Thorac Cardiovasc Surg 1999;117:54–63 [discussion: 5].

15. Richards WG, Godleski JJ, Yeap BY, et al. Proposed adjustments to pathologic staging of epithelial malignant pleural mesothelioma based on analysis of 354 cases. Cancer 2010;116:1510–7.
16. Brims FJ, Meniawy TM, Duffus I, et al. A novel clinical prediction model for prognosis in malignant pleural mesothelioma using decision tree analysis. J Thorac Oncol 2016;11:573–82.
17. (UICC) IUAC. TNM atlas. 4th edition. Berlin: Springer; 1992.
18. Bears OH, Henson DE. Fourth edition of the AJCC manual for staging of cancer. Philadelphia: J. B. Lippincott; 1992.
19. Rusch VW. A proposed new international TNM staging system for malignant pleural mesothelioma. From the International Mesothelioma Interest Group. Chest 1995;108:1122–8.
20. Pass H, Giroux D, Kennedy C, et al. The IASLC mesothelioma staging project: improving staging of a rare disease through international participation. J Thorac Oncol 2016;11:2082–8.
21. Pass HI, Giroux D, Kennedy C, et al. Supplementary prognostic variables for pleural mesothelioma: a report from the IASLC staging committee. J Thorac Oncol 2014;9:856–64.
22. Friedberg JS, Culligan MJ, Tsao AS, et al. A proposed system toward standardizing surgical-based treatments for malignant pleural mesothelioma, from the Joint National Cancer Institute-International Association for the Study of Lung Cancer-Mesothelioma Applied Research Foundation Taskforce. J Thorac Oncol 2019;14:1343–53.
23. Flores RM. The role of PET in the surgical management of malignant pleural mesothelioma. Lung Cancer 2005;49(Suppl 1):S27–32.
24. Flores RM, Routledge T, Seshan VE, et al. The impact of lymph node station on survival in 348 patients with surgically resected malignant pleural mesothelioma: implications for revision of the American Joint Committee on Cancer staging system. J Thorac Cardiovasc Surg 2008;136:605–10.
25. Sugarbaker DJ, Richards WG, Bueno R. Extrapleural pneumonectomy in the treatment of epithelioid malignant pleural mesothelioma: novel prognostic implications of combined N1 and N2 nodal involvement based on experience in 529 patients. Ann Surg 2014;260:577–80 [discussion: 80–2].
26. Patz EF Jr, Shaffer K, Piwnica-Worms DR, et al. Malignant pleural mesothelioma: value of CT and MR imaging in predicting resectability. AJR Am J Roentgenol 1992;159:961–6.
27. Flores RM, Riedel E, Donington JS, et al. Frequency of use and predictors of cancer-directed surgery in the management of malignant pleural mesothelioma in a community-based (Surveillance, Epidemiology, and End Results [SEER]) population. J Thorac Oncol 2010;5:1649–54.
28. Taioli E, Wolf AS, Moline JM, et al. Frequency of surgery in black patients with malignant pleural mesothelioma. Dis Markers 2015;2015:282145.
29. Flores RM, Krug LM, Rosenzweig KE, et al. Induction chemotherapy, extrapleural pneumonectomy, and postoperative high-dose radiotherapy for locally advanced malignant pleural mesothelioma: a phase II trial. J Thorac Oncol 2006;1:289–95.
30. Weder W, Kestenholz P, Taverna C, et al. Neoadjuvant chemotherapy followed by extrapleural pneumonectomy in malignant pleural mesothelioma. J Clin Oncol 2004;22:3451–7.
31. Richards WG, Zellos L, Bueno R, et al. Phase I to II study of pleurectomy/decortication and intraoperative intracavitary hyperthermic cisplatin lavage for mesothelioma. J Clin Oncol 2006;24:1561–7.

32. Pass HI, Temeck BK, Kranda K, et al. Phase III randomized trial of surgery with or without intraoperative photodynamic therapy and postoperative immunochemotherapy for malignant pleural mesothelioma. Ann Surg Oncol 1997;4:628–33.

33. de Perrot M, Feld R, Leighl NB, et al. Accelerated hemithoracic radiation followed by extrapleural pneumonectomy for malignant pleural mesothelioma. J Thorac Cardiovasc Surg 2016;151(2):468–73.

34. Kindler HL, Karrison TG, Gandara DR, et al. Multicenter, double-blind, placebo-controlled, randomized phase II trial of gemcitabine/cisplatin plus bevacizumab or placebo in patients with malignant mesothelioma. J Clin Oncol 2012;30:2509–15.

35. Tano ZE, Chintala NK, Li X, et al. Novel immunotherapy clinical trials in malignant pleural mesothelioma. Ann Transl Med 2017;5(11):245.

36. Flores RM, Zakowski M, Venkatraman E, et al. Prognostic factors in the treatment of malignant pleural mesothelioma at a large tertiary referral center. J Thorac Oncol 2007;2:957–65.

37. Wolf AS, Daniel J, Sugarbaker DJ. Surgical techniques for multimodality treatment of malignant pleural mesothelioma: extrapleural pneumonectomy and pleurectomy/decortication. Semin Thorac Cardiovasc Surg 2009;21:132–48.

38. Sarot IA. Extrapleural pneumonectomy and pleurectomy in pulmonary tuberculosis. Thorax 1949;4:173–223.

39. Sugarbaker DJ, Gill RR, Yeap BY, et al. Hyperthermic intraoperative pleural cisplatin chemotherapy extends interval to recurrence and survival among low-risk patients with malignant pleural mesothelioma undergoing surgical macroscopic complete resection. J Thorac Cardiovasc Surg 2013;145:955–63.

40. Tilleman TR, Richards WG, Zellos L, et al. Extrapleural pneumonectomy followed by intracavitary intraoperative hyperthermic cisplatin with pharmacologic cytoprotection for treatment of malignant pleural mesothelioma: a phase II prospective study. J Thorac Cardiovasc Surg 2009;138:405–11.

41. Aziz T, Jilaihawi A, Prakash D. The management of malignant pleural mesothelioma; single centre experience in 10 years. Eur J Cardiothorac Surg 2002;22:298–305.

42. Batirel HF, Metintas M, Caglar HB, et al. Trimodality treatment of malignant pleural mesothelioma. J Thorac Oncol 2008;3:499–504.

43. Weder W, Stahel RA, Bernhard J, et al. Multicenter trial of neo-adjuvant chemotherapy followed by extrapleural pneumonectomy in malignant pleural mesothelioma. Ann Oncol 2007;18:1196–202.

44. Krug LM, Pass HI, Rusch VW, et al. Multicenter phase II trial of neoadjuvant pemetrexed plus cisplatin followed by extrapleural pneumonectomy and radiation for malignant pleural mesothelioma. J Clin Oncol 2009;27:3007–13.

45. de Perrot M, Feld R, Cho BC, et al. Trimodality therapy with induction chemotherapy followed by extrapleural pneumonectomy and adjuvant high-dose hemithoracic radiation for malignant pleural mesothelioma. J Clin Oncol 2009;27:1413–8.

46. Cho BC, Feld R, Leighl N, et al. A feasibility study evaluating surgery for mesothelioma after radiation therapy: the "SMART" approach for resectable malignant pleural mesothelioma. J Thorac Oncol 2014;9:397–402.

47. Baldini EH, Richards WG, Gill RR, et al. Updated patterns of failure after multimodality therapy for malignant pleural mesothelioma. J Thorac Cardiovasc Surg 2015;149:1374–81.

48. Flores RM, Pass HI, Seshan VE, et al. Extrapleural pneumonectomy versus pleurectomy/decortication in the surgical management of malignant pleural mesothelioma: results in 663 patients. J Thorac Cardiovasc Surg 2008;135:620–6, 626.e1–3.

49. Flores RM. Surgical options in malignant pleural mesothelioma: extrapleural pneumonectomy or pleurectomy/decortication. Semin Thorac Cardiovasc Surg 2009;21:149–53.

50. McCormack PM, Nagasaki F, Hilaris BS, et al. Surgical treatment of pleural mesothelioma. J Thorac Cardiovasc Surg 1982;84:834–42.

51. Flores RM. Pleurectomy decortication for mesothelioma: the procedure of choice when possible. J Thorac Cardiovasc Surg 2016;151(2):310–2.

52. Gupta V, Mychalczak B, Krug L, et al. Hemithoracic radiation therapy after pleurectomy/decortication for malignant pleural mesothelioma. Int J Radiat Oncol Biol Phys 2005;63:1045–52.

53. Rosenzweig KE, Zauderer MG, Laser B, et al. Pleural intensity-modulated radiotherapy for malignant pleural mesothelioma. Int J Radiat Oncol Biol Phys 2012;83: 1278–83.

54. Wolf AS, Gill RR, Baldini EH, et al. Patterns of recurrence following pleurectomy/decortication for malignant pleural mesothelioma. 11th International Conference of the International Mesothelioma Interest Group:Boston, MA, USA;Sept. 12, 2012.

55. Burt BM, Cameron RB, Mollberg NM, et al. Malignant pleural mesothelioma and the Society of Thoracic Surgeons Database: an analysis of surgical morbidity and mortality. J Thorac Cardiovasc Surg 2014;148:30–5.

56. Cao C, Tian D, Park J, et al. A systematic review and meta-analysis of surgical treatments for malignant pleural mesothelioma. Lung Cancer 2014;83:240–5.

57. Taioli E, Wolf AS, Flores RM. Meta-analysis of survival after pleurectomy decortication versus extrapleural pneumonectomy in mesothelioma. Ann Thorac Surg 2015;99:472–80.

58. Wolf AS, Jacobson FL, Tilleman TR, et al. Managing the pneumonectomy space after extrapleural pneumonectomy: postoperative intrathoracic pressure monitoring. Eur J Cardiothorac Surg 2010;37:770–5.

59. Treasure T, Lang-Lazdunski L, Waller D, et al. Extra-pleural pneumonectomy versus no extra-pleural pneumonectomy for patients with malignant pleural mesothelioma: clinical outcomes of the Mesothelioma and Radical Surgery (MARS) randomised feasibility study. Lancet Oncol 2011;12:763–72.

60. Waller DA, Dawson AG. Randomized controlled trials in malignant pleural mesothelioma surgery—mistakes made and lessons learned. Ann Transl Med 2017; 5(11):240.

61. Garon EB, Rizvi NA, Hui R, et al. Pembrolizumab for the treatment of non-small-cell lung cancer. N Engl J Med 2015;372:2018–28.

62. Inahuma S, Lasota J, Czapiewski P, et al. CD70 expression correlates with a worse prognosis in malignant pleural mesothelioma patients via immune evasion and enhanced invasiveness. J Pathol 2020;250(2):205–2016.

63. Desai A, Karrison T, Rose B, et al. Phase II trial of pembrolizumab (NCT02399371) in previously-treated malignant mesothelioma (MM): final analysis. J Thorac Oncol 2018;13(10 Suppl).10.1016/j.jtho.2018.08.277.

64. Desai A, Nakano T, Okada M, et al. Long-term efficacy and safety of nivolumab in second-or third-line japanese malignant pleural mesothelioma patients (phase II: MERIT study). J Thorac Oncol 2018;13(10 Suppl). 10.1016/j.jtho.2018.08.275.

65. Antonia SJ, Villegas A, Daniel D, et al. Durvalumab after chemoradiotherapy in stage III non-small-cell lung cancer. N Engl J Med 2017;377:1919–19298.

66. Langer CJ, Gadgeel SM, Borghaei H, et al. Carboplatin and pemetrexed with or without pembrolizumab for advanced, non-squamous non-small-cell lung cancer: a randomised, phase 2 cohort of the open-label KEYNOTE-021 study. Lancet Oncol 2016;17(11):1497–508.

Multidisciplinary Evaluation and Management of Early Stage Esophageal Cancer

Amit Bhatt, MD[a],*, Suneel Kamath, MD[b],
Sudish C. Murthy, MD, PhD[c], Siva Raja, MD, PhD[c]

KEYWORDS

- Esophageal cancer • Endoscopic submucosal dissection
- Endoscopic mucosal resection • Esophagectomy

KEY POINTS

- Endoscopic submucosal dissection allows for en-bloc resection of early esophageal cancer, despite the size or associated fibrosis of a lesion.
- Poor differentiation, lymphovascular invasion, and deep submucosal invasion are high-risk features, and even if margin-negative endoscopic resection is achieved, additional therapy should be considered.
- For patients with high-risk pathology after endoscopic submucosal dissection, we recommend esophagectomy for medically fit patients; for nonsurgical candidates, we recommend discussing the risks and benefits of radiation and/or chemotherapy.
- One the limitations of endoscopic resection is that the at-risk organ is left in place, and patients are at risk of developing local and metachronous recurrence.
- Modern surgical and perioperative care has significantly improved morbidity and mortality after esophagectomy; despite these improvements, the risk of perioperative mortality remains approximately 3.4%.

INTRODUCTION

Esophageal cancer is the sixth leading cause of cancer related mortality worldwide, with a 5-year survival rate of approximately 20%.[1,2] There are 2 main histologic subtypes, esophageal squamous cell cancer (SCC) and esophageal adenocarcinoma (EAC). SCC is the predominant subtype worldwide, representing 87% of all

Conflict of Interest: A. Bhatt: Consultant Boston Scientific, Lumendi, Aries Pharmaceuticals, Medtronics. Royalties Medtronics. S. Kamath: None. S. Murthy: None. S. Raja: Consultant Smiths Medical.
Funding source: None.
[a] Department of Gastroenterology and Hepatology, A31 desk, Cleveland, Ohio 44195, USA; [b] Taussig Cancer Institute, 9500 Euclid Avenue, Cleveland, OH 44195, USA; [c] Department of Thoracic and Cardiovascular Surgery, J4-1, 9500 Euclid Ave, Cleveland, Ohio 44195, USA
* Corresponding author.
E-mail address: BHATTA3@ccf.org

esophageal cancer cases.[3] The incidence of EAC in the West has increased rapidly over the last few decades and it has become the predominant form of esophageal cancer in Western countries.[4–6] The majority of esophageal cancer is diagnosed at a late stage with a dismal prognosis. In contrast, early stage esophageal cancer has a more favorable prognosis.[7–9] Early stage esophageal cancer is defined as a cancer involving the mucosal or submucosal layer of the esophagus, encompassing Tis, T1a, and T1b tumors.[10] The management of early esophageal cancer requires a multidisciplinary approach, and management should be tailored to the individual patient. Management involves accurate tumor staging, treatment, and surveillance. Treatment options include endoscopic mucosal resection (EMR), endoscopic submucosal dissection (ESD), esophagectomy, radiation therapy, brachytherapy, and chemotherapy. Although endoscopic resection has become the preferred method for management of early stage esophageal cancer, it is not feasible or sufficient in all early stage esophageal cancers. Therefore, an upfront multidisciplinary evaluation can help to orchestrate appropriate local therapy based on patient and tumor characteristics and available institutional expertise.

CLINICAL PRESENTATION

Although advanced esophageal tumors commonly present with dysphagia or bleeding, the majority of early esophageal are asymptomatic and found incidentally on upper endoscopy while investigating upper gastrointestinal symptoms, or surveillance of Barrett's esophagus (BE). Owing to the distensible nature of the esophagus, obstructive symptoms do not develop until late in the disease, and any patient referred with a reported early esophageal cancer with dysphagia should be evaluated for potentially more advanced disease versus a concomitant nonmalignant cause, such as a stricture, that can complicate local therapy.

STAGING OF EARLY ESOPHAGEAL CANCER

Stage directed therapies are used in esophageal cancer and accurate staging is paramount. Endoscopic ultrasound (EUS) examination is best for assessing the depth of tumor invasion and locoregional lymph node involvement. PET scan identifies incrementally more metastases than a computed tomography (CT) scan alone, and hybrid scanners that perform both PET and CT scan are increasingly being used.[11] The 2 techniques are complementary and the National Comprehensive Cancer Network (NCCN) recommends clinical staging with combination of integrated PET/CT scan and EUS before initiating therapy for esophageal cancer.[10]

ENDOSCOPIC ULTRASOUND EXAMINATION

Since the introduction of EUS examination in the early 1980s, it has played a vital role in esophageal cancer staging. EUS examination is able to visualize the individual wall layers of the esophagus, and is superior to cross-sectional imaging in determining the T stage and locoregional lymph involvement.[12–14] Although the benefits of EUS in advanced esophageal cancer are established, the role of EUS examination in early stage esophageal cancer is more controversial. Multiple studies have now shown that EUS examination can be unreliable in differentiating T1a from T1b tumors, raising doubts about the usefulness of EUS examination in early stage esophageal cancer. The recently published American Society for Gastrointestinal Endoscopy guideline on screening and surveillance of BE, has recommended against the routine use of EUS examination in BE patients with early EAC (**Fig. 1**).[15–18]

In our experience, we see usefulness in EUS assessment of early esophageal cancer. EUS assessment of depth of invasion becomes particularly important when selecting patients for ESD. To perform ESD, there needs to be some submucosal plane to expand and dissect through, when the submucosal layer cannot be clearly delineated on EUS examination, we find it is unlikely a plane for submucosal dissection will be present. In the ESD era, larger tumors are being referred for endoscopic resection and EUS examination allows us to rule out invasion of the muscularis propria and local lymph node involvement before endoscopic resection is undertaken.

PET/COMPUTED TOMOGRAPHY SCANS

Although the PET/CT scan is a staple in staging advanced esophageal cancer, its role in early esophageal cancer is less clear. Two studies have shown that PET/CT scan does not reliably detect early esophageal cancer and is unable to differentiate T1a from T1b tumors.[19,20] In addition, and of more concern, in 1 study on patients with early esophageal cancer undergoing PET/CT scan, all 18 fluorodeoxyglucose-avid nodes seen were false positives, with biopsies showing no metastatic disease.[19] In clinical practice, this could lead to overtreatment of early esophageal cancer. These limitations have to be weighed against the limitations of performing PET/CT scan after endoscopic resection, where the inflammation from the postendoscopic resection site limits PET/CT scan's diagnostic usefulness. This can lead to diagnostic uncertainty in patients after endoscopic resection with a high-risk pathology who require additional treatment. In our practice, when performing staging endoscopic resection for bulkier esophageal tumors that may undergo surgery if a high-risk pathology is found, we perform a PET scan before ESD, while being cognizant of its limitations.

ENDOSCOPIC TREATMENT OPTIONS
Risk of Lymph Node Metastasis in Early Esophageal Cancer

The main difference between the endoscopic and surgical resection of a tumor is the absence of lymph node dissection with endoscopic techniques. Thus, endoscopic resection should only be considered in tumors with a very low risk of lymph node

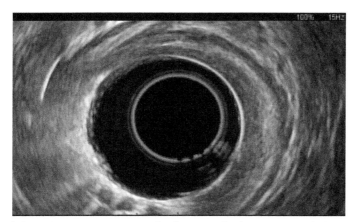

Fig. 1. Radial EUS imaging suggestive of T1b cancer, final resection pathology T1a, highlighting the limitations of EUS examination in early esophageal cancer.

metastasis, or an estimated risk that is lower than the acceptable morbidity and mortality of esophagectomy. The assessment of risk of lymph node metastases is based on the depth of tumor invasion, the presence of poorly differentiated pathology, and/or the presence of lymphovascular invasion (LVI). The esophageal wall is unique in the gastrointestinal tract, in that the lymphatics penetrate through the muscularis mucosa and are present in the lamina propria, giving even T1a esophageal cancer a theoretic risk of lymph node metastasis (**Fig. 2**).[21] In BE-related neoplasia, 1 systemic review showed mucosal-based tumors had a risk of lymph node metastasis of 1% to 2%.[22] As EAC invades deeper in the submucosa, the risk of lymph node metastasis increases. In a surgical series involving primarily EAC, the risk of lymph node metastasis in tumors involving SM1 (superficial submucosal invasion) was 7.5%, SM2 (middle third of SM layer) was 10%, and SM3 (deep submucosal invasion) was 45%.[21] In surgical series of esophageal SCC, M1 (intraepithelial) and M2 (invading the lamina propria) tumors were not associated with lymph node metastasis, M3 (reaching or infiltrating the muscularis mucosae) tumors had a risk of lymph node metastasis of 8% to 18%, tumors with submucosal invasion of less than 200 microns had a risk of lymph node metastasis risk of 11% to 53%, and tumors with SM invasion of more than 200 microns were associated with a lymph node metastasis risk of 30% to 54%.[23–26] Deciding between endoscopic and surgical resection of a tumor is done by weighing the risk of lymph node metastasis versus the mortality and morbidity associated with esophagectomy in a patient.

Endoscopic Mucosal Resection

The first endoscopic polypectomy was performed in Japan in 1974, and since then there have been several advances in endoscopic resection of gastrointestinal tract lesions. EMR is one of the most widely used and successful techniques. It involves raising a lesion with either injection of fluid or suction then removing it with a snare.[27] In the esophagus, the most commonly used EMR techniques are the band ligation

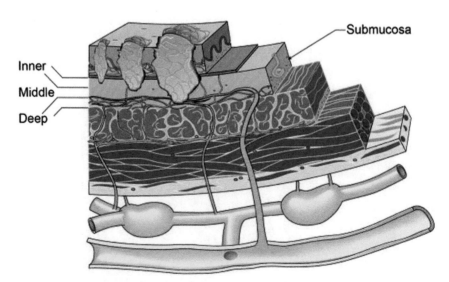

Fig. 2. Wall layers and lymphatics of the esophageal wall. (*From* Raja S, Rice TW, Goldblum JR, et al. Esophageal submucosa: the watershed for esophageal cancer. The Journal of thoracic and cardiovascular surgery. 2011;142(6):1403-1411 e1401.)

method and the cap snare method. A randomized trial between the techniques showed no significant differences in area of the resected specimens, efficacy or safety.[28] Band ligation EMR is more commonly used owing to its lower cost and shorter procedure time.[29]

Among the first investigators to describe EMR in EAC were Ell and colleagues,[30] who reported EMR results in 64 patients; 61 with EAC and 3 with high-grade dysplasia. In the low-risk tumor group, based on tumor size, macroscopic appearance, and tumor grade, 49 EMR procedures were performed and achieved complete resection in 34 of 35 patients, with recurrence noted in 6 of 35 patients (17%) during an average follow-up of 12 ± 7 months. In the high-risk tumor group, 71 EMR procedures were performed and achieved complete resection in 13 of 22 patients, with recurrence noted in 3 of 22 patients (14%) during an average follow-up of 10 ± 8 months. A hallmark study that secured the role of EMR in EAC, was performed by Pech and colleagues,[31] that evaluated EMR in 1000 patients with T1a EAC tumors. A total of 2687 EMR procedures were performed and achieved complete remission in 963 of 1000 patients (96.3%) with T1a EAC, with recurrence noted in 140 of 963 (14.5%) patients during a median follow-up of 26.5 months, with 115 of 140 recurrences (82%) successfully treated endoscopically. The long-term complete remission rate was 93.8% after a mean follow-up period of 56.6 ± 33.4 months.

Esophageal EMR has a low risk of adverse events, including bleeding (1.2%), stricture formation (1.0%), and perforation (with rates varying from 0.2% to 1.3%). The safety profile, technical ease, and success rate of EMR has led to its widespread use in the treatment of early esophageal cancer.

EMR is not without its flaws. It can only achieve en bloc resection of lesions less than 15 to 20 mm; larger lesions require piecemeal resection, which is associated with a higher risk of recurrence.[32,33] This finding was seen in the studies from Pech and colleagues[31] and Ell and colleagues,[30] as discussed elsewhere in this article, where numerous EMR procedures were sometimes required to achieve complete resection, and there was a high rate of recurrence noted on follow-up.

Endoscopic Submucosal Dissection

ESD was developed in Japan in the 1990s to overcome the limitations of EMR. ESD is an advanced endoscopic technique with precise control of both lateral and deep margin dissection allowing for en bloc resection of a lesion despite its size or associated fibrosis (**Fig. 3**).[34] Achieving en bloc resection results in higher curative resection rates, lower recurrence rates, and allows for precise histopathologic analysis. The basic steps to perform ESD are shown in **Fig. 4** and include:

- Marking the periphery of the lesion with cautery marks
- Expanding the submucosal layer with the injection of a viscous solution
- Performing a circumferential mucosal incision around the lesion with an electro-cautery knife
- Dissecting the submucosal layer beneath the lesion with an electrocautery knife releasing the lesion in one en bloc piece

Although the steps of performing ESD are relatively straightforward, ESD is technically challenging to perform, has a flat (difficult) learning curve, and can be time consuming, especially while learning the procedure. A study in a porcine model from our group showed with expert video-based supervision 2 trainees reached technical competency in ESD within a porcine model after 25 procedures. Although initial human cases performed after this training were technically successful, they had long procedure times, highlighting the challenges of learning ESD.[35] Performing ESD in the

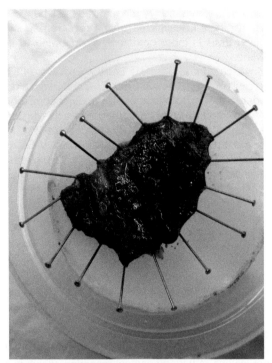

Fig. 3. En bloc ESD resection specimen pinned to wax.

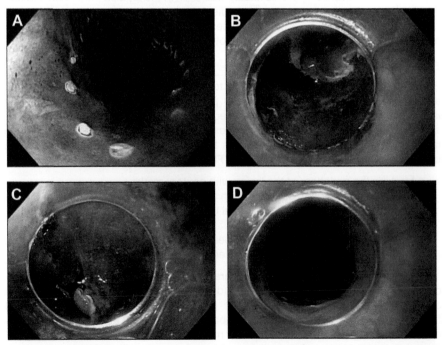

Fig. 4. Steps of ESD resection. (*A*) Marking, (*B*) mucosal incision, and (*C*) submucosal dissection. (*D*) Completed resection.

esophagus has its unique challenges. (1) The specimen retracts distally making orientation and traction difficult to maintain. (2) The thin muscularis propria of the esophageal wall increases the risk of perforation. (3) Finally, the narrow esophageal lumen limits scope maneuverability and gravity counter-traction.[36] Innovations in technique have helped to address the unique challenges of performing ESD in the esophagus. Yoshida and colleagues[37] showed in a randomized multicenter trial that clip line traction assisted ESD resulted in significantly shorter procedure time than conventional ESD (44.5 minutes vs 60.5 minutes, respectively; P<.001). Our group recently evaluated a new esophageal ESD technique—an insulated-tip knife tunneling technique with C-shaped incision—and achieved excellent technical results with an en bloc resection rate of 97.6%, R0 resection rate of 88.1%, and 0% perforations.[38]

   The majority of the initial literature on ESD originated from Japan, where ESD was developed, but primarily focused on SCC, because EAC is rare in Japan. More recently, major studies have been published in the West evaluating ESD in BE-related neoplasia. A multicenter retrospective study from 5 academic tertiary referral centers in the United States that evaluated 46 patients with BE-related neoplasia (high-grade dysplasia and EAC) who underwent ESD, reported en bloc and curative resection rates of 96% and 70%, respectively, with 1 perforation that was managed endoscopically.[39] The European Barrett's Endoscopic Submucosal Dissection Trial performed a retrospective analysis of 143 ESDs for BE-related neoplasia in 3 tertiary referral centers; the en bloc resection rate was 90.8%, R0 resection rate of 79%, and 0 perforations.[40] It should be noted that these studies were performed during the introductory phase of ESD in the West and likely reflected the early learning period of the procedure. Despite this factor, the results are respectable and show the efficacy and safety of esophageal ESD in the West. This finding was further confirmed in a meta-analysis of 11 studies including 524 BE-related neoplasia lesions that underwent ESD, the en bloc resection rate was 92.9%, the R0 resection rate was 74.5%, the perforation rate was 1.5%, and the bleeding rate was 1.7%.[41] The reported benefits of ESD over EMR also include more precise histopathologic analysis, and this was evaluated in a recent study by Podboy and colleagues[42] (**Fig. 5**). They evaluated 31 EMR and 20 ESD BE-related neoplasia specimens and found more equivocal lateral

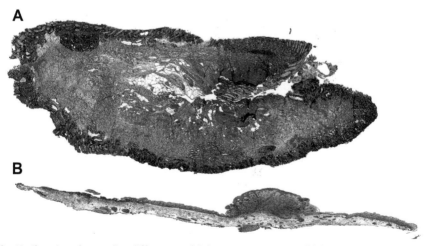

Fig. 5. Showing the quality difference of (*A*). EMR specimen and (*B*) ESD specimen.

margins (EMR 13/31 [41.9%] vs ESD 1/20 [5%]; *P*<.05) and vertical margins (EMR 13/31 [41.9%] vs ESD 0/20 [0%]; *P*<.05) in the EMR group. This process led to diagnostic uncertainty in 13 EMR patients, with 4 of the 13 undergoing esophagectomy owing to unclear diagnosis.

The results of the only Western randomized controlled trial on ESD versus EMR has questioned the role of ESD in BE-related neoplasia.[43] They evaluated 40 patient with BE-related neoplasia, 20 randomized to ESD, and 20 to EMR. Although the ESD arm had higher en bloc (ESD 20/20 [100%] vs EMR 3/20 [15%]) resection rates, and higher R0 resection rates (ESD 10/17 [58.8%] vs EMR 2/17 [11%]), it also had an alarmingly higher perforation rate (ESD 2/20 [10%] vs EMR 0/20 [0%]). In addition, there was no difference in complete remission from neoplasia at 3 months (ESD 15/16 vs EMR 16/17). The authors concluded ESD does not seem to offer clinical advantages over EMR, was more time consuming, and may cause more severe adverse events. The limitations of the study are that the outcomes in the ESD arm are significantly worse than what has been presented in numerous other studies on esophageal ESD, and the study was neither powered or had appropriate length of follow-up to properly assess for complete remission or recurrence rates. In contrast, the preliminary results of our retrospective multicenter study of ESD versus EMR for BE-related neoplasia showed not only that ESD had higher en bloc (ESD 96% vs EMR 33%; *P*<.0001) and R0 resection rates (ESD 76% vs EMR 54%; *P* = .0009), but that ESD had lower recurrence rates (ESD 3% vs EMR 39%; *P*<.0001) and required significantly fewer endoscopic resection procedures (ESD 0 [0,2] versus EMR 0.5 [0,8]; *P*<.001) to acquire complete remission than EMR.[44] These study results suggest ESD results in more definitive treatment of BE-related neoplasia than EMR.

INDICATIONS FOR ENDOSCOPIC SUBMUCOSAL DISSECTION
Barrett's-Related Neoplasia

As outlined in the European Society of Gastrointestinal Endoscopy ESD guideline and American Gastroenterological Association ESD practice update, ESD should be considered in superficial visible lesions with EAC or high-grade dysplasia in BE, when[45,46]

- Lesion size is greater 15 mm
- There are poorly lifting lesions
- Lesions are at risk of submucosal invasion

ESD should be considered in lesions greater than 15 mm, because EMR may not be able to achieve en bloc resection. Poorly lifting lesions with fibrosis may not be amenable to complete resection with EMR, but ESD is able to dissect through a fibrotic submucosal layer and remove these lesions en bloc, although this procedure can be technically challenging. In lesions at risk for submucosal invasion, ESD allows for precise histopathologic analysis and precise measurement of depth of submucosal invasion, differentiating superficial from deep submucosal invasion. Lesions less than 15 mm, without features suggestive of submucosal involvement or fibrosis, should be treated with EMR, because it performs well in this group of lesions.

Squamous Cell Cancer and Dysplasia

In SCC and dysplasia, ESD should be considered in[45] superficial lesions greater than 10 mm in size. The reason for the smaller lesion size recommendation in SCC than EAC is that, in a meta-analysis of 12 studies, ESD had higher en-bloc resection rates than EMR even in lesions 10 mm in size.[47]

POSTENDOSCOPIC RESECTION PATHOLOGIC RESULTS

The European Society of Gastrointestinal Endoscopy ESD guidelines define histologic outcomes as discussed in this section.[45]

Esophageal Adenocarcinoma

Curative criteria
- En bloc R0 resection of mucosal EAC well-differentiated or moderately differentiated tumors without LVI

Low-risk lesion
- En bloc R0 resection of sm1 lesions ($\leq$500 μm) with well-differentiated or moderately differentiated pathology and no LVI.

Noncurative lesion
- Lesions with LVI, poorly differentiated tumors, submucosal invasion greater than 500 μm, or positive vertical margins.

Squamous Cell Cancer

Curative criteria
- En bloc R0 resection of superficial well-differentiated SCC with histology no more advanced than m2 SCC, with no LVI

Low-risk lesion
- En bloc R0 resection of well differentiated m3/sm1 ($\leq$200 μm) without LVI

Noncurative lesions
- Lesions with greater than 200 μm submucosal invasion, poorly differentiated tumor, LVI, or positive vertical margin.

Patients with tumors within the curative criteria should undergo surveillance. Patient with low-risk tumors should undergo multidisciplinary discussion to weigh the risk of lymph node metastasis with surveillance versus the risks of morbidity and mortality with surgery. Surgery is recommended in patients with noncurative resections. If the patient is not a surgical candidate, other adjuvant treatment like chemotherapy and/or radiation should be considered.

SURGERY FOR EARLY ESOPHAGEAL CANCER

Until this decade, the treatment for all esophageal cancer was limited to some combination of esophagectomy, chemotherapy and radiation. Even the treatment of BE, a premalignant condition, involved surgical resection. Although the treatment of locally advanced esophageal cancer in the modern era is relegated to these aggressive modalities, earlier cancers are at times treated with less intensive therapies.

Lymph node metastasis, or the risk of spread, seems to be the watershed that separates aggressive disease requiring aggressive therapy and localized disease amenable to local therapy. With the unchanged goal of potential cure, lesser or local therapies are aimed only at esophageal cancers that are localized. Early attempts to define early cancers had been hindered by confusing early cancers with superficial cancers. Traditionally, tumors limited to the mucosa (T1a) and submucosa (T1b) were considered superficial cancers based on the limited depth of invasion. However, we have since identified, as previously noted, T1b cancers as having around a 25% risk of lymph node metastasis, making it an advanced stage.[21] In contrast, T1a cancers can have a less than 1% risk of local-regional spread making a perfect candidate of local therapies such as EMR or ESD.[7,48]

Within superficial cancers, recent works have been aimed at risk stratification within superficial cancers. Typically, poorly differentiated cancers with lymphatic invasion are considered high risk of local-regional metastasis.[21] As such, T1a cancers with high risk factors may be considered for radical surgery and T1b cancers without high risk features can be considered for local therapy.[22,49]

Local therapy for clinical mucosal (cT1a) cancers has quickly replaced esophagectomy as the treatment of choice. For cT1a cancers, esophagectomy is limited to medically fit patients with multifocal disease, patients with positive margins, and those patients with recurrent disease after local therapy.

Esophagectomy for patients with cT1a cancers is indeed a subject of debate. The dearth of information about the true risk of lymph node metastasis in this clinical entity is the underlying cause of this debate. At our institution, surgery is offered to patients whose T1a cancers show high-risk features on pathology after endoscopic resection after discussion in a multidisciplinary conference and a thorough evaluation for fitness to undergo surgery. The role of esophagectomy is accepted in clinical submucosal cancers (cT1b) cancers and is the treatment of choice for this stage of disease in medically fit patients.

Contemporary surgical and perioperative care has significantly improved morbidity and mortality after esophagectomy. Despite these improvement the risk of perioperative mortality remains at approximately 3.4%.[50] As such, when the risk of regional spread is between 3% and 4%, it can be difficult to justify a therapy that carries a 3% to 4% mortality rate. Furthermore, this is a procedure that can carry a 33% perioperative major morbidity. Long-term sequelae such as regurgitation, aspiration, and dumping syndrome are also not inconsequential. Therefore, when clinically appropriate, an organ-preserving strategy should be the preferred approach.

CHEMOTHERAPY AND RADIATION IN EARLY ESOPHAGEAL CANCER

Although the optimal management of early esophageal cancer is primarily endoscopic or surgical resection, there is a role for chemotherapy and radiation in patients who are not candidates for resection or those who choose nonresection therapy. The majority of the data come from nonrandomized studies conducted in Japan that included older patients with esophageal squamous cell carcinoma and multiple comorbidities. The data for chemoradiation for patients with early EAC are lacking.

Chemoradiation

One study enrolled 320 patients between 2001 and 2011 with T1bN0M0 esophageal squamous cell carcinoma who underwent either esophagectomy (102 patients) or definitive chemoradiation (dCRT) with 5-fluoracil and cisplatin combined with 60 Gy radiation in 30 fractions (218 patients). It showed superior 5-year overall survival with esophagectomy compared with dCRT (88.2% vs 80.2%; $P = .004$).[51] The Japan Clinical Oncology Group (JCOG)0502 trial also prospectively compared esophagectomy with dCRT in patients with stage T1bN0M0 esophageal squamous cell carcinoma, although in a nonrandomized fashion. The study included 368 evaluable patients, most of whom were older men. Of the 209 patients who underwent esophagectomy versus 159 patients who received dCRT (5-fluoracil and cisplatin combined with 60 Gy radiation in 30 fractions), overall survival was similar at 3 years (94.7% vs 93.1%) and 5 years (86.5% vs 85.5%) (adjusted hazard ratio, 1.05; 95% CI, 0.67–1.64). Two patients who underwent esophagectomy died; there were no deaths in the dCRT group.[52] Several other smaller studies, including the JCOG9708 trial, have shown that esophagectomy leads to improved local recurrence rates and better disease-free survival, but overall survival is comparable between esophagectomy and dCRT.[53–57] Of note, a radiation dose of 50.4 Gy seems to be noninferior and less toxic for patients with noncervical esophagus cancer based on multiple studies and is the recommended dose by the NCCN.[10,58–60]

Chemoradiation can also be used after ESD for nonsurgical candidates, particularly for patients with high-risk features such as LVI, poorly differentiated histology, a positive margin, and tumors greater than 2 cm in size.[10] The JCOG0508 study examined the role of chemoradiation after ESD in 2 groups: patients with pT1b tumors with a negative resection margin or pT1a tumors with LVI (group B) or with a positive vertical resection margin (group C). Group A patients had pT1a tumors with a negative resection margin and no LVI and were observed. They found the 3-year overall survival rate was 90.7% for group B patients and 92.6% for all included patients. Toxicities overall were expected and manageable, with only 1 patient experiencing a grade 3 esophageal stricture and 1 patient experiencing late grade 4 cardiac ischemia. Of note, 7 patients underwent salvage surgery for local recurrence.[61] Multiple other series support these findings, although prospective, randomized studies are lacking.[62–64] However, the data consistently show that esophagectomy offers significantly improved disease-free survival and local control over chemoradiation and should remain the standard of care for surgical candidates.[52,62–65] Radiotherapy alone after ESD may also improve local control, particularly in those with resection defects involving more than 75% of the esophageal circumference.[66]

Radiation Therapy

Radiotherapy alone is also a reasonable approach for older patients who are not candidates for surgery or endoscopic resection and would not tolerate concurrent chemotherapy. One retrospective study that compared 29 patients who underwent esophagectomy with 38 patients who received definitive radiation (of note 14 received brachytherapy and 15 received concurrent chemotherapy) found that the 3-year overall survival was similar between the groups, but 3-year relapse-free survival was significantly better with esophagectomy. For patients with T1a tumors, the 3-year overall survival and relapse-free survival in the surgery group were 83% and 83%, respectively, versus 77.8% and 55.6%, respectively, in the radiation group. For patients with T1b tumors, the 3-year overall survival and relapse-free survival in the surgery group were 76.2% and 73%, respectively, versus 73.1% and 52.3%, respectively, in the radiation group ($P = .0219$).[64] Data from other small series support these findings; however, their retrospective designs and lack of standardization in radiation dose and use of concurrent chemotherapy and/or brachytherapy make it challenging to draw definitive conclusions.[18–20] Another propensity score matching study of 185 patients age 80 or older treated with either concurrent chemoradiation or radiation alone showed there was no difference in the 3-year overall survival, cause-specific survival, or progression-free survival between the groups, suggesting that chemotherapy can safely be omitted in this elderly population.[67]

Brachytherapy

The role for brachytherapy in early-stage esophageal cancer remains unclear. The data for brachytherapy alone are limited, with 1 series of 13 patients treated with high dose rate brachytherapy showing a high initial treatment failure rate of 39%.[68] One study of 59 patients with T1 esophageal cancers evaluated the benefit of brachytherapy in addition to external beam radiation therapy (EBRT) compared with EBRT alone. There was no improvement in the response rate and although the locoregional recurrence rate was numerically better in the EBRT + brachytherapy group compared with EBRT alone (17% vs 35%), this difference did not reach statistical significance (P = .2). The 5-year cause-specific survival rate was improved in the EBRT + brachytherapy group compared with the EBRT alone group (86% vs 62%).[69] Late complications including esophageal fistula can be a major concern with brachytherapy.[69–71] For example, the Radiation Therapy Oncology Group (RTOG) 9207 study showed a 12% incidence of esophageal fistula, a complication that seems to be exacerbated when concurrent chemotherapy is used.[70] Overall, brachytherapy likely has a limited role in this setting that remains poorly defined.

We use dCRT for patients with T1b tumors that are not amenable to surgery or endoscopic resection. For patients with high-risk pathology after ESD (LVI, poorly differentiated histology, positive margin, and tumors >2 cm in size), we recommend esophagectomy for those who are surgical candidates. For nonsurgical candidates, chemoradiation is an appropriate alternative. Radiation alone is also a reasonable approach for older patients with multiple comorbidities to achieve local control and prevent local complications.

SURVEILLANCE

One of the limitations of organ preserving endoscopic resection for esophageal cancer is that the at-risk tissue remains in situ. This remnant might be in the form of the adjacent mucosa that may be subject to a field defect or in the form of regional lymph nodes that can harbor undetected spread. As such, there is a risk of developing local as well as regional recurrence and surveillance should address both. There is a lack of evidence to define the most effective follow-up after endoscopic resection of esophageal cancer, and Western gastroenterology guidelines have not provided specific recommendations. It is clear that, after ESD resection of EAC, patients should undergo radiofrequency ablation of any residual BE to decrease the risk of developing metachronous cancer. We wait 3 months for the ESD scar to heal, before starting radiofrequency ablation of BE. Regarding surveillance intervals, for T1a cancers, the NCCN guidelines recommend upper endoscopy surveillance be performed every 3 months for the first year, then every 6 months for the second year, and then annually indefinitely; imaging studies are not recommended.[10] For T1b cancers, the NCCN recommends upper endoscopy every 3 months for the first year, every 4 to 6 months for the second year, then annually indefinitely. They also state that EUS examination may be considered in conjunction with EGD, and CT chest/abdomen scans with contrast may be consider every 12 months for 3 years.[10] It should be stated, however, that the NCCN does not give any references to support these recommendation. The recently published Japan Gastroenterological Endoscopy Society ESD/EMR guidelines for esophageal cancer have strongly recommended patients undergo endoscopic examination at least once a year after endoscopic resection of SCC. For patients who underwent endoscopic resection of SCC with muscularis mucosa or submucosal involvement, they weakly recommend a CT scan at least once a year.[72] They make no specific recommendations in regard to EAC, given its rarity in Japan.

In our practice, we follow the NCCN recommended guidelines on upper endoscopy surveillance for low-risk small esophageal cancer lesions that undergo EMR resection. Because ESD resection of larger and more aggressive EAC tumors is a newer phenomenon, and there are no established data yet to help guide surveillance, we proceed cautiously with close observation. We perform an upper endoscopy with EUS examination every 6 months for the first 2 years, then yearly indefinitely. For higher risk tumors that do not undergo surgical resection, we perform even closer

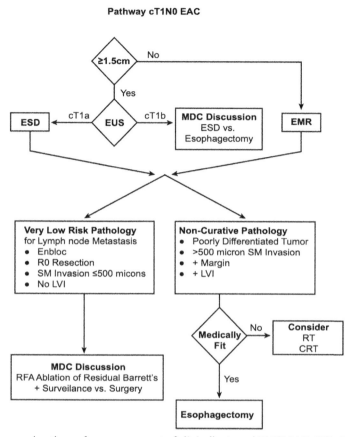

Pathway cT1N0 EAC

Fig. 6. Proposed pathway for management of clinically staged T1 N0 EAC. CRT, chemoradiation therapy; MDC, multidisciplinary committee; RT, radiation therapy; SM, submucosal.

surveillance, every 3 months for the first year. We also perform CT scans annually for 4 to 5 years based on our own data showing recurrences after esophagectomy for pT1aN0M0 cancers for can happen in the first 4 years.[7]

SUMMARY

The management paradigms for early esophageal cancer continue to evolve in favor of organ-preserving local therapies. However, early stage esophageal cancers can be a heterogeneous group that is best managed through a multidisciplinary approach to diagnosis, management and therapy (**Fig. 6**). As such, achieving optimal outcomes for patients with these cancers requires aligning the cancer characteristics with patient characteristics and institutional expertise.

REFERENCES

1. Bray F, Ferlay J, Soerjomataram I, et al. Global cancer statistics 2018: GLOBO-CAN estimates of incidence and mortality worldwide for 36 cancers in 185 countries. CA Cancer J Clin 2018;68(6):394–424.

2. Miller KD, Nogueira L, Mariotto AB, et al. Cancer treatment and survivorship statistics, 2019. CA Cancer J Clin 2019;69(5):363–85.

3. Arnold M, Soerjomataram I, Ferlay J, et al. Global incidence of oesophageal cancer by histological subtype in 2012. Gut 2015;64(3):381–7.

4. Abrams JA, Sharaiha RZ, Gonsalves L, et al. Dating the rise of esophageal adenocarcinoma: analysis of Connecticut Tumor Registry data, 1940-2007. Cancer Epidemiol Biomarkers Prev 2011. https://doi.org/10.1158/1055-9965.EPI-10-0802.

5. Trivers KF, Sabatino SA, Stewart SL. Trends in esophageal cancer incidence by histology, United States, 1998–2003. Int J Cancer 2008;123(6):1422–8.

6. Devesa SS, Blot WJ, Fraumeni JF. Changing patterns in the incidence of esophageal and gastric carcinoma in the United States. Cancer 1998;83(10):2049–53.

7. Li Z, Rice TW, Liu X, et al. Intramucosal esophageal adenocarcinoma: primum non nocere. J Thorac Cardiovasc Surg 2013;145(6):1519–24, 1524.e1-3.

8. Zhang Y, Ding H, Chen T, et al. Outcomes of endoscopic submucosal dissection vs esophagectomy for T1 esophageal squamous cell carcinoma in a real-world cohort. Clin Gastroenterol Hepatol 2019;17(1):73–81.e3.

9. Wani S, Drahos J, Cook MB, et al. Comparison of endoscopic therapies and surgical resection in patients with early esophageal cancer: a population-based study. Available at: http://www.seer.cancer.gov. Accessed March 30, 2020.

10. Ajani JA, D'Amico TA, Bentrem DJ, et al. Esophageal and esophagogastric junction cancers, Version 2.2019. JNCCN J Natl Compr Cancer Netw 2019;17(7):855–83.

11. Van Vliet EPM, Heijenbrok-Kal MH, Hunink MGM, et al. Staging investigations for oesophageal cancer: a meta-analysis. Br J Cancer 2008;98(3):547–57.

12. Kimmey MB, Martin RW, Haggitt RC, et al. Histologic correlates of gastrointestinal ultrasound images. Gastroenterology 1989;96(2 Pt 1):433–41.

13. Takizawa K, Matsuda T, Kozu T, et al. Lymph node staging in esophageal squamous cell carcinoma: a comparative study of endoscopic ultrasonography versus computed tomography. J Gastroenterol Hepatol 2009;24(10):1687–91.

14. Akdamar MK, Cerfolio RJ, Ojha B, et al. A prospective comparison of computerized tomography(CT), 18 fluoro-deoxyglucose positron emission tomography(FDG-PED) and endoscopic ultrasonography (EUS) in the preoperative evaluation of potentially operable esophageal cancer patients. Am J Gastroenterol 2003;98:S5–6.

15. May A, Günter E, Roth F, et al. Accuracy of staging in early oesophageal cancer using high resolution endoscopy and high resolution endosonography: a comparative, prospective, and blinded trial. Gut 2004;53(5):634–40.

16. Thomas T, Gilbert D, Kaye PV, et al. High-resolution endoscopy and endoscopic ultrasound for evaluation of early neoplasia in Barrett's esophagus. Surg Endosc 2010;24(5):1110–6.

17. Rampado S, Bocus P, Battaglia G, et al. Endoscopic ultrasound: accuracy in staging superficial carcinomas of the esophagus. Ann Thorac Surg 2008;85(1):251–6.

18. ASGE Standards of Practice Committee, Qumseya B, Sultan S, et al. ASGE guideline on screening and surveillance of Barrett's esophagus. Gastrointest Endosc 2019;90(3):335–59.e2.

19. Betancourt Cuellar SL, Carter BW, Macapinlac HA, et al. Clinical staging of patients with early esophageal adenocarcinoma: does FDG-PET/CT have a role? J Thorac Oncol 2014;9(8):1202–6.

20. Little SG, Rice TW, Bybel B, et al. Is FDG-PET indicated for superficial esophageal cancer? Eur J Cardiothorac Surg 2007;31(5):792–7.

21. Raja S, Rice TW, Goldblum JR, et al. Esophageal submucosa: the watershed for esophageal cancer. J Thorac Cardiovasc Surg 2011;142(6):1403–11.e1.

22. Dunbar KB, Spechler SJ. The risk of lymph-node metastases in patients with high-grade dysplasia or intramucosal carcinoma in Barrett's esophagus: a systematic review. Am J Gastroenterol 2012;107(6):850–62 [quiz: 863].

23. Tajima Y, Nakanishi Y, Tachimori Y, et al. Significance of involvement by squamous cell carcinoma of the ducts of esophageal submucosal glands. Analysis of 201 surgically resected superficial squamous cell carcinomas. Cancer 2000; 89(2):248–54.

24. Yachida T, Oda I, Abe S, et al. Risk of lymph node metastasis in patients with the superficial spreading type of esophageal squamous cell carcinoma. Digestion 2019. https://doi.org/10.1159/000499017.

25. Natsugoe S, Baba M, Yoshinaka H, et al. Mucosal squamous cell carcinoma of the esophagus: a clinicopathologic study of 30 cases. Oncology 1998;55(3): 235–41.

26. Bollschweiler E, Baldus SE, Schröder W, et al. High rate of lymph-node metastasis in submucosal esophageal squamous-cell carcinomas and adenocarcinomas. Endoscopy 2006;38(2):149–56.

27. Mejía-Pérez LK, Abe S, Stevens T, et al. A minimally invasive treatment for early GI cancers. Cleve Clin J Med 2017;84(9):707–17.

28. May A, Gossner L, Behrens A, et al. A prospective randomized trial of two different endoscopic resection techniques for early stage cancer of the esophagus. Gastrointest Endosc 2003;58(2):167–75.

29. Pouw RE, van Vilsteren FGI, Peters FP, et al. Randomized trial on endoscopic resection-cap versus multiband mucosectomy for piecemeal endoscopic resection of early Barrett's neoplasia. Gastrointest Endosc 2011;74(1):35–43.

30. Ell C, May A, Gossner L, et al. Endoscopic mucosal resection of early cancer and high-grade dysplasia in Barrett's esophagus. Gastroenterology 2000;118:670–7.

31. Pech O, May A, Manner H, et al. Long-term efficacy and safety of endoscopic resection for patients with mucosal adenocarcinoma of the esophagus. Gastroenterology 2014;146(3):652–60.e1.

32. Katada C, Muto M, Manabe T, et al. Local recurrence of squamous-cell carcinoma of the esophagus after EMR. Gastrointest Endosc 2005;61(2):219–25.

33. Tanabe S, Koizumi W, Higuchi K, et al. Clinical outcomes of endoscopic oblique aspiration mucosectomy for superficial esophageal cancer. Gastrointest Endosc 2008;67(6):814–20.

34. Bhatt A, Abe S, Kumaravel A, et al. Indications and Techniques for Endoscopic Submucosal Dissection. Am J Gastroenterol 2015;110(6):784–91.

35. Bhatt A, Abe S, Kumaravel A, et al. Video-based supervision for training of endoscopic submucosal dissection. Endoscopy 2016;48(8). https://doi.org/10.1055/s-0042-106722.

36. Abe S, Oda I, Suzuki H, et al. Insulated tip knife tunneling technique with clip line traction for safe endoscopic submucosal dissection of large circumferential esophageal cancer. VideoGIE 2017;2(12):342–5.

37. Yoshida M, Takizawa K, Nonaka S, et al. Conventional versus traction-assisted endoscopic submucosal dissection for large esophageal cancers: a multicenter, randomized controlled trial (with video). Gastrointest Endosc 2020;91(1): 55–65.e2.

38. Mehta N, Abushahin A, Sarvepalli S, et al. Tu1189 insulated-tip knife tunneling technique for esophageal endoscopic submucosal dissection: an initial western experience. Gastrointest Endosc 2018;87(6):AB561.

39. Yang D, Coman RM, Kahaleh M, et al. Endoscopic submucosal dissection for Barrett's early neoplasia: a multicenter study in the United States. Gastrointest Endosc 2017;86(4):600–7.

40. Subramaniam S, Chedgy F, Longcroft-Wheaton G, et al. Complex early Barrett's neoplasia at 3 Western centers: European Barrett's Endoscopic Submucosal Dissection Trial (E-BEST). Gastrointest Endosc 2017;86(4):608–18.

41. Yang D, Zou F, Xiong S, et al. Endoscopic submucosal dissection for early Barrett's neoplasia: a meta-analysis. Gastrointest Endosc 2018;87(6):1383–93.

42. Podboy A, Kolahi KS, Friedland S, et al. Endoscopic submucosal dissection is associated with less pathologic uncertainty than endoscopic mucosal resection in diagnosing and staging Barrett's-related neoplasia. Dig Endosc 2020;32(3):346–54.

43. Terheggen G, Horn EM, Vieth M, et al. A randomised trial of endoscopic submucosal dissection versus endoscopic mucosal resection for early Barrett's neoplasia. Gut 2017;66(5):783–93.

44. Mejia Perez LK, Alaber OA, Jawaid S, et al. Endoscopic submucosal dissection vs. endoscopic mucosal resection for treatment of Barrett's related superficial esophageal neoplasia. Am J Gastroenterol 2019;114(Supplement):S209.

45. Pimentel-Nunes P, Dinis-Ribeiro M, Ponchon T, et al. Endoscopic submucosal dissection: European Society of Gastrointestinal Endoscopy (ESGE) Guideline. Endoscopy 2015;47:829–54.

46. Draganov PV, Wang AY, Othman MO, et al. AGA institute clinical practice update: endoscopic submucosal dissection in the United States. Clin Gastroenterol Hepatol 2019;17(1):16–25.e1.

47. Cao Y, Liao C, Tan A, et al. Meta-analysis of endoscopic submucosal dissection versus endoscopic mucosal resection for tumors of the gastrointestinal tract. Endoscopy 2009;41(9):751–7.

48. Ancona E, Rampado S, Cassaro M, et al. Prediction of lymph node status in superficial esophageal carcinoma. Ann Surg Oncol 2008;15(11):3278–88.

49. Manner H, May A, Pech O, et al. Early Barrett's carcinoma with "low-risk" submucosal invasion: long-term results of endoscopic resection with a curative intent. Am J Gastroenterol 2008;103(10):2589–97.

50. Raymond DP, Seder CW, Wright CD, et al. Predictors of major morbidity or mortality after resection for esophageal cancer: a society of thoracic surgeons general thoracic surgery database risk adjustment model. Ann Thorac Surg 2016;102(1):207–14.

51. Zhao H, Koyanagi K, Kato K, et al. Comparison of long-term outcomes between radical esophagectomy and definitive chemoradiotherapy in patients with clinical T1bN0M0 esophageal squamous cell carcinoma. J Thorac Dis 2019;11(11):4654–62.

52. Kato K, Igaki H, Ito Y, et al. Parallel-group controlled trial of esophagectomy versus chemoradiotherapy in patients with clinical stage I esophageal carcinoma (JCOG0502). J Clin Oncol 2019;37(4_suppl):7.

53. Jethwa KR, Deng W, Gonuguntla K, et al. Multi-Institutional Evaluation of Curative Intent Chemoradiotherapy for Patients with Clinical T1N0 Esophageal Adenocarcinoma. Int J Radiat Oncol 2019;105(1):E186–7.

54. Kato H, Sato A, Fukuda H, et al. A Phase II Trial of Chemoradiotherapy for Stage I Esophageal Squamous Cell Carcinoma: Japan Clinical Oncology Group Study (JCOG9708). Jpn J Clin Oncol 2009;39(10):638–43.
55. Motoori M, Yano M, Ishihara R, et al. Comparison between radical esophagectomy and definitive chemoradiotherapy in patients with clinical T1bN0M0 esophageal cancer. Ann Surg Oncol 2012;19(7):2135–41.
56. Koide Y, Kodaira T, Tachibana H, et al. Clinical outcome of definitive radiation therapy for superficial esophageal cancer. Jpn J Clin Oncol 2017;47(5):393–400.
57. Yamamoto S, Ishihara R, Motoori M, et al. Comparison between definitive chemoradiotherapy and esophagectomy in patients with clinical stage I esophageal squamous cell carcinoma. Am J Gastroenterol 2011;106(6):1048–54.
58. Minsky BD, Pajak TF, Ginsberg RJ, et al. INT 0123 (Radiation Therapy Oncology Group 94-05) Phase III trial of combined-modality therapy for esophageal cancer: high-dose versus standard-dose radiation therapy. J Clin Oncol 2002;20(5):1167–74.
59. Nemoto K, Kawashiro S, Toh Y, et al. Comparison of the effects of radiotherapy doses of 50.4 Gy and 60 Gy on outcomes of chemoradiotherapy for thoracic esophageal cancer: subgroup analysis based on the Comprehensive Registry of Esophageal Cancer in Japan from 2009 to 2011 by the Japan Esophageal Society. Esophagus 2020;17(2):122–6.
60. Wang S, Liao Z, Chen Y, et al. Esophageal cancer located at the neck and upper thorax treated with concurrent chemoradiation: a single-institution experience. J Thorac Oncol 2006;1(3):252–9.
61. Minashi K, Nihei K, Mizusawa J, et al. Efficacy of endoscopic resection and selective chemoradiotherapy for stage I esophageal squamous cell carcinoma. Gastroenterology 2019;157(2):382–90.e3.
62. Hamada K, Ishihara R, Yamasaki Y, et al. Efficacy and safety of endoscopic resection followed by chemoradiotherapy for superficial esophageal squamous cell carcinoma: a retrospective study. Clin Transl Gastroenterol 2017;8(8):e110.
63. Kawaguchi G, Sasamoto R, Abe E, et al. The effectiveness of endoscopic submucosal dissection followed by chemoradiotherapy for superficial esophageal cancer. Radiat Oncol 2015;10(1). https://doi.org/10.1186/s13014-015-0337-4.
64. Matsumoto S, Takayama T, Tamamoto T, et al. A comparison of surgery and radiation therapy for cT1 esophageal squamous cell carcinoma. Dis Esophagus 2011;24(6):411–7.
65. Suzuki G, Yamazaki H, Aibe N, et al. Endoscopic submucosal dissection followed by chemoradiotherapy for superficial esophageal cancer: choice of new approach. Radiat Oncol 2018;13(1):246.
66. Hisano O, Nonoshita T, Hirata H, et al. Additional radiotherapy following endoscopic submucosal dissection for T1a-MM/T1b-SM esophageal squamous cell carcinoma improves locoregional control. Radiat Oncol 2018;13(1):14.
67. Jingu K, Takahashi N, Murakami Y, et al. Is concurrent chemotherapy with radiotherapy for esophageal cancer beneficial in patients aged 80 years or older? Anticancer Res 2019;39(8):4279–83.
68. Maingon P, D'Hombres A, Truc G, et al. High dose rate brachytherapy for superficial cancer of the esophagus. Int J Radiat Oncol Biol Phys 2000;46(1):71–6.
69. Ishikawa H, Nonaka T, Sakurai H, et al. Usefulness of intraluminal brachytherapy combined with external beam radiation therapy for submucosal esophageal cancer: long-term follow-up results. Int J Radiat Oncol Biol Phys 2010;76(2):452–9.
70. Gaspar LE, Winter K, Kocha WI, et al. A phase I/II study of external beam radiation, brachytherapy, and concurrent chemotherapy for patients with localized

carcinoma of the esophagus (Radiation Therapy Oncology Group Study 9207): final report. Cancer 2000;88(5):988–95.

71. Pasquier D, Mirabel X, Adenis A, et al. External beam radiation therapy followed by high-dose-rate brachytherapy for inoperable superficial esophageal carcinoma. Int J Radiat Oncol Biol Phys 2006;65(5):1456–61.

72. Ishihara R, Arima M, Iizuka T, et al. Endoscopic submucosal dissection/endoscopic mucosal resection guidelines for esophageal cancer. Dig Endosc 2020. https://doi.org/10.1111/den.13654.

Management of Locally Advanced Esophageal Cancer

Nicolas Zhou, DO, Ravi Rajaram, MD, MSc,
Wayne L. Hofstetter, MD*

KEYWORDS

- Esophageal cancer • Adenocarcinoma • Squamous cell carcinoma
- Chemoradiation • Salvage • MSI • PD-L1 • HER2

KEY POINTS

- Trimodality therapy should be preferred over bimodality therapy as the gold standard for locally advanced esophageal cancers in patients who are candidates.
- Chemoradiation or chemotherapy before esophagectomy provides better oncologic outcomes and improves overall survival compared with surgery alone.
- Hybrid or minimally invasive esophagectomy should be considered in appropriate patients.
- In patients with unresectable or metastatic disease, novel therapies should be considered for tumor profiles positive for HER2, MSI-H/dMMR, and PD-L1 positive.

BACKGROUND

Esophageal cancer is one of the most common causes of cancer deaths worldwide. However, in the United States and other western societies, it is a relatively uncommon disease. In the United States, esophageal cancer represented 17,650 (1%) of diagnosed tumors, and 16,080 (2.6%) of cancer deaths in 2019.[1] From 2007 to 2016, localized disease accounted for 20% of cases compared with 32% with regional involvement.[2] Most cases are advanced beyond local disease at time of diagnosis, due to the insidious onset of symptoms. Upward of 90% of patients present with dysphagia, secondary to progressive obstruction of the esophageal lumen. Other symptoms include weight loss, odynophagia, emesis, cough, regurgitation, anemia, hematemesis, and aspiration pneumonia.

Department of Thoracic and Cardiovascular Surgery, University of Texas MD Anderson Cancer Center, 1515 Holcombe Blvd, Houston, TX 77005, USA
* Corresponding author.
E-mail address: WHofstetter@MDAnderson.org

Surg Oncol Clin N Am 29 (2020) 631–646
https://doi.org/10.1016/j.soc.2020.06.003
1055-3207/20/© 2020 Elsevier Inc. All rights reserved.

surgonc.theclinics.com

The current range of therapies differs based on stage, histology, and performance status of the patient. While early, intramucosal disease can be locally controlled and potentially cured through endoscopic resection techniques, tumor invasion into or beyond the deep submucosa has considerable risk of lymphatic involvement, often necessitating a multimodality approach for treatments. For example, in a study of 90 patients with superficial esophageal adenocarcinoma (EAC), tumor confinement to the lamina propria had 0% lymphatic invasion, while tumors with deep submucosal involvement had 36% regional lymph node metastasis on surgical pathology.[3] More advanced stages with nodal involvement portends a poor prognosis in esophageal cancer with a 5-year overall survival (OS) of 25% in those with regional disease compared with 47% in patients with localized disease.[2]

Upfront esophagectomy was common in the past, but evidence has accumulated that this approach does not achieve cure in most locally advanced cases. Several studies have demonstrated significant benefits with a multimodality approach. Chemotherapy followed by surgery, trimodality with neoadjuvant chemoradiation followed by surgery, and bimodality therapy with definitive chemoradiation have all shown efficacy in randomized controlled trials. However, there are nuances to the findings of these studies. For patients in whom surgical resection is not an option, there are some completed studies and other ongoing trials exploring the benefit of HER2 targeted therapy and immune checkpoint inhibitors (ICI) in select patients. This article describes the current trends and controversies in the management of locally advanced esophageal cancer, and provides insight into optimal treatment strategies based on available evidence.

DEFINITION OF LOCALLY ADVANCED

For the purposes of this discussion, the definition of locally advanced disease will mainly include patients with disease that is resectable, lacks metastasis, but is beyond the superficial layers of the esophagus. According to the 8th edition of the AJCC/UICC staging manual,[4] this would include more advanced cT2N0 and cT3-4aN0-3M0. Tumors clinically staged cT2N0 fall into an intermediate stage, where some smaller tumors that are well to moderately differentiated and lack lymphovascular invasion (LVI) would be considered for upfront surgery. While others who have poor prognostic features, such as longer length (3.5 cm), poor differentiation, or LVI would typically be considered locally advanced and candidates for multimodality therapy based on risk of lymph node metastasis.[5]

SURGICAL APPROACHES FOR ESOPHAGECTOMY

Comparisons of transhiatal versus transthoracic approaches for esophagectomy have been extensively discussed within the literature.[6–9] Our institutional preference for locally advanced esophageal cancer is a transthoracic Ivor Lewis approach for several reasons. First, this affords direct visualization of the involved esophagus, which by definition has significant depth of tumor invasion and/or associated lymphadenopathy. Given the improved exposure, the likelihood of an R1/R2 resection may be reduced compared with a transhiatal approach.[10] In addition, an extensive lymphadenectomy can be performed for not only staging purposes, but also to provide excellent locoregional control of the disease which may translate into improved survival.[10] Moreover, the historically significant morbidity of an intrathoracic anastomotic leak with associated mediastinitis has been cited as a considerable disadvantage when compared with the relatively low risk of a cervical leak. However, surgical techniques, such as pedicled omental flaps have mitigated much of the risk associated with an intrathoracic leak. Rescue strategies, including an endovacuum sponge, covered stents, and thoracoscopic or percutaneous chest drainage have also facilitated the management of perioperative conduit leaks.[11–19] Finally, enhanced recovery pathways, minimally invasive surgery, and multimodal analgesic regimens may further reduce the pulmonary morbidity associated with a transthoracic approach.[20,21]

In recent years, several studies have been published regarding minimally invasive esophagectomy (MIE). This surgical experience primarily focuses on either complete MIE, using conventional laparoscopy/thoracoscopy or robotic-assisted surgery, or a hybrid approach with laparoscopy combined with an open thoracotomy. Although our discussion centers on the aforementioned techniques, we should note that additional variations have been described, such as robotic-assisted transhiatal esophagectomy, and so forth.[22] Studies to date suggest that any form of MIE performed in selected patients is associated with fewer complications, less pain, and reduced lengths of stay with equivalent oncologic outcomes as compared with open esophagectomy.[23–26] In addition, in a major multicenter randomized controlled trial comparing hybrid Ivor Lewis esophagectomy with open surgery, Mariette and colleagues[27] found that a hybrid approach was associated with a 77% reduction in the rate of major intraoperative and postoperative complications compared with open esophagectomy. This decrease in overall complications was in large part attributed to a 50% reduction in pulmonary complications in the hybrid group. We should note that the definition of a major complication included Clavien-Dindo grade II or higher events. Given the broad range of this definition, the sequelae of these complications to patients in this study encompasses a wide range of outcomes. There were no differences between cohorts in the number of lymph nodes resected or surgical margin positivity. In addition, 3-year OS was 67% in the hybrid group compared with 55% in the open group, although this difference did not reach statistical significance.[27] Considering the potential for lower morbidity reported within the literature, MIE or hybrid esophagectomy may be associated with improved perioperative outcomes in centers with experience in using these approaches.

NEOADJUVANT CHEMOTHERAPY

Due to the difficulty of patients tolerating adjuvant chemotherapy and rather disappointing outcomes with upfront surgery in patients with locally advanced disease, much of the attention has been shifted to neoadjuvant therapies. Early trials comparing neoadjuvant chemotherapy plus surgery with surgery alone have reported mixed results, with the European MRC trial showing survival benefit in the neoadjuvant chemotherapy group at both 2 years[28] (43% versus 34%) and 5 years[29] (23% versus 17%; $P = .03$), while the US Intergroup-113 trial[30,31] showed no difference in 2- or 5-year survival. In a meta-analysis of 8 trials comparing neoadjuvant chemotherapy versus surgery alone, there was a significant 2-year OS benefit of 7% (hazard ratio [HR] = 0.90; 95% CI, 0.81–1.00; $P = .05$) in the neoadjuvant chemotherapy group. By histology, the benefit appears to be significant for EAC (HR = 0.78; 95% CI, 0.64–0.95; $P = .014$), but not esophageal squamous cell carcinoma (ESCC). The benefit of neoadjuvant chemotherapy has also been observed in large trials, including MAGIC[32] and ACCORD,[33] where 26% and 75% of the tumors, respectively, are located in the lower esophagus or gastroesophageal junction (GEJ). Recent data on neoadjuvant chemotherapy regimen consisting of fluorouracil, leucovorin, oxaliplatin, and docetaxel (FLOT) have also shown promising results, where 30% of patients with GEJ EAC had pathologic complete response (pCR: ypT0N0M0) upon resection[34] and up to 78% of patients achieved 2-year survival.[35] These trials have focused on EAC of the lower esophagus and GEJ, and results should not be extrapolated to ESCC.

TRIMODALITY THERAPY

In one of the most referenced studies, the CROSS trial[36] evaluated 366 patients (75% EAC and 22% ESCC) comparing neoadjuvant chemotherapy followed by surgery versus surgery alone. Neoadjuvant chemotherapy consisted of 5 cycles of intravenous carboplatin and paclitaxel with concurrent radiation (41.4 Gy in 23 fractions) followed by esophagectomy within 4 to 6 weeks after chemoradiation. With a medium follow-up period of 45 months, the chemoradiation plus surgery group had a higher proportion of OS compared with those who had surgery alone (49.4% versus 24%; $P = .003$). In addition, patients who underwent neoadjuvant chemoradiation had a sustained reduction in both locoregional disease (22% versus 38%; $P<.001$) and distant disease recurrences (49% versus 66%; $P = .004$). An R0 resection was achieved in 92% of the chemoradiation–surgery group compared with 69% in the surgery-only group ($P<.001$). pCR was observed in 23% of the EAC and 49% of the ESCC. While the number of nodes resected was not different between the 2 groups, 75% of the patients in the surgery-only group had positive nodes compared with 31% in the chemoradiation–surgery group ($P<.001$). These results were echoed by the NEO-CRTEC 20150 trial,[37] where 451 ESCC cases were evaluated. There was an improved OS in the neoadjuvant group (100 versus 67 months; $P = .025$), a higher rate of R0 resections, and a 43.2% pCR rate. These 2 large trials showed the benefit of trimodality therapy in both EAC and ESCC, and the results suggest that chemoradiation before surgery offers not only a survival benefit for patients, but results in more frequent R0 resection compared with upfront surgery. Currently, trimodality therapy consisting of neoadjuvant chemoradiation followed by surgery or chemotherapy followed by surgery should be the standard of care in locally advanced esophageal carcinomas.

NEOADJUVANT CHEMOTHERAPY VERSUS NEOADJUVANT CHEMORADIATION

The decision of neoadjuvant chemotherapy or chemoradiation is a topic for debate as available trial data are still inconclusive. The POET trial[38] evaluated neoadjuvant chemotherapy versus neoadjuvant chemoradiation in locally advanced GEJ EAC. Neoadjuvant chemoradiation showed an improved pCR and tumor-free lymph nodes. Despite not being statistically significant, there was a survival benefit at 3 years in the chemoradiation group (47.4% versus 27.7%; $P = .07$). The NeoRes trial[39] compared the 2 neoadjuvant treatments in both EAC and ESCC. While the chemoradiation group had better pCR (28% versus 9%; $P = .002$), lower lymph node disease, and better R0 resection, there were no differences in OS. It is important to note that, in this trial, both EAC and ESCC were included, and may have diluted the benefit of a particular neoadjuvant modality for a specific histologic type. Another important consideration is the method of achieving locoregional control. NeoRes had a higher rate of 2- or 3-field approach compared with POET or CROSS, potentially negating the benefit of radiation in locoregional control. In patients who could not tolerate such an approach, perhaps radiation helps to obtain locoregional control. Nevertheless, it is important to distinguish which patient population would benefit from neoadjuvant chemotherapy versus chemoradiation. Currently there are 2 ongoing clinical trials—ESOPEC[40] using the FLOT protocol, and NEO-AEGIS[41] using the MAGIC or FLOT protocol in comparison with the neoadjuvant chemoradiation protocol used in the CROSS trial to evaluate survival, morbidity and quality of life.

BIMODALITY THERAPY (DEFINITIVE CHEMORADIATION)

Although trimodality therapy offers improved survival and locoregional disease control, there are many who achieve pCR after chemoradiation, especially in ESCC. The value of surgery in these patients is controversial. While it is generally agreed upon that surgery should only be offered to selected patients, the optimal selection criteria are unclear. There are 2 studies that offer some support for bimodality therapy (definitive chemoradiation) versus trimodality therapy in patients with ESCC. A randomized trial by Stahl and colleagues[42] compared 172 patients in cohorts of planned surgery versus observation. After induction chemotherapy, trimodality patients were treated with neoadjuvant chemoradiation (40 Gy) followed by surgery, and bimodality patients completed their definitive chemoradiation (50–60 Gy). Patients had a median follow-up of 6 years. At 2 years, the median survival time for chemoradiation with surgery was 16.4 months compared with 14.9 months without surgery, and the authors did not find a difference in OS between the 2 groups (39.9% versus. 35.4%; test for equivalence $\delta = -0.15$, $P = .007$). They did, however, find a lower local disease recurrence rate in patients who completed trimodality therapy, as well as lower use of palliative procedures, such as dysphagia during follow-up. Criticisms of the study include inappropriate statistical method for the given conclusion,[43] an unusually high 11.3% in-hospital surgical mortality, and survival trend favoring surgery in the Kaplan-Meier curve after 2 years.

The FFCD 9102 study[44] also reported equivalence in the outcomes of these 2 treatment arms; survival analysis at 2 years for trimodality (33.6% $\pm$ 4.5%) and bimodality (39.8% $\pm$ 4.5%) showed no statistical difference in the intent-to-treat analysis, with median survival times of 17.7 and 19.3 months, respectively. In contrast to the Stahl trial, this trial design randomized only those with excellent clinical response to chemoradiation. In an analysis by Vincent and colleagues,[45] patients excluded from the FFCD 9102 trial due to no response to chemoradiation, but who subsequently underwent surgery, had equivalent OS to the trial patients. The message is that, for patients who achieve clinical response, outcomes may be equivocal, but for those who have no response, surgery is still an important component of treatment of ESCC. Long-term results have not been published on this trial, which would be important to see the maintenance of equipoise beyond 2 years for this treatment strategy.

Recent, retrospective data for bimodality and trimodality therapy have not reflected the conclusions of the 2 trials. Barbetta and colleagues[46] compared 124 bimodality and 108 trimodality patients with locally advanced ESCC. The analysis of 5-year OS in a propensity score-matched cohort showed OS of 45% (95% CI, 33–62) for trimodality therapy compared with 29% (95% CI, 18–49) in the bimodality group, with surgery being an independent predictor of survival. The study is limited in its retrospective nature, and selection bias is inherent in the 2 groups, even after matching for known variables. Nevertheless, this further suggests that surgery should not be dismissed as part of the decision-making process for ESCC after chemoradiation.

SELECTIVE SURGERY STRATEGY

With pCR observed in 23% of EAC[47] and 35%–49% of ESCC[37,42,47] from chemoradiation alone, efforts have been made to differentiate those who would benefit from an esophagectomy and those who would not with either histology. Hence, strategies of selective esophageal resection after chemoradiation have been used by many centers.

The phase II RTOG 0246[48] study by Swisher and colleagues was designed to assess the feasibility of a selective resection strategy. After chemoradiation with fluorouracil and cisplatin along with 50.4 Gy radiation, patients are restaged to determine clinical complete response (cCR) or clinical noncomplete response. The study was designed to detect a survival of 77.5% or greater at 1 year in patients who underwent selective or salvage esophagectomy. Study sample consisted of 72% EAC, and more than 70% T3 or N1 disease. Out of 41 eligible patients, 37 completed chemoradiation, of the 21 patients who underwent selected surgery, 17 had residual disease, 3 had recurrent disease, and 1 due to personal choice after achieving cCR. The 1-year survival was 71%, and did not reach the 77.5% hypothesized. In the long-term follow-up,[48] the 5- and 7-year OS was 36.6% (95% CI, 22.3–51.0) and 31.7% (95% CI, 18.3–46.0), respectively. Important to this trial was that the decision to go to surgery was based on the surgeon's assessment of less than complete response. Of interest, albeit a small trial, the surgeon's decision to operate was always confirmed by a pathology report showing residual disease. Unmeasured variables that are observed by experienced esophageal surgeons should not be overlooked; the outcomes of mucosal biopsy and positron emission tomographic maximum standard uptake value cannot and should not be the sole determination of need for surgery. All patients completing bimodality therapy should be seen by a surgeon and discussed in a multidisciplinary setting.

Nonetheless, further study is warranted. The ongoing SANO trial is a phase III, multicenter stepped-wedge cluster randomized controlled trial.[49] Designed as a noninferiority trial, the study compares active surveillance versus planned esophagectomy in 300 patients with EAC or ESCC. After chemoradiation, patients undergo 2 rounds of assessment for cCR at 4 to 6 weeks and then at 10 to 14 weeks after the end of chemoradiation, as described in the Pre-SANO trial.[50] Patients with cCR after both rounds are randomized to surgery or active surveillance group. This trial is powered to detect noninferiority by no lower than 15% of the expected 67% survival at 3 years. There is much interest for the outcomes of this study in determining who would benefit from an esophagectomy after neoadjuvant chemoradiation.

SALVAGE ESOPHAGECTOMY

In patients who have completed definitive chemotherapy and experienced recurrence of disease, restaging and surgical evaluation is warranted. Salvage esophagectomy is a viable option for select patients who failed with locoregional recurrence, however, outcomes of salvage esophagectomy may differ depending on histology and timing of recurrence. There is no universally accepted definition for salvage esophagectomy, most published studies define salvage esophagectomy as either esophagectomy more than 90 days after the end of chemoradiation for persistent disease, or radiographic and clinical evidence of disease-free interval before recurrence of disease. In a meta-analysis by Faiz and colleagues,[51] comprising a total of 28 studies and 1076 patients who received a salvage esophagectomy, the pooled 3-year survival rate for salvage patients was at 39%. In our experience of comparing salvage esophagectomy with those who had planned trimodality therapy, salvage patients had a 3-year OS (48% versus 55%) and 5-year OS (32% versus 45%) that were comparable with the planned surgery cohort.[52] One-third of patients in both groups had postoperative complications, although salvage patients had significantly more postoperative blood transfusions and intensive care unit admissions. Overall, salvage esophagectomy for EAC has an acceptable outcome compared with trimodality therapy, and patients who failed bimodality therapy should be considered for a salvage esophagectomy.

For ESCC, outcomes after salvage may not be comparable with trimodality therapy. In our experience of evaluating 41 patients who were planned to undergo salvage esophagectomy and 35 patients who underwent actual salvage esophagectomy, there was a 90-day mortality of 9.8% versus 17.1%, respectively.[53] Postoperative events (a summation of major pulmonary events, cardiovascular complications, and clinically significant anastomotic leaks) occurred in 36.6% of planned salvage esophagectomies and 71.4% of actual salvage esophagectomies. Three-year OS was 73% for planned and 46% for salvage groups. These results are limited to a single-center experience, and we caution against drawing conclusions directly from these 2 groups as selection bias is inherent. Nevertheless, should bimodality fail with locoregional recurrence, patients may not achieve the same durable survival with salvage esophagectomy as they would in EAC.

Outcomes in salvage esophagectomy in ESCC also seem to differ based on whether it is performed for persistent or recurrent disease. Wang and colleagues[54] found that patients who underwent salvage esophagectomy for recurrent disease have an improved 3-year survival compared with those with persistent disease (56% versus 30%). Taniyama and colleagues[55] reported similar findings in their 5-year survival rates in recurrent versus persistent disease (47% versus 13%). These studies were limited to small sample size, lack of adjustment for confounders, and should be interpreted with caution. Nevertheless, this finding may indicate the aggressive nature of the underlying biology in persistent disease, and may play a role in the decision-making process for surgeons considering salvage esophagectomy.

SURVEILLANCE AFTER DEFINITIVE TREATMENT

Following locoregional control with either definitive chemoradiation or trimodality therapy, surveillance is a necessary component of long-term patient care. This is particularly true in the first 2 to 3 years after treatment as 80% to over 90% of recurrences occur during this time period.[56–58] In recently published data from 2 prospective phase II trials by the Swiss Group for Clinical Cancer Research, the median event-free survival time was 2.7 (95% CI, 1.9–6.8) years in patients undergoing trimodality therapy.[57] Viewed alternatively, data from a multi-institutional analysis reported the 5-year recurrence-free survival to be 54.9% in this patient population.[58] Both of these studies reported that pCR was significantly associated with not only recurrence-free survival, but OS as well.[57,58] However, regardless of tumor histoviability, surveillance is an important aspect of evaluating not only for recurrent disease, but for perioperative events, such as diaphragm hernia and metachronous cancers in the remnant esophagus.

Guidelines published by the National Comprehensive Cancer Network (NCCN) recommend that surveillance for patients with esophageal cancer should be dictated by both the stage of their disease and the type of definitive treatment administered.[59] In patients with T2-T4/N0-N3 disease treated with definitive chemoradiation, computed tomography of the chest and abdomen should be performed every 6 months for 2 years. In addition, because locoregional recurrences are frequently seen in these patients, an upper endoscopy should also be performed every 3 to 6 months for the first 2 years, followed by every 6 months in the third year, with clinical re-evaluation as required going forward. In some instances, patients with recurrent local disease may be candidates for salvage esophagectomy as discussed previously. In contrast, patients completing trimodality therapy do not require routine upper endoscopy surveillance due to the low incidence of local recurrence. Rather, these patients should undergo computed tomography of the chest and abdomen every

6 months for 2 years similar to bimodality patients. Beyond 2 years, both bimodality and trimodality patients should be imaged annually for at least 5 years after treatment.[59]

TARGETED THERAPY

When disease recurs and resection is not an option, tumor biology may provide targets for additional treatment options. HER2/neu is a tyrosine kinase receptor that acts as a growth factor. Its role is well understood in breast cancer, and HER2 is also prevalent in esophageal cancers. HER2-positive status is determined most commonly by a combination of immunohistochemistry (IHC) and fluorescent in situ hybridization.[60] Recently, next-generation sequencing has also been used to determine HER2 status in tumors with high concordance rate with the traditional system.[61] In available literature, approximately 15% to 32% of EAC,[62–65] and 2% to 11% of ESCC[62,63,66] overexpress HER2. HER2 portends a poor prognosis in breast cancer, but the prognostic value of HER2 is controversial in EAC; while some studies found HER2 to be prognostic for poor outcomes,[67–69] others find it to be a favorable prognosis.[65,70,71] Nevertheless, tyrosine kinase inhibitors targeting HER2 have been shown to prolong survival in esophagogastric adenocarcinoma.

The ToGA trial was a major phase III randomized control trial evaluating trastuzumab in addition to standard chemotherapy as first-line agent for treatment of HER2-positive advanced gastric or GEJ carcinomas. Patients with the addition of trastuzumab had longer OS than those who received chemotherapy alone (13.8 versus 11.1 months, HR = 0.74; 95% CI, 0.60–0.91, P = .0046), subgroup analysis showed those with higher HER2 positivity derived greater survival benefit from the treatment. Trastuzumab was approved by Food and Drug Administration (FDA), and the current NCCN guidelines[72] advocate for the addition of trastuzumab to chemotherapy as standard therapy for HER2-positive tumors in unresectable locally advanced, recurrent, or metastatic gastroesophageal adenocarcinoma where local therapy is not indicated.

IMMUNE CHECKPOINT INHIBITORS

Recent development of ICI targeting programmed death protein 1 (PD-1)/programmed death-ligand 1 (PD-L1) pathway has shown promising results in patients who have exhausted standard therapies. PD-L1 positivity is determined by the so-called combined positive score (CPS), which is calculated as the number of PD-L1 expressing cells (tumor cells, lymphocytes, macrophages) divided by the total tumor cells, multiplied by 100. In most clinical trials, PD-L1 positivity is defined as CPS greater than 1 on IHC.[73–75] Pembrolizumab and nivolumab are the 2 anti-PD-1 antibody therapies that have been approved for use in the United States and Japan, respectively.

Results from the KEYNOTE-012[75] and KEYNOTE 059[76] trials granted FDA approval for the use of pembrolizumab for PD-L1-positive recurrent or metastatic esophagogastric junction (EGJ) adenocarcinomas. In Japan, nivolumab was approved for treatment of EGJ and gastric cancers regardless of PD-L1 status because of positive results from the ATTRACTION-2[77] study. In addition, a first-ever site-agnostic approval by the FDA was granted to pembrolizumab in 2017 to treat tumors expressing high microsatellite instability (MSI-H)/defective mismatch repair (dMMR),[78] therefore, MSI-H/dMMR status should also be determined in patients with metastatic disease or where local treatment is not feasible.

As second-line agents, ATTRACTION-3[79] phase III trial compared nivolumab to chemotherapy in 419 ESCC patients who were treatment refractory to previous chemotherapy, and showed a better OS than the chemotherapy group (10.9 versus 8.4 months, P = .019). For pembrolizumab, the KEYNOTE-180[80] phase II trial evaluated 121 heavily pretreated patients; the objective response rate was 9.9% (95% CI, 5.2–16.7) and 13.8% (95% CI, 6.1–25.4) in PD-L1-positive patients. In the follow-up study, phase III KEYNOTE-181 trial,[81] 628 patients were randomized to either pembrolizumab or investigator choice of chemotherapy. Although there was no difference in OS in the cohort, pembrolizumab had a better safety profile than chemotherapy. Of importance, in patients with CPS $\geq$ 10, pembrolizumab demonstrated improved OS (9.3 versus 6.7 months, P = .0074). This led to the approval of pembrolizumab for previously treated, recurrent locally advanced or metastatic cancer in patients with CPS $\geq$ 10. The currently ongoing KEYNOTE-590 trial[82] (NCT03189719) will evaluate pembrolizumab plus chemotherapy as first-line therapy for locally advanced or metastatic esophageal cancer.

Although relatively new on the market, ICI seems to be providing select patients with durable responses who have no other treatment options. The nuances of incorporating immunotherapy into current treatment regimen will likely continue to evolve in the coming years. Regardless, ICI will likely become adopted due to observed survival benefit in these trials, and its safety profile in comparison with standard chemotherapy. At the least, it provides another tool in the armamentarium of treatment of esophageal cancers.

PALLIATION OF LOCALLY ADVANCED ESOPHAGEAL CANCER

In patients who are not candidates for definitive therapy, palliative care focuses primarily on symptom management. Patients with locoregionally advanced esophageal cancer suffer almost uniformly from dysphagia. Utilization of dysphagia grading scales may be helpful in classifying symptomology and assessing the response to treatment.[83] The degree of dysphagia often depends on the depth of tumor invasion at the time of diagnosis. In a study by Fang and colleagues,[84] a dysphagia grade of 3 or greater, indicating the ability to tolerate only liquids or those with complete dysphagia to liquids/saliva, had a positive predictive value of 100% for T3 disease, although sensitivity was only 36% in this study. Several different strategies have been used to address not only the inherent quality of life limitations from dysphagia, but also the malnutrition and weight loss that inevitably follow. First-line management of dysphagia in this patient population has traditionally been stenting.[85,86] Self-expanding metal stents (SEMS) are preferable to plastic stents and can typically be placed with minimal adverse events, with or without the use of fluoroscopy, and allow patients to swallow effectively immediately after procedure in most instances. Stent-related complications can occur and primarily include chest discomfort, migration of the stent, gastroesophageal reflux, or in rare cases esophageal perforation.[85,86] Long-term complications include the need for multiple stent exchanges and the possibility of fistula formation to the nearby airway. In our practice, we typically place partially covered SEMS, which prevents tumor ingrowth into the stent aiding future retrievability, while at the same time affording some granulation tissue within the stent's exposed metal flange to limit migration. Of note, in patients with significant dysphagia in whom future definitive surgical resection is planned, evidence suggests that stents may reduce the likelihood of an R0 resection and worsen both locoregional control and OS compared with patients not undergoing stent placement.[59,87,88] Consequently, stents should be avoided as a bridge to surgery, regardless of whether neoadjuvant chemoradiotherapy is planned, because of poorer oncologic outcomes.

In addition to stent placement, several other methods have been used to address dysphagia in this population. These primarily include chemotherapy, external radiation therapy, brachytherapy, photodynamic therapy, and laser or ablative therapy.[85,86,89] Aside from relieving dysphagia, surgeons should also consider the need for additional nutritional support with placement of feeding tubes. Percutaneous endoscopic gastrostomy tubes with bolus feedings are typically preferred to jejunostomy tubes in most patients.

Additional palliative considerations in this population include control of pain, chronic nausea, and psychosocial distress given the prognosis of their disease. The NCCN provides resources specific to these issues, which may be helpful in the management of these challenging situations. In addition, early involvement of supportive or palliative care services significantly aids in the management of both symptoms and discussions regarding goals of care.

SUMMARY

Treatment of locally advanced esophageal cancer requires a multimodality approach. Neoadjuvant chemotherapy or chemotherapy with concurrent radiation followed by surgery is the standard of care for both EAC and ESCC. In select patients who achieve cCR, definitive chemoradiation with close surveillance within the first 2 to 3 years is currently under scrutiny. Minimally invasive or hybrid approaches to esophagectomy show equivalent oncologic resection, while reducing perioperative risks, and should be considered. Patients with locoregional recurrences warrant a surgical evaluation for a salvage esophagectomy; however, in our experience, while morbidity and mortality seem equivalent for planned and salvage esophagectomy in EAC, salvage esophagectomy in ESCC shows a higher risk of major cardiopulmonary complications and significant anastomotic leaks. In patients with unresectable local disease or distal metastasis, tumor profiling can identify those who would benefit from novel targeted therapy and immunotherapy. Palliative goals for patients should be focused on symptomatic relief, mainly dysphagia, with an emphasis on early involvement in supportive care services to manage symptoms and discussion of goals of care.

DISCLOSURE

The authors have no relevant affiliations or financial involvement with any organization or entity with a financial interest in or financial conflict with the subject matter or materials discussed in the article. This includes employment, consultancies, honoraria, stock ownership or options, expert testimony, grants or patents received or pending, or royalties.

REFERENCES

1. Howlander NNA, Krapcho M, Miller D, et al. SEER cancer statistics review, 1975-2017. Bethesda (MD): National Cancer Institute; 2019. Available at: https://seer.cancer.gov/csr/1975_2017/.

2. Surveillance Research Program. SEER*Explorer software. Bethesda (MD): National Cancer Institute; 2019. Available at: seer.cancer.gov/seerstat.

3. Liu L, Hofstetter WL, Rashid A, et al. Significance of the depth of tumor invasion and lymph node metastasis in superficially invasive (t1) esophageal adenocarcinoma. Am J Surg Pathol 2005;29(8):1079–85.

4. Rice TW, Patil DT, Blackstone EH. AJCC/UICC staging of cancers of the esophagus and esophagogastric junction: application to clinical practice. Ann Cardiothorac Surg 2017;6(2):119.

5. Atay SM, Correa A, Hofstetter WL, et al. Predictors of staging accuracy, pathologic nodal involvement, and overall survival for cT2N0 carcinoma of the esophagus. J Thorac Cardiovasc Surg 2019;157(3):1264–72.e6.

6. Chang AC, Ji H, Birkmeyer NJ, et al. Outcomes after transhiatal and transthoracic esophagectomy for cancer. Ann Thorac Surg 2008;85(2):424–9.

7. Connors RC, Reuben BC, Neumayer LA, et al. Comparing outcomes after transthoracic and transhiatal esophagectomy: a 5-year prospective cohort of 17,395 patients. J Am Coll Surg 2007;205(6):735–40.

8. Hulscher JB, van Sandick JW, de Boer AG, et al. Extended transthoracic resection compared with limited transhiatal resection for adenocarcinoma of the esophagus. N Engl J Med 2002;347(21):1662–9.

9. Omloo JM, Lagarde SM, Hulscher JB, et al. Extended transthoracic resection compared with limited transhiatal resection for adenocarcinoma of the mid/distal esophagus: five-year survival of a randomized clinical trial. Ann Surg 2007; 246(6):992–1000 [discussion:1].

10. Kutup A, Nentwich MF, Bollschweiler E, et al. What should be the gold standard for the surgical component in the treatment of locally advanced esophageal cancer: transthoracic versus transhiatal esophagectomy. Ann Surg 2014;260(6): 1016–22.

11. Dasari BV, Neely D, Kennedy A, et al. The role of esophageal stents in the management of esophageal anastomotic leaks and benign esophageal perforations. Ann Surg 2014;259(5):852–60.

12. Heits N, Bernsmeier A, Reichert B, et al. Long-term quality of life after endovactherapy in anastomotic leakages after esophagectomy. J Thorac Dis 2018;10(1): 228–40.

13. Heits N, Stapel L, Reichert B, et al. Endoscopic endoluminal vacuum therapy in esophageal perforation. Ann Thorac Surg 2014;97(3):1029–35.

14. Hwang JJ, Jeong YS, Park YS, et al. Comparison of endoscopic vacuum therapy and endoscopic stent implantation with self-expandable metal stent in treating postsurgical gastroesophageal leakage. Medicine (Baltimore) 2016;95(16): e3416.

15. Martin LW, Swisher SG, Hofstetter W, et al. Intrathoracic leaks following esophagectomy are no longer associated with increased mortality. Ann Surg 2005; 242(3):392–9 [discussion:399–402].

16. Mennigen R, Senninger N, Laukoetter MG. Novel treatment options for perforations of the upper gastrointestinal tract: endoscopic vacuum therapy and over-the-scope clips. World J Gastroenterol 2014;20(24):7767–76.

17. Schaheen L, Blackmon SH, Nason KS. Optimal approach to the management of intrathoracic esophageal leak following esophagectomy: a systematic review. Am J Surg 2014;208(4):536–43.

18. Schorsch T, Muller C, Loske G. Endoscopic vacuum therapy of perforations and anastomotic insufficiency of the esophagus. Chirurg 2014;85(12):1081–93 [in German].

19. Sepesi B, Swisher SG, Walsh GL, et al. Omental reinforcement of the thoracic esophagogastric anastomosis: an analysis of leak and reintervention rates in patients undergoing planned and salvage esophagectomy. J Thorac Cardiovasc Surg 2012;144(5):1146–50.

20. Markar SR, Karthikesalingam A, Low DE. Enhanced recovery pathways lead to an improvement in postoperative outcomes following esophagectomy: systematic review and pooled analysis. Dis Esophagus 2015;28(5):468–75.

21. Van Haren RM, Mehran RJ, Mena GE, et al. Enhanced recovery decreases pulmonary and cardiac complications after thoracotomy for lung cancer. Ann Thorac Surg 2018;106(1):272–9.

22. Dunn DH, Johnson EM, Morphew JA, et al. Robot-assisted transhiatal esophagectomy: a 3-year single-center experience. Dis Esophagus 2013;26(2):159–66.

23. Luketich JD, Pennathur A, Franchetti Y, et al. Minimally invasive esophagectomy: results of a prospective phase II multicenter trial-the eastern cooperative oncology group (E2202) study. Ann Surg 2015;261(4):702–7.

24. Ruurda JP, van der Sluis PC, van der Horst S, et al. Robot-assisted minimally invasive esophagectomy for esophageal cancer: a systematic review. J Surg Oncol 2015;112(3):257–65.

25. van der Sluis PC, van der Horst S, May AM, et al. Robot-assisted minimally invasive thoracolaparoscopic esophagectomy versus open transthoracic esophagectomy for resectable esophageal cancer: a randomized controlled trial. Ann Surg 2019;269(4):621–30.

26. Yerokun BA, Sun Z, Yang CJ, et al. Minimally invasive versus open esophagectomy for esophageal cancer: a population-based analysis. Ann Thorac Surg 2016;102(2):416–23.

27. Mariette C, Markar SR, Dabakuyo-Yonli TS, et al. Hybrid minimally invasive esophagectomy for esophageal cancer. N Engl J Med 2019;380(2):152–62.

28. Medical Research Council Oesophageal Cancer Working Party. Surgical resection with or without preoperative chemotherapy in oesophageal cancer: a randomised controlled trial. Lancet 2002;359(9319):1727–33.

29. Allum WH, Stenning SP, Bancewicz J, et al. Long-term results of a randomized trial of surgery with or without preoperative chemotherapy in esophageal cancer. J Clin Oncol 2009;27(30):5062–7.

30. Kelsen DP, Ginsberg R, Pajak TF, et al. Chemotherapy followed by surgery compared with surgery alone for localized esophageal cancer. N Engl J Med 1998;339(27):1979–84.

31. Kelsen DP, Winter KA, Gunderson LL, et al. Long-term results of RTOG trial 8911 (USA Intergroup 113): a random assignment trial comparison of chemotherapy followed by surgery compared with surgery alone for esophageal cancer. J Clin Oncol 2007;25(24):3719–25.

32. Cunningham D, Allum WH, Stenning SP, et al. Perioperative chemotherapy versus surgery alone for resectable gastroesophageal cancer. N Engl J Med 2006;355(1):11–20.

33. Ychou M, Boige V, Pignon J-P, et al. Perioperative chemotherapy compared with surgery alone for resectable gastroesophageal adenocarcinoma: an FNCLCC and FFCD multicenter phase III trial. J Clin Oncol 2011;29(13):1715–21.

34. Homann N, Pauligk C, Luley K, et al. Pathological complete remission in patients with oesophagogastric cancer receiving preoperative 5-fluorouracil, oxaliplatin and docetaxel. Int J Cancer 2012;130(7):1706–13.

35. Lorenzen S, Pauligk C, Homann N, et al. Feasibility of perioperative chemotherapy with infusional 5-FU, leucovorin, and oxaliplatin with (FLOT) or without (FLO) docetaxel in elderly patients with locally advanced esophagogastric cancer. Br J Cancer 2013;108(3):519–26.

36. Shapiro J, van Lanschot JJB, Hulshof MCCM, et al. Neoadjuvant chemoradiotherapy plus surgery versus surgery alone for oesophageal or junctional cancer

(CROSS): long-term results of a randomised controlled trial. Lancet Oncol 2015; 16(9):1090–8.

37. Yang H, Liu H, Chen Y, et al. Neoadjuvant chemoradiotherapy followed by surgery versus surgery alone for locally advanced squamous cell carcinoma of the esophagus (NEOCRTEC5010): a phase III multicenter, randomized, open-label clinical trial. J Clin Oncol 2018;36(27):2796–803.

38. Stahl M, Walz MK, Stuschke M, et al. Phase III comparison of preoperative chemotherapy compared with chemoradiotherapy in patients with locally advanced adenocarcinoma of the esophagogastric junction. J Clin Oncol 2009; 27(6):851–6.

39. Klevebro F, Alexandersson von Döbeln G, Wang N, et al. A randomized clinical trial of neoadjuvant chemotherapy versus neoadjuvant chemoradiotherapy for cancer of the oesophagus or gastro-oesophageal junction. Ann Oncol 2016; 27(4):660–7.

40. Hoeppner J, Lordick F, Brunner T, et al. ESOPEC: prospective randomized controlled multicenter phase III trial comparing perioperative chemotherapy (FLOT protocol) to neoadjuvant chemoradiation (CROSS protocol) in patients with adenocarcinoma of the esophagus (NCT02509286). BMC Cancer 2016; 16:503.

41. Reynolds JV, Preston SR, O'Neill B, et al. ICORG 10-14: NEOadjuvant trial in Adenocarcinoma of the oEsophagus and oesophagoGastric junction International Study (Neo-AEGIS). BMC Cancer 2017;17(1):401.

42. Stahl M, Stuschke M, Lehmann N, et al. Chemoradiation with and without surgery in patients with locally advanced squamous cell carcinoma of the esophagus. J Clin Oncol 2005;23(10):2310–7.

43. Ruhstaller T, Mueller A, Koeberle D, et al. Is there really enough evidence to abandon surgery after radiation chemotherapy in esophageal cancer? J Clin Oncol 2005;23(33):8547–8.

44. Bedenne L, Michel P, Bouche O, et al. Chemoradiation followed by surgery compared with chemoradiation alone in squamous cancer of the esophagus: FFCD 9102. J Clin Oncol 2007;25(10):1160–8.

45. Vincent J, Mariette C, Pezet D, et al. Early surgery for failure after chemoradiation in operable thoracic oesophageal cancer. Analysis of the non-randomised patients in FFCD 9102 phase III trial: chemoradiation followed by surgery versus chemoradiation alone. Eur J Cancer 2015;51(13):1683–93.

46. Barbetta A, Hsu M, Tan KS, et al. Definitive chemoradiotherapy versus neoadjuvant chemoradiotherapy followed by surgery for stage II to III esophageal squamous cell carcinoma. J Thorac Cardiovasc Surg 2018;155(6):2710–21.e3.

47. van Hagen P, Hulshof MCCM, van Lanschot JJB, et al. Preoperative chemoradiotherapy for esophageal or junctional cancer. N Engl J Med 2012;366(22): 2074–84.

48. Swisher SG, Winter KA, Komaki RU, et al. A phase II study of a paclitaxel-based chemoradiation regimen with selective surgical salvage for resectable locoregionally advanced esophageal cancer: initial reporting of RTOG 0246. Int J Radiat Oncol Biol Phys 2012;82(5):1967–72.

49. Noordman BJ, Wijnhoven BPL, Lagarde SM, et al. Neoadjuvant chemoradiotherapy plus surgery versus active surveillance for oesophageal cancer: a stepped-wedge cluster randomised trial. BMC Cancer 2018;18(1):142.

50. Noordman BJ, Spaander MCW, Valkema R, et al. Detection of residual disease after neoadjuvant chemoradiotherapy for oesophageal cancer (preSANO): a prospective multicentre, diagnostic cohort study. Lancet Oncol 2018;19(7):965–74.

51. Faiz Z, Dijksterhuis WPM, Burgerhof JGM, et al. A meta-analysis on salvage surgery as a potentially curative procedure in patients with isolated local recurrent or persistent esophageal cancer after chemoradiotherapy. Eur J Surg Oncol 2019; 45(6):931–40.

52. Marks JL, Hofstetter W, Correa AM, et al. Salvage esophagectomy after failed definitive chemoradiation for esophageal adenocarcinoma. Ann Thorac Surg 2012;94(4):1126–32.

53. Mitchell KG, Nelson DB, Corsini EM, et al. Morbidity following salvage esophagectomy for squamous cell carcinoma: the MD Anderson experience. Dis Esophagus 2020;33(3):doz067.

54. Wang S, Tachimori Y, Hokamura N, et al. Prognostic analysis of salvage esophagectomy after definitive chemoradiotherapy for esophageal squamous cell carcinoma: the importance of lymphadenectomy. J Thorac Cardiovasc Surg 2014; 147(6):1805–11.

55. Taniyama Y, Sakurai T, Heishi T, et al. Different strategy of salvage esophagectomy between residual and recurrent esophageal cancer after definitive chemoradiotherapy. J Thorac Dis 2018;10(3):1554–62.

56. Lou F, Sima CS, Adusumilli PS, et al. Esophageal cancer recurrence patterns and implications for surveillance. J Thorac Oncol 2013;8(12):1558–62.

57. Steffen T, Dietrich D, Schnider A, et al. Recurrence patterns and long-term results after induction chemotherapy, chemoradiotherapy, and curative surgery in patients with locally advanced esophageal cancer. Ann Surg 2019;269(1):83–7.

58. Xi M, Yang Y, Zhang L, et al. Multi-institutional analysis of recurrence and survival after neoadjuvant chemoradiotherapy of esophageal cancer: impact of histology on recurrence patterns and outcomes. Ann Surg 2019;269(4):663–70.

59. Esophageal and esophagogastric junction cancers - version 2.2019. National Comprehensive Cancer Network - Clinical Practice Guidelines in Oncology; 2019.

60. Hofmann M, Stoss O, Shi D, et al. Assessment of a HER2 scoring system for gastric cancer: results from a validation study. Histopathology 2008;52(7): 797–805.

61. Janjigian YY, Sanchez-Vega F, Jonsson P, et al. Genetic predictors of response to systemic therapy in esophagogastric cancer. Cancer Discov 2018;8(1):49–58.

62. The Cancer Genome Atlas Research N, Kim J, Bowlby R, et al. Integrated genomic characterization of oesophageal carcinoma. Nature 2017;541:169.

63. Reichelt U, Duesedau P, Tsourlakis MC, et al. Frequent homogeneous HER-2 amplification in primary and metastatic adenocarcinoma of the esophagus. Mod Pathol 2007;20(1):120–9.

64. Yoon HH, Shi Q, Sukov WR, et al. Association of HER2/ErbB2 expression and gene amplification with pathologic features and prognosis in esophageal adenocarcinomas. Clin Cancer Res 2012;18(2):546–54.

65. Janjigian YY, Werner D, Pauligk C, et al. Prognosis of metastatic gastric and gastroesophageal junction cancer by HER2 status: a European and USA International collaborative analysis. Ann Oncol 2012;23(10):2656–62.

66. Gibault L, Metges JP, Conan-Charlet V, et al. Diffuse EGFR staining is associated with reduced overall survival in locally advanced oesophageal squamous cell cancer. Br J Cancer 2005;93(1):107–15.

67. Yoon HH, Shi Q, Sukov WR, et al. Adverse prognostic impact of intratumor heterogeneous HER2 gene amplification in patients with esophageal adenocarcinoma. J Clin Oncol 2012;30(32):3932–8.

68. Tanner M, Hollmen M, Junttila TT, et al. Amplification of HER-2 in gastric carcinoma: association with topoisomerase IIalpha gene amplification, intestinal type, poor prognosis and sensitivity to trastuzumab. Ann Oncol 2005;16(2): 273–8.

69. Brien TP, Odze RD, Sheehan CE, et al. HER-2/neu gene amplification by FISH predicts poor survival in Barrett's esophagus-associated adenocarcinoma. Hum Pathol 2000;31(1):35–9.

70. Plum PS, Gebauer F, Krämer M, et al. HER2/neu (ERBB2) expression and gene amplification correlates with better survival in esophageal adenocarcinoma. BMC Cancer 2019;19(1):38.

71. Duhaylongsod FG, Gottfried MR, Iglehart JD, et al. The significance of c-erb B-2 and p53 immunoreactivity in patients with adenocarcinoma of the esophagus. Ann Surg 1995;221(6):677–84.

72. Ajani JA, D'Amico TA, Bentrem DJ, et al. Esophageal and esophagogastric junction cancers, version 2.2019, NCCN clinical practice guidelines in oncology. J Natl Compr Cancer Netw 2019;17(7):855–83.

73. Bang YJ, Ruiz EY, Van Cutsem E, et al. Phase III, randomised trial of avelumab versus physician's choice of chemotherapy as third-line treatment of patients with advanced gastric or gastro-oesophageal junction cancer: primary analysis of JAVELIN Gastric 300. Ann Oncol 2018;29(10):2052–60.

74. Janjigian YY, Bendell J, Calvo E, et al. CheckMate-032 study: efficacy and safety of nivolumab and nivolumab plus ipilimumab in patients with metastatic esophagogastric cancer. J Clin Oncol 2018;36(28):2836–44.

75. Muro K, Chung HC, Shankaran V, et al. Pembrolizumab for patients with PD-L1-positive advanced gastric cancer (KEYNOTE-012): a multicentre, open-label, phase 1b trial. Lancet Oncol 2016;17(6):717–26.

76. Fuchs CS, Doi T, Jang RW, et al. Safety and efficacy of pembrolizumab monotherapy in patients with previously treated advanced gastric and gastroesophageal junction cancer: phase 2 clinical KEYNOTE-059 trial. JAMA Oncol 2018;4(5): e180013.

77. Kang Y-K, Boku N, Satoh T, et al. Nivolumab in patients with advanced gastric or gastro-oesophageal junction cancer refractory to, or intolerant of, at least two previous chemotherapy regimens (ONO-4538-12, ATTRACTION-2): a randomised, double-blind, placebo-controlled, phase 3 trial. Lancet 2017; 390(10111):2461–71.

78. Prasad V, Kaestner V, Mailankody S. Cancer drugs approved based on biomarkers and not tumor type—FDA approval of pembrolizumab for mismatch repair-deficient solid cancers. JAMA Oncol 2018;4(2):157–8.

79. Kato K, Cho BC, Takahashi M, et al. Nivolumab versus chemotherapy in patients with advanced oesophageal squamous cell carcinoma refractory or intolerant to previous chemotherapy (ATTRACTION-3): a multicentre, randomised, open-label, phase 3 trial. Lancet Oncol 2019;20(11):1506–17.

80. Shah MA, Kojima T, Hochhauser D, et al. Efficacy and safety of pembrolizumab for heavily pretreated patients with advanced, metastatic adenocarcinoma or squamous cell carcinoma of the esophagus: the phase 2 KEYNOTE-180 study. JAMA Oncol 2019;5(4):546–50.

81. Kojima T, Muro K, Francois E, et al. Pembrolizumab versus chemotherapy as second-line therapy for advanced esophageal cancer: phase III KEYNOTE-181 study. J Clin Oncol 2019;37(4_suppl):2.

82. Kato K, Shah MA, Enzinger P, et al. KEYNOTE-590: phase III study of first-line chemotherapy with or without pembrolizumab for advanced esophageal cancer. Future Oncol 2019;15(10):1057–66.
83. Blazeby JM, Williams MH, Brookes ST, et al. Quality of life measurement in patients with oesophageal cancer. Gut 1995;37(4):505–8.
84. Fang TC, Oh YS, Szabo A, et al. Utility of dysphagia grade in predicting endoscopic ultrasound T-stage of non-metastatic esophageal cancer. Dis Esophagus 2016;29(6):642–8.
85. Pavlidis TE, Pavlidis ET. Role of stenting in the palliation of gastroesophageal junction cancer: a brief review. World J Gastrointest Surg 2014;6(3):38–41.
86. Spaander MC, Baron TH, Siersema PD, et al. Esophageal stenting for benign and malignant disease: European Society of Gastrointestinal Endoscopy (ESGE) Clinical Guideline. Endoscopy 2016;48(10):939–48.
87. Ahmed O, Bolger JC, O'Neill B, et al. Use of esophageal stents to relieve dysphagia during neoadjuvant therapy prior to esophageal resection: a systematic review. Dis Esophagus 2020;33(1):doz090.
88. Mariette C, Gronnier C, Duhamel A, et al. Self-expanding covered metallic stent as a bridge to surgery in esophageal cancer: impact on oncologic outcomes. J Am Coll Surg 2015;220(3):287–96.
89. Fuccio L, Mandolesi D, Farioli A, et al. Brachytherapy for the palliation of dysphagia owing to esophageal cancer: a systematic review and meta-analysis of prospective studies. Radiother Oncol 2017;122(3):332–9.

Siewert III Adenocarcinoma
Still Searching for the Right Treatment Combination

Andrew Tang, MD[a], Davendra Sohal, MD, MPH[b],
Michael McNamara, MD[c], Sudish C. Murthy, MD, PhD[a],
Siva Raja, MD, PhD[a],*

KEYWORDS

- Siewert tumor • Esophageal cancer • Gastric cancer • Neoadjuvant chemoradiation
- Esophagectomy • Gastrectomy

KEY POINTS

- It remains uncertain whether Siewert III tumors should be treated as esophageal or gastric cancers.
- Neoadjuvant therapy has been shown to improve survival in both esophageal and gastric trials. Randomized control trials comparing neoadjuvant chemotherapy versus chemoradiation should help define the most optimal treatment regimen.
- Surgical treatment follows general oncology principals: resect to negative margins with complete lymph node dissection, and, the extent of resection often extends more proximal onto the esophagus in addition to the total/subtotal gastrectomy.

INTRODUCTION

Borders invite contest. Not too differently from geopolitical divides, our attempts to classify gastroesophageal junction (GEJ) tumors based on arbitrary borders have met similar discourse. Siewert and Stein were the first to propose a map of this territory, drawing the confines of the esophagus and the stomach (**Fig. 1**).[1] However, from this map, it is difficult to determine which parts of the GEJ belong to the esophagus and which belong to the stomach. This debate generally involves the Siewert III tumor, which was originally described as a "subcardial gastric carcinoma which infiltrates the

[a] Thoracic and Cardiovascular Surgery, Cleveland Clinic, 9500 Euclid Avenue, J4-1, Cleveland, OH 44195, USA; [b] Solid Tumor Oncology, Lerner College of Medicine, Cleveland Clinic, 9500 Euclid Avenue, R35, Cleveland, OH 44195, USA; [c] Cleveland Clinic, 9500 Euclid Avenue, R35, Cleveland, OH 44195, USA
* Corresponding author. Department of Thoracic and Cardiovascular Surgery, Heart, Vascular, and Thoracic Institute, Cleveland Clinic Foundation, J4-1, 9500 Euclid Ave, Cleveland, OH 44195, USA
E-mail address: rajas@ccf.org

Surg Oncol Clin N Am 29 (2020) 647–653
https://doi.org/10.1016/j.soc.2020.07.002
1055-3207/20/© 2020 Elsevier Inc. All rights reserved.
surgonc.theclinics.com

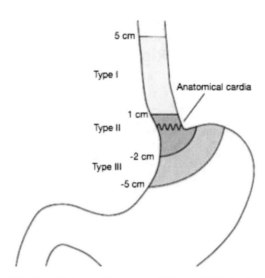

Fig. 1. Siewert classification. (*Adapted from* Yang Z, Wang J, Wu D, Zheng J, Li Y. Retrospectively analysis of the pathology and prognosis of 131 cases of adenocarcinoma of the esophagogastric junction (Siewert type II/III). *Transl Cancer Res.* 2017;6(5):949-959. https://doi.org/10.21037/tcr.2017.09.18.)

esophagogastric junction and distal esophagus from below" (see **Fig. 1**).[1] Even now, it remains unclear if this tumor is in the domain of the esophagus or the stomach, and not surprisingly, it remains controversial how to best treat Siewert III tumors- as esophageal cancers or as gastric cancers.

CURRENT DEFINITIONS: AMERICAN JOINT COMMISSION ON CANCER 7 VERSUS AMERICAN JOINT COMMISSION ON CANCER 8

Tumor location can be difficult to determine clinically and precisely how much extension into the esophagus is necessary for a gastric cardia tumor to be classified as a Siewert III tumor is nebulous. In the seventh edition of the American Joint Commission on Cancer (AJCC), tumors extending from the lower esophagus to within the first 5 cm of the gastric cardia were classified as Siewert III and staged as esophageal cancers.[2] This definition was adjusted in the eighth edition of the AJCC, which classifies tumor location by its epicenter regardless of how far proximally or distally the tumor extends.[3] Different from 7th AJCC, the eighth edition categorizes Siewert III tumors as gastric carcinomas. Admittedly, the authors of the eighth edition AJCC esophageal cancer staging state that this anatomic boundary is more of a placeholder until the pathogenesis and molecular differences between esophageal and gastric carcinomas are better understood in this region.[4]

LANDMARK CLINICAL TRIALS: NEOADJUVANT THERAPY? IF SO, WHICH ONE?

As ruling jurisdictions over territories change, governing laws become jumbled over time. This confusion has fostered Siewert III tumors inclusion into both esophageal and gastric cancer trials.

The Radiation Therapy Oncology Group trial 8911 (RTOG 8911) trial randomized patients with epidermoid (squamous cell carcinoma) and adenocarcinomas of the esophagus and GEJ to undergo either neoadjuvant cisplatin and fluorouracil and surgery versus surgery alone (**Table 1**).[5] Unfortunately, the authors did not specify how many patients had GEJ tumors. They were only able to show the importance of a complete resection (R0) on overall survival but did not find neoadjuvant chemotherapy improved overall survival.[5]

Role for neoadjuvant chemotherapy in esophageal and GEJ cancers was demonstrated by the Medical Research Council Oesophageal Cancer Working Group (OEO2) trial, which definitively proved a survival benefit for neoadjuvant chemotherapy.[6] However, while the OEO2 trial demonstrated the importance of neoadjuvant chemotherapy, only 10% of patients in that study had cardia tumors (see **Table 1**). There was no description of proximal tumor extent or tumor epicenter.[6] The OEO2 trial dovetailed into the Medical Research Council Adjuvant Gastric Infusional Chemotherapy (MAGIC) trial, which randomized patients with clinical T2 and greater biopsy proven adenocarcinoma of the stomach/lower third of the esophagus. Patients were randomized to 6 cycles of perioperative chemotherapy and surgery versus surgery alone (see **Table 1**).[7] This landmark trial was originally designed for gastric cancers; however, due to the increasing incidence of lower esophageal adenocarcinomas in addition to the positive findings from the OEO2 trial, the authors extended eligibility criteria to include esophageal and GEJ carcinomas.[6,7] While the MAGIC trial showed survival benefits in the group that received perioperative epirubicin, cisplatin, and fluorouracil (ECF), only 11.5% of patients had tumors in the GEJ. In the chemotherapy arm, 90% of patients completed all 3 cycles of neoadjuvant chemotherapy; however, only 42% tolerated all 6 perioperative cycles. While these trials demonstrate survival benefits of neoadjuvant chemotherapy for both esophageal and gastric cancer, only a small minority of patients actually had Siewert III cancers. The question therefore remains: do we treat Siewert III tumors as esophageal or gastric cancers?

The ChemoRadiotherapy for Esophageal cancer followed by Surgery Study (CROSS) trial served to solve this question (see **Table 1**). Patients with clinically resectable, locally advanced esophagus or GEJ cancers (clinical T1–3N0–1M0, according to AJCC 6) were randomized to receive either weekly administration of 5 cycles of neoadjuvant chemoradiotherapy (intravenous carboplatin [area under the curve 2 mg/mL per min] and intravenous paclitaxel [50 mg/m of body-surface area] for 23 days) with concurrent radiotherapy (41.4 Gy, given in 23 fractions of 1.8 Gy 5 days per week) followed by surgery, or surgery alone. In contrast to previous trials, nearly a quarter of patients enrolled in the CROSS trial had GEJ tumors. Neoadjuvant chemoradiation was generally well tolerated, as 95% of patients in the chemoradiation arm completed their full course. Patients in the chemoradiation arm had improved overall survival and 29% of patients even had a complete pathologic response.[8]

Although the data strongly favored neoadjuvant therapy, a persistent question that remains is which regimen is better? One study tried to answer the question of neoadjuvant chemotherapy versus chemoradiation for patients with GEJ tumors, however, it was closed due to low recruitment.[9] Patients with locally advanced GEJ adenocarcinomas (cT3-4NXM0) were randomized to undergo either 15 weeks of neoadjuvant chemotherapy or 12 weeks of neoadjuvant chemotherapy and 3 weeks of radiation followed by surgery.[10] Although there was no difference in overall survival, patients who underwent neoadjuvant chemoradiation had more pathologic complete response (15.6% vs 2.0%) and tumor-free lymph nodes (64.4% vs 37.7%) at resection.[10] The study was unfortunately underpowered to demonstrate a difference in overall survival.

Currently, there are multiple randomized control trials comparing neoadjuvant chemotherapy to neoadjuvant chemoradiation.[11–13] The NEOadjuvant Trial in Adenocarcinoma of the oEsophagus and oesophagoGastric Junction International Study (NEO-AEGIS) trial randomizes patients with cT2-3N0-3M0 esophageal and GEJ adenocarcinomas to

Table 1
Landmark trials

Study	Study Population	Study Arms	Results	Limitations
RTOG 8911	Esophageal squamous and adenocarcinoma	Neoadjuvant cisplatin and fluorouracil + surgery (n = 216) vs surgery (n = 227)	No survival difference between groups. R0 resection most important for survival.	Did not specify how many patients had GEJ tumors.
OEO2	Esophageal squamous and adenocarcinoma	Neoadjuvant cisplatin and fluorouracil + surgery (n = 400) vs surgery (n = 402)	Neoadjuvant chemotherapy hazard ratio for death 0.84 (95% CI, 0.72–0.98; P = .03).	10% cardia tumors
MAGIC	Gastric and lower esophageal adenocarcinoma	Perioperative epirubicin, cisplatin and fluorouracil + surgery (n = 250) vs surgery (n = 253)	Perioperative chemotherapy hazard ratio for death, 0.75 (95% CI, 0.60–0.93; P = .009).	11.5% GEJ tumors. Only 42% patients tolerated all 6 perioperative cycles.
CROSS	Esophageal squamous and adenocarcinoma	Neoadjuvant carboplatin and paclitaxel with 41.4 Gy + surgery (n = 178) vs surgery (n = 188)	Neoadjuvant chemoradiation hazard ratio for death 0.657; (95% CI, 0.495–0.871; P = .003). 29% complete response rate.	24% GEJ tumors

Abbreviations: CI, confidence interval; GEJ, gastroesophageal junction.

receive either a modified version of the MAGIC trial chemotherapy or the CROSS regimen.[11] Similarly, the ESOPEC trial is randomizing patients with cT1N + M0 or cT2-4aNxM0 esophageal and GEJ adenocarcinoma to either receive neoadjuvant FLOT (5-fluorouracil/leucovorin/oxaliplatin/docetaxel) or the CROSS regimen.[13] Finally, the Trial Of Preoperative therapy for Gastric and Esophagogastric junction AdenocaRcinoma (TOPGEAR) is grouping Siewert III tumors with gastric cancers and randomizing patients to undergo either neoadjuvant ECF or neoadjuvant ECF with radiation (45 Gy) followed by surgery.[12] Subanalyses of results from these trials, focusing on patients with Siewert III hopefully will help us better understand how to best treat these tumors: as esophageal or gastric cancers.

SURGICAL APPROACH: HOW HIGH SHOULD WE GO?

Although GEJ tumor location influences the choice of neoadjuvant regimen, anatomic location becomes even more important in choosing the optimal surgical approach. Where the tumor originates determines the extent of resection and which region encompasses the lymphatic drainage basin. In their institutional series, Siewert and colleagues[14,15] performed extended gastrectomy on 97% of patients with type III GEJ adenocarcinomas. Their extended gastrectomy consists of total gastrectomy with D2-level lymph node dissection and lower posterior mediastinum lymph node dissection. Occasionally these tumors extend higher into up the thoracic esophagus. It may be beneficial to sample subcarinal lymph nodes to ensure that there is no locoregional tumor metastases to thoracic lymph nodes. A proximal resection margin of ≥6 cm may be required to achieve a microscopically negative proximal margin, therefore mandating additional dissection from the thoracic cavity.[16] This may require a thoracoabdominal approach versus a transhiatal approach, depending on the level of surgeon comfort in the chest.[16] One randomized control trial suggested that the left thoracoabdominal approach was associated with worse survival and worse perioperative morbidity.[17] However, on closer examination of the complications, the investigators note that the left thoracoabdominal approaches was associated with worse pancreatic fistula, abdominal abscess, pneumonia, anastomotic, leak, empyemas, and mediastinitis. Pancreatic fistulas and abdominal abscesses atypically occur after a left thoracoabdominal approach; however, this finding is likely due to the investigators' aggressive D2 dissections that included splenectomy, which has been shown to increase perioperative morbidity and overall mortality.[18]

SUMMARY

Our understanding of gastroesophageal junction tumors is limited to our clinical determination of where the tumor lies and how far it extends. This has hindered our ability to develop more targeted treatment regimens. While neoadjuvant regimens have been shown to be beneficial in treating Siewert III tumors, it is unclear if a course of neoadjuvant chemotherapy is sufficient or if the addition of neoadjuvant radiation helps improve survival. Depending on the proximal extent of the tumor, there are different approaches for resection. Outcomes from these resections can differ depending on the degree of lymphadenectomy performed, as well as the surgeon level of comfort in the thoracic cavity. Results from ongoing randomized control trials hopefully will shed more light on the true biologic behavior of the Siewert III tumor.

FUTURE DIRECTIONS

As cancer care moves toward targeted molecular therapies, immunotherapy is being added to the arsenal of treatment. For patients with metastatic gastric and GEJ cancers adenocarcinoma, the KEYNOTE-059 phase II trial showed that pembrolizumab 200 mg, administered intravenously every 3 weeks until disease progression, or patient withdrawal, provided 11.6% of patients with objective response and 2.3% with complete response.[19] Similarly, the KEYNOTE-180 study showed that patients with metastatic esophageal squamous cell carcinoma and adenocarcinoma could similarly derive some radiologic improvement in tumor response.[20] Although pembrolizumab is a monoclonal antibody targeting programmed death 1 ligand (PD-L1), both studies found objective tumor response to pembrolizumab even in patients with PD-L1–negative tumors. This suggests that the mechanism behind these targeted therapies may involve multiple pathways that are yet fully understood. However, the response to these therapies may help us better understand the true cell origin of Siewert III tumors in this contested anatomic region. Immunotherapy may also potentially bring previously unresectable tumors into the fold of resectability.

DISCLOSURE

The authors have nothing to disclose.

REFERENCES

1. Siewert JR, Stein HJ. Classification of adenocarcinoma of the oesophagogastric junction. Br J Surg 1998;85(11):1457–9.
2. Rice TW, Blackstone EH, Rusch VW. Editorial: 7th edition of the AJCC cancer staging manual: esophagus and esophagogastric junction. Ann Surg Oncol 2010;17(7):1721–4.
3. Rice TW, Ishwaran H, Ferguson MK, et al. Cancer of the esophagus and esophagogastric junction: an eighth edition staging primer. J Thorac Oncol 2016;12(1): 36–42.
4. Rice TW, Gress DM, Patil DT, et al. Cancer of the esophagus and esophagogastric junction-major changes in the American Joint Committee on Cancer eighth edition cancer staging manual. CA Cancer J Clin 2017;67(4):304–17.
5. Kelsen DP, Winter KA, Gunderson LL, et al. Long-term results of RTOG trial 8911 (USA intergroup 113): A random assignment trial comparison of chemotherapy followed by surgery compared with surgery alone for esophageal cancer. J Clin Oncol 2007;25(24):3719–25.
6. Allum WH, Stenning SP, Bancewicz J, et al. Long-term results of a randomized trial of surgery with or without preoperative chemotherapy in esophageal cancer. J Clin Oncol 2009;27(30):5062–7.
7. Cunningham D, Allum WH, Stenning SP, et al. Perioperative chemotherapy versus surgery alone for resectable gastroesophageal cancer. N Engl J Med 2006; 335(1):11–20.
8. Van Hagen P, Hulshof MCCM, Van Lanschot JJB, et al. Preoperative chemoradiotherapy for esophageal or junctional cancer. N Engl J Med 2012;366(22): 2074–84.
9. Stahl M, Walz MK, Stuschke M, et al. Phase III comparison of preoperative chemotherapy compared with chemoradiotherapy in patients with locally advanced adenocarcinoma of the esophagogastric junction. J Clin Oncol 2009; 27(6):851–6.

10. Stahl M, Walz MK, Riera-Knorrenschild J, et al. Preoperative chemotherapy versus chemoradiotherapy in locally advanced adenocarcinomas of the oesophagogastric junction (POET): Long-term results of a controlled randomised trial. Eur J Cancer 2017;81:183–90.

11. Reynolds JV, Preston SR, O'Neill B, et al. ICORG 10-14: NEOadjuvant trial in Adenocarcinoma of the oEsophagus and oesophagoGastric junction International Study (Neo-AEGIS). BMC Cancer 2017;17(1):1–10.

12. Leong T, Smithers BM, Haustermans K, et al. TOPGEAR: a randomized, phase III trial of perioperative ECF chemotherapy with or without preoperative chemoradiation for resectable gastric cancer: interim results from an International, Intergroup Trial of the AGITG, TROG, EORTC and CCTG. Ann Surg Oncol 2017;24(8):2252–8.

13. Hoeppner J, Lordick F, Brunner T, et al. ESOPEC: Prospective randomized controlled multicenter phase III trial comparing perioperative chemotherapy (FLOT protocol) to neoadjuvant chemoradiation (CROSS protocol) in patients with adenocarcinoma of the esophagus (NCT02509286). BMC Cancer 2016;16(1):1–10.

14. Siewert JR, Stein HJ, Feith M. Adenocarcinoma of the esophagogastric junction. Scand J Surg 2006;95:260–9.

15. Siewert JR, Feith M, Stein HJ. Biologic and clinical variations of adenocarcinoma at the esophago-gastric junction: relevance of a topographic-anatomic subclassification. J Surg Oncol 2005;90(3):139–46.

16. Ito H, Clancy TE, Osteen RT, et al. Adenocarcinoma of the gastric cardia: What is the optimal surgical approach? J Am Coll Surg 2004;199(6):880–6.

17. Kurokawa Y, Sasako M, Sano T, et al. Ten-year follow-up results of a randomized clinical trial comparing left thoracoabdominal and abdominal transhiatal approaches to total gastrectomy for adenocarcinoma of the oesophagogastric junction or gastric cardia. Br J Surg 2015;102(4). https://doi.org/10.1002/bjs.9764.

18. Schmidt B, Yoon SS. D1 versus D2 lymphadenectomy for gastric cancer. J Surg Oncol 2013;107(3):259–64.

19. Fuchs CS, Doi T, Jang RW, et al. Safety and efficacy of pembrolizumab monotherapy in patients with previously treated advanced gastric and gastroesophageal junction cancer: Phase 2 clinical KEYNOTE-059 trial. JAMA Oncol 2018;4(5):2–9.

20. Shah MA, Kojima T, Hochhauser D, et al. Efficacy and safety of pembrolizumab for heavily pretreated patients with advanced, metastatic adenocarcinoma or squamous cell carcinoma of the esophagus: the phase 2 KEYNOTE-180 study. JAMA Oncol 2019;5(4):546–50.

Surgical Management of Chest Wall Sarcoma

Nathan W. Mesko, MD[a], Alejandro C. Bribriesco, MD[b], Daniel P. Raymond, MD[b],*

KEYWORDS

- Chest wall sarcoma • Chondrosarcoma • Osteosarcoma • Ewing sarcoma
- Chest wall resection

KEY POINTS

- Chest wall sarcoma is a rare cancer due to a heterogenous collection of histologies. Multidisciplinary management in centers experienced in these pathologies is optimal.
- There are many opportunities for scientific investigation to answer basic questions about chest wall sarcoma management including treatment components, treatment sequence, optimal margin, and optimal reconstruction.
- Incomplete excisions, often during incisional biopsies, require reexcision of the entire surgical bed, and radiation should be considered as an adjuvant.
- The general principle of 2 cm margin for low-grade tumors and 4 cm margins for high-grade tumors still applies, although data supporting this approach are very limited.

INTRODUCTION

In 2020, there will be an estimated 13,130 cases of soft tissue sarcoma and 3600 cases of bone sarcoma (BS) in adults and children in the United States, with approximately 7100 deaths.[1,2] Overall, sarcoma cancers account for less than 1% of adult malignancies and 15% to 20% of pediatric malignancies. Most sarcomas arise de novo and not from premalignant lesions. A review of 4500 soft tissue sarcomas suggested that approximately 1 in 5 soft tissue sarcomas occur in chest wall/torso location, with the majority presenting in the lower and upper extremities.[3] Those patients presenting with chest wall tumors can present in a variety of ways, with the most common presentation being that of a palpable and symptomatic mass. The manner of treatment is largely dictated on tumor location, biological risk (ie, tumor size, grade, histology), and metastatic status at presentation. Risk factors that have been associated with lower overall survival include margin status, age, grade of the tumor, and radiation-associated histology.[4,5] Although BS and soft tissue sarcoma histologies

[a] Dept of Orthopaedic Surgery, Cleveland Clinic, 9500 Euclid Ave, Crile Bldg, A41, Cleveland, OH 44195, USA; [b] Department of Thoracic & Cardiovascular Surgery, Cleveland Clinic, 9500 Euclid Avenue, J4-1, Cleveland, OH 44195, USA
* Corresponding author.
E-mail address: raymond3@ccf.org

Surg Oncol Clin N Am 29 (2020) 655–672
https://doi.org/10.1016/j.soc.2020.06.008
1055-3207/20/© 2020 Elsevier Inc. All rights reserved.
surgonc.theclinics.com

follow many commonalities with regard to diagnosis and treatment, a variety of histologies should be highlighted and will be a focus in this review.

More common in the chest wall are nonsarcoma etiology malignancies (direct invasion breast cancers, metastatic disease, plasmacytomas) and benign entities (enchondroma, fibrous dysplasia, osteochondroma, aneurysmal bone cysts, eosinophilic granulomas, desmoid fibromatosis) that comprise additional chest wall neoplastic processes.[6] Although surgical intervention can be entertained in many of these diagnoses, understanding the natural history of common chest wall nonsarcoma origin tumors is important when guiding treatment considerations.

The purpose of this review is to highlight chest wall malignancies (and select benign entities) with a focus on chest wall sarcoma and discuss appropriate preoperative workup, neoadjuvant therapy, the oncologic resection, and definitive reconstructive methods.

Initial Evaluation

Imaging
An magnetic resonance scan (MRI) of the primary site of concern (with and without intravenous contrast) is best for extremity sarcoma, whereas computed tomography (CT) scan has long been advocated as an appropriate choice in chest wall and retroperitoneal sarcoma investigation. MRI of the chest wall can be considered when assessing for soft tissue edema. This may help delineate the "reactive zone" of a sarcoma where microscopic "satellite" cells may be found or may have utility for identify "skip" lesions in the ribs or sternomanubrial/clavicular anatomy in the setting of BS. A CT of the chest should be obtained for staging of all soft tissue sarcomas and BS. Intravenous contrast is useful in studying the relationship of a tumor with vascular structures, as well as delineating possible hilar or mediastinal lymphadenopathy. PET scans should not be obtained routinely in patients with isolated or metastatic soft tissue sarcoma, although PET imaging has been shown to be useful in prognostication, grading, and determining response to chemotherapy in tumors greater than 3 cm, high grade, and deep to fascia.[7] Trends are shifting in Ewing sarcoma toward higher utilization of PET-CT imaging, with recent literature suggesting that PET-CT scan imaging may be able to avoid the need for bone marrow biopsy in Ewing sarcoma staging.[8,9] PET-CT has also been shown to add insight into distinguished neurofibromas from possible transformed malignant peripheral nerve sheath tumors (MPNST) in the setting of NF-1.[10–12] The role of PET scan should be discussed at a multidisciplinary sarcoma conference in individual cases.

A nonexhaustive list of previously described common entities for chest wall sarcomas include liposarcoma, rhabdomyosarcoma, leiomyosarcoma, synovial sarcoma, undifferentiated pleomorphic sarcoma (formerly malignant fibrous histiocytoma), angiosarcoma, MPNST, Ewing sarcoma, osteosarcoma, and chondrosarcoma. Special circumstances for advanced imaging do apply for certain tumor histologies[13,14]:

- Myxoid/round cell/liposarcoma—as per National Comprehensive Cancer Network guidelines, a dedicated spine imaging (MRI or CT) is recommended. PET-CT imaging as a standalone has lacked as a sufficiency screening tool in this variant, which has tendency for extrapulmonary metastases.[15] Contrast is recommended to decipher enhancement pattern of possible metastasis versus benign elements such as a Schmorl node or hemangioma. CT abdomen/pelvis is also recommended for these subtypes. Evidence does suggest that PET-CT scans and MRIs alone can be useful in finding metastatic foci. An argument can be made that combining a whole-body MRI and PET capability with a PET-MRI can look not only at the spine but also at other extrapulmonary locations that myxoid liposarcoma can be predisposed toward.[15–19]

- Angiosarcoma—historically, central nervous system imaging has been recommended, in the form of either a CT head or a brain MRI. A recommendation is to obtain an MRI of the brain (or CT head if MRI is contraindicated) based on clinical suspicion. A CT abdomen/pelvis is recommended, in addition to a CT chest.
- Dedifferentiated liposarcoma—a CT chest/abdomen/pelvis is recommended.
- Leiomyosarcoma—CT abdomen/pelvis imaging is recommended. PET-CT imaging can be ordered on a case by case basis due to clinical concerns. These will be taking origin from smooth muscle, likely of vascular origin in the chest. Vascular invasion on final pathology review is an important prognostic detail.
- "RACES" sarcomas—although uncommonly noted to disseminate through lymphatic channels as hematopoietic dissemination is mainstay for sarcoma histologies, several sarcomas have a rare but known predisposition toward lymph node dissemination (*RACES—R*habdomyosarcoma, *A*ngiosarcoma, *C*lear Cell Sarcoma, *E*pithelioid Sarcoma, *S*ynovial Sarcoma). A clinical lymph node examination is mandatory, as well as CT abdomen/pelvis imaging. Any suspicion on clinical examination should mandate a sentinel lymph node biopsy and PET-CT imaging (whole body).
- Ewing sarcoma—evolving evidence supports the use of PET-CT whole-body imaging as part of the preoperative workup, in addition to a CT chest. If the PET-CT does not show increased avidity in the marrow, then a bone marrow biopsy is not necessary. If a PET-CT is either not approved or shows marrow avidity, then a Bone marrow biopsy is necessary to prove marrow dissemination.
- Osteosarcoma—whole-body bone scan is recommended, in addition to the CT chest. An MRI chest with and without contrast may be helpful in looking for "skip" metastases in the bone or for soft tissue edema extent when planning oncologic resection margins.
- Chondrosarcoma—whole-body bone scan is recommended, in addition to the CT Chest. An MRI chest with and without contrast may be helpful in looking for "skip" metastases in the bone or for soft tissue edema extent when planning oncologic resection margins.
- Plasmacytoma—a skeletal survey is recommended over a whole-body bone scan, in order to appropriately understand distant bony involvement.

Several benign and nonsarcoma malignant tumors should also have special considerations when determining an appropriate preoperative workup:

- Osteochondroma—in the setting of multiple osteochondromas, suspicion for multiple hereditary exostosis (MHE) should be had. A skeletal survey can be ordered to look at all major bones (long and flat bones) in order to obtain a baseline for comparison purposes in the future. The risk of malignant transformation, even in syndromic MHE, is low ($\sim$1%).[20] A CT chest can help prove marrow confluence between the tumor and the adjacent bone.
- Desmoid tumor—in the young patient, Lynch syndrome/familial adenomatous polyposis should be ruled out with germline testing and tumor genetic testing. A family history with suspicion for colon cancer should trigger a referral for colonoscopy. An MRI with and without contrast is helpful for looking at characteristic "dark T1, dark T2" signal suggested for fibrotic makeup of the tumor.

- Aneurysmal bone cyst—an MRI with and without contrast is helpful when suspected. This can show "fluid-fluid" levels characteristic of this diagnosis, as well as look for more aggressive features that may suggest concern for a telangiectatic osteosarcoma.
- Solitary fibrous tumor—a CT chest is recommended, and if pathology is concerning for a high-risk stratification (**Box 1**), then a CT abdomen/pelvis is recommended.[21]

Echocardiogram

All patients with anticipated anthracycline-based agents (ie, doxorubicin or adriamycin) should have an echocardiogram to assess left ventricular ejection fraction (before receiving doxorubicin) due to the risk of development or worsening of congestive heart failure.

Laboratory assessment

Baseline laboratories, specifically a complete metabolic panel and complete blood count should be performed on all patients. In addition, suspicion for a plasmacytoma should also include a serum and urine electrophoresis.

Biopsy

If imaging does not clearly delineate a diagnosis (ie, benign lipoma, osteochondroma, fibrous dysplasia, chondrosarcoma, etc.), then a carefully planned biopsy is necessary. Importantly, such interventions should be performed along planned the future resection axis with minimal dissection and careful attention to hemostasis. Although tumor tract seeding is extremely rare with needle biopsy and correlates with the size of the needle,[22] large hematoma formation by a poorly planned biopsy has the potential to affect surgical planning and functional outcome. Strictly for diagnostic purposes, a needle biopsy is favored over an incisional or excisional biopsy in most of the cases.

Best practice for all potential sarcomas (retroperitoneal, head and heck, extremity/trunk) supports biopsy procedures at the facility where definitive care will most likely take place, in an effort to prevent complication.[23,24] The literature strongly favors treatment of sarcomas in a "centralized" fashion, where referral to a high-volume center has lower local recurrence risk, more reliable margin status, lower amputation rates, improved survival with high-grade tumors, lower complication and mortality rates, and more reliable administration of appropriate adjuvant therapies.[23–25] Given the rarity of this disease, pathologic diagnosis should be confirmed by a pathologist who is an expert in the assessment of sarcoma due to concerns regarding higher false-negative rates from less-experienced pathologists.[26]

Box 1
Features associated with malignant behavior for solitary fibrous tumors

Size greater than 10 cm

Greater than 4 mitoses/10 HPFs

Increased nuclear pleomorphism

Increased cellularity

Tumor necrosis

Abbreviation: HPF, high-power field.

Data from Refs.[73,74]

With regard to those soft tissue sarcomas that have a higher predisposition to lymph node metastases (**Box 2**), a sentinel lymph node (SLN) biopsy should be performed on all patients with palpable lymphadenopathy or advanced imaging showing pathologic enlargement of lymph nodes in the same drainage pattern as the sarcoma in question. Those patients without clinical or radiographic evidence of lymphadenopathy with the aforementioned diagnoses should be decided upon on a case-by-case basis, given lack of good evidence for an SLN biopsy as a routine practice.

Pathology

Sarcomas are rare cancers with more than 50 to 75 different histologic subtypes classified by the World Health Organization. Soft tissue and bone malignancies are graded by the FNCLCC grading system, which is a 3-grade system (low, intermediate, and high).

Immunohistochemistry and molecular genetic studies are frequently used to classify bone and soft tissue sarcomas. Immunohistochemistry is generally useful in delineating the line of differentiation of the tumor, which is the basis of classifying bone and soft tissue tumors (eg, skeletal muscle differentiation for rhabdomyosarcoma). In addition, some immunohistochemical markers (eg, STAT6 in malignant/benign solitary fibrous tumor, MUC-4 in low-grade fibromyxoid sarcoma, INI-1 loss in epithelioid sarcoma) and gene fusions (eg, *EWSR1-FLI1* in Ewing sarcoma) are pathognomonic or strongly suggest many entities. Looking for additional fusion partners in order to aid with diagnosis, as well as to identify potential targets with immunotherapy or targeted therapy should be discussed on a case-by-case basis. Specific to chest wall sarcomas, past studies show most of the chest wall tumors undergoing surgical excision to be high-grade malignancies.[4]

Preoperative Planning

The foundation of an effective treatment plan begins with appropriate preoperative assessment. The cornerstone of this assessment is obtaining the correct diagnosis. As mentioned previously, the use of core needle biopsies as opposed to incisional biopsies is desirable, as it limits potential spillage of tumor cells and contamination of surrounding tissue. Once the diagnosis is determined, discussion in a multidisciplinary setting specializing in sarcoma is important to assure the appropriate staging evaluation and treatment sequence. This process can be facilitated by the use of institution- or society-derived care paths to assure standardization of care and avoidance of unnecessary tests.

Physiologic assessment of the patient can be performed as a concurrent process. A standard thoracic surgical evaluation including pulmonary function tests, a functional test such as a 6-minute walk test, and cardiac risk assessment is advisable. Functional

---

Box 2
Sarcomas requiring lymph node assessment

Rhabdomyosarcoma

Angiosarcoma

Clear cell sarcoma

Epithelioid sarcoma

Synovial sarcoma

testing is desirable to assess the patient's strength and ability to recover from a significant physiologic insult including loss of chest wall function. Assessment of secretion management, diaphragm function, and patient vigor are required to counsel the patient on risks of postoperative atelectasis, which could lead to repeated invasive procedures such as toilet bronchoscopy, reintubation, and respiratory failure. A history of vocal cord dysfunction or aspiration should be investigated to identify patients at higher risk for postoperative respiratory complications.

Surgical planning revolves around determining the size of the chest wall defect, the skin defect, the means of reconstruction, and the need for additional soft-tissue coverage. Consultation with a Plastic Surgeon may be necessary to plan out various soft tissue coverage strategies including rotational flaps and free flaps with muscle and skin.

Surgical Treatment—Soft Tissue Sarcoma

The generally accepted rule of thumb for resection of chest wall sarcomas is based on tumor grade: 4 cm margins for high-grade lesions and 2 cm margins for low-grade lesions (with some exceptions such as desmoid tumors).[27] The data, however, to support this rule of thumb are rather sparse. One of the early landmark studies is a single-center retrospective series from the Mayo Clinic where King and colleagues[28] demonstrated that a greater than 4 cm margin was associated with a 5-year survival of 56% as opposed to 29% in patients with a 2 cm margin ($P<.06$). This univariate analysis did not account for tumor size, grade, or histology (nor did it reach statistical significance) yet the 4 cm margin became widely accepted, given the paucity of available data. A more contemporary series from Shewale and colleagues[4] included 121 patients with primary chest wall sarcoma over a 15-year period. This study did not specifically study margin length but rather divided patients into 3 groups: R0, R1, and R2 resections. Multivariable analysis identified tumor grade (hazard ratio [HR] 15.21; 95% confidence interval [CI] 3.57–64.87; $P<.001$), incomplete resection (R1; HR 3.10; 95% CI 1.40–6.86; $P = .005$; R2 HR 5.18; 95% CI 1.91–14.01; $P = .001$), and increasing age (HR 1.02; 95% CI 1.01–1.03; $P = .002$) to be independently associated with worsened overall survival. Interestingly, in this analysis, tumor histology, induction chemotherapy, and large tumor size did not achieve significance. An analysis by Scarnecchia and colleagues[29] similarly identified R0 resection to be an independent predictor of survival following chest wall resection (HR 5.6; 95% CI 2.95–11.93; $P<.001$). This analysis notably combined primary tumors of the chest wall with lung cancer with chest wall involvement, primary tumors being roughly 25% of the entire population. A 2015 cohort of 65 chest wall sarcomas (Ewing sarcoma and chondrosarcoma histologies excluded) showed a reduction of local recurrence and distant metastases in patients with stage IIb and stage III disease with the addition of radiation therapy and chemotherapy, respectively, at 5- and 10-year endpoints.[30]

Histology-dependent soft tissue sarcoma excisions and margin measurements are controversial. Histologies that are more infiltrative in nature, such as myxofibrosarcoma, dedifferentiated liposarcoma, or dermatofibrosarcoma protuberans variants, may require more extensive margin planning at the offset to account for the microscopic infiltrative extensions.

Although other studies exist on this topic, generally the small size, retrospective nature, heterogeneity of histologies included in the studies and heterogeneity of variables included in analyses make it challenging to draw definitive conclusions regarding optimal margin determination. What should be noted, however, is the currently accepted practice in extremity soft tissue sarcoma to pursue limb salvage over radical resection, thus potentially sacrificing the traditional "wide margins."

This approach has been noted to be associated with higher rates of local recurrence but not overall survival, thus emphasizing the importance of systemic control of the disease with evolving systemic therapies.[31,32]

A further challenge in the chest is the lack of data on long-term functional outcome, which is well described in the orthopedic population. This prevents analysis of risk:benefit with radical resections. We are therefore left to conclude that there are no data that strongly recommend a change in the generally accepted practice of 2 cm for low-grade and 4 cm for high-grade chest wall tumor resection. The authors suspect that broader margins are more likely to assure an R0 resection, as we have limited capability to perform frozen section analysis of chest wall specimens. Conceptually, a reasonable alternative would be a delayed reconstruction with "fast tracked" pathologic analysis; however, this could potentially increase risk of prosthetic infection, a potentially devastating complication. Better imaging and understanding of different histologies may allow us, in the future, to tailor margins more effectively and thus potentially decrease postoperative respiratory complications and improve long-term functional results.

Surgical Treatment—Bone Sarcoma

For BS excision, a negative surgical margin has been reported as a key indicator toward effecting both local recurrence and overall survival prognosis. Literature has suggested tumor necrosis following neoadjuvant chemotherapy and pleural involvement to be potentially predictive for overall survival outcome, but due to the rare nature of this histology previous studies are not statistically powered to definitively answer the question of factors that are clearly linked to overall survival.[33] Histology-specific considerations are as follows:

- *Chondrosarcoma* is traditionally considered a radio-resistant and chemo-resistant histology, with up front wide surgical margin excision the standard of care. Prior studies have shown excellent survival with R0 excision in chondrosarcoma. With achieved negative margins (R0), chondrosarcoma has shown 5-year overall survival of up to 100% in grade 1 and 2 tumors.[34] Overall 10-year survival is affected when a local recurrence occurs.[35]
- *Ewing sarcoma* has generally been thought of as a histology that benefits from multimodal treatment, including surgery in combination with either radiation therapy or chemotherapy. In the large chest wall Ewing sarcoma multicentric German registry study, surgery versus radiation and surgery treatment did not show benefit from local recurrence if the initial excision was R0.[36] Radiation has shown benefit as an adjuvant treatment with chemotherapy and surgery in those patients who were identified to have low tumor necrosis following en bloc excision pathology review.[33,37] Controversy exists as to whether or not the entire rib seen as the epicenter should be excised, although no definitive evidence has pointed toward a survival advantage with full rib resection versus partial rib resection.
- *Osteosarcoma* is generally a histology where surgery and chemotherapy are a mainstay. Low-grade osteosarcomas are rare in the chest wall, with additional histologies such as chondroblastic osteosarcoma showing little anticipated response to induction chemotherapy (behaving similar to chondrosarcoma histologies). Generally, a survival advantage exists with skeletal osteosarcoma by combining surgery and chemotherapy. The role of radiation therapy is more controversial with osteosarcoma, generally reserved for palliative situations. No literature specifically looking at a homogenous osteosarcoma chest wall population exists.

- *Radiation-induced sarcomas* (RIS) generally occurs in the setting of radiation to the chest wall for breast cancer, lung cancer, or non-Hodgkin lymphoma, in as short a latency period as 3 years following radiation and a median of 10 to 15 years.[33,37–39] Wide excision is the gold-standard treatment of RIS of the chest wall, with relatively poor local recurrence and overall survival prognosis. The role of chemotherapy and radiation therapy are controversial, and literature is limited in proving their benefit.

Incomplete Excisions

When a sarcoma is incompletely removed, oftentimes because a sarcoma is not suspected at the time of surgery, an immediate referral to a tertiary care sarcoma center is recommended. No prior studies evaluating this scenario in chest wall tumors exist, but a mixture of extremity and trunk populations has been published. Current rates of incomplete excision rates range from 18% to 53%, with most literature ~30%. Depending on location of the lesion, these will require reexcision of the contaminated sarcoma bed ± radiation therapy used as an adjuvant treatment. Without reexcision, those sarcomas with microscopically or macroscopic positive margins may have recurrence rates as high as 70% to 90%.[40–42] Microscopic disease has been noted in 14% to 74% of reexcised tumor specimens.[43] Although a properly reexcised soft tissue sarcoma bed has not been reliably linked with adverse overall survival effect, reexcision is generally associated with greater financial burden cost and more morbidity at the time of surgery.[44,45]

Surgical treatment—nonsarcoma neoplasms

Surgical resection considerations should be taken into account for different histologies.

- *Benign tumors* such as fibrous dysplasia, enchondromas, or osteochondromas can be safely observed to prove stability. Surgical excision is considered for symptomatic tumors or tumors that show aggressive feature transformation with serial imaging. Eosinophilic granulomas (aka Langerhans cell histocytosis) often can seem aggressive and may require biopsy. The biopsy manipulation itself has been shown to be curative, as well as observation, steroid injections, or surgical curettage.[46]
- *Desmoid tumors (extraabdominal)* generally should not undergo surgical intervention, given the prohibitively high risk of local recurrence that approaches 100% after even an R0 resection. R0 and R1 margins have not shown a predictable difference in determining local recurrence risk. Consensus and recent publications have pushed toward nonoperative, and even observation, treatments.[47,48] Antiinflammatories, antihormonal medications, and a variety of chemotherapy regimens have all shown sporadic benefit. Surgery and radiation are often reserved as last-line treatments unless there is an impending life-threatening mass effect on a nearby vital structure. Minimally invasive options, such as cryoablation or magnetic resonance–guided high-frequency ultrasound have been described as showing benefit from presenting progression.[49,50]
- *Plasmacytomas*, if identified to be isolated (normal bloodwork, bone survey, and/or marrow studies), should be considered for a side excision. Sarcoma margin literature cannot be extrapolated to this histology, and consideration of preserving as much anatomy as possible while still obtaining an R0 resection should be made.
- *Aneurysmal bone cysts* have historically been described in extremity and spine literature as being amendable to open intralesional approaches and bone

grafting. The "curopsy" has also been described, as similar to an eosinophilic granuloma, where the simple irritation from the biopsy can stimulate resolution of the lesion.[51] Recently, CT-guided injections of doxycycline—an agent that acts as a sclerosing/irritant chemical—has shown great promise in preventing the need for surgery.[52,53]

Surgical Reconstruction

Large, single-center case series from major institutions such as Mayo Clinic,[54,55] Emory University,[56] Memorial Sloan Kettering,[57] and MD Anderson[58,59] comprise the most often referenced studies on chest wall resection and reconstruction. Each center has developed a particular and nuanced approach with some overlapping similarities, but in general there is no unified consensus or clear superiority regarding many of the technical aspects such as type of mesh to implant or the use of rigid versus flexible prosthesis for chest wall stabilization (**Table 1**).

There is general agreement in underlying guiding principles behind chest wall reconstruction should be to stabilize the thorax to achieve (1) optimal respiratory function; (2) protection of underlying organs; and (3) acceptable cosmetic outcome. A multidisciplinary approach to these often complex patients is essential. Below is a stepwise approach to devising a plan for chest wall resection, which will ultimately be colored by surgeon preference and available resources.

Is reconstruction necessary?

Some chest wall defects do not necessarily require reconstruction. The 2 major, interrelated factors are size and location of the defect. Many investigators agree that reconstruction is not necessary for defects smaller than 5 cm in any location or up to 10 cm if protected by the scapula and there is no risk of scapular entrapment. With respect to location, Scarnecchia and colleagues[29] defined "critical areas" of the chest that require skeletal reconstruction as anterior or lateral chest wall and defects of 3 or more ribs not covered by scapula. In their study of 71 patients undergoing chest wall resection, 41 had a defect in a critical area. Skeletal stabilization was inversely correlated with acute respiratory complications and flail chest. Without reconstruction in a critical area, 100% of patients had respiratory complications versus 5.7% in reconstructed patients.

Should rigid or flexible material be used?

The ideal characteristics of a prosthesis include the following: (1) sufficient stability to abolish paradoxic chest movement; (2) malleable to allow shaping; (3) ability for host tissue ingrowth/incorporation; (4) resistant to infection; (5) radiolucent; (6) cost permissive; and (7) durable with long-term mechanical integrity.[60,61] In addition, choice of prosthesis is an important component in the concept of "biomimesis" where the natural biological form and function of the chest wall are recreated.[62]

The only definitive conclusions that can be summed from the literature are that there is no perfect prosthetic material (**Table 2**) currently available and that any type of prosthetic material (rigid or flexible) can be used successfully in experienced hands.[54,57,59,61]

Flexible materials are the simplest to implant but sacrifice rigidity, which is optimal for preservation of respiratory mechanics. Porous materials seem to have the advantage of the capability for tissue ingrowth and thus greater resistance to infection. In the authors' experience, the lack of tissue incorporation of polytetrafluoroethylene (PTFE) leads to more frequent reintervention for infection. Methacrylate is the most common material used for rigid reconstruction of the chest wall. The creation of a composite of

Table 1
Examples of center-dependent preferences for chest wall resection

	# Pts	Prosthesis Flexible/ Rigid/ None	Skeletal Rsxn Rib Rsxn Sternal Rsxn	Pulmonary Complications	ID Complications	
Scarnecchia et al,[29] 2018, JTD	71	Prosthesis: 33 (49.3%) None: 36 (41 critical/30 noncritical)	Ribs mean 3 (2–6) Sternal rsxn: Total: 6 Partial: 4	10 pts (14%) In critical area: Recon: 5.7% Non: 100% Flail: 9 (6 non-recon)	No infection of chest wall prosthesis observed/ reported	Periop mortality: NR Morbidity: 45% R0 = 76%, 5-y OS 67% R1 = 24%, 5-y OS: 15%
Spicer et al,[59] 2016, Annals	427	Flex: 345 Rigid: 82 None: 20	Ribs—median Flex: 3 (1–6) Rigid: 3 (1–8) Sternal rsxn: Flex: 24 (6.9%) Rigid: 9 (11%)	102 (24%) Flex: 78 (22%) Rigid: 24 (29.3%) P=NS	Wound infect 12 (2.8%) Empyema 3 (0.7%)	30 d mortality: 1% 60 d mortality: 6% Median survival: 40 mo Preop: 12 • None for infected mesh • 1 broken strut • 11 = recurrence
Kachroo et al,[75] 2012, J Thor Oncol	51	Flex: 24 Rigid: 18 None: 9	Ribs—avg 3.7 (1–10)	2 (3.9%) Combo lung: 14 pt (27%)	Wound infection 2 (4%) Empyema 1 (2%)	Mortality: 0% Morbidity: 10 (20%)
Hanna et al,[76] 2011, Surgery	37	Flex: 18 Rigid: 0 None: 19	Ribs 3 or more: 38% Sternal rsxn: Total: 8 pt (22%) Partial: 1 pt (3%)	Combo lung rsxn: 3 pt (8%)	Wound infection 2 pt (5%) Remove prosthesis: 1 pt (5.5%)	Mortality: 0%

Study	N	Resection type	Resection details	Outcome	Complications	Mortality/Morbidity
Weyant et al,[57] 2006, Annals	262	Flex: 97 Rigid 112 None: 53	Ribs—median Flex: 3 (1-6) Rigid: 3 (1-8) None: 3 (1-4) Sternum: 49 pts Total: 6 (2.3%) Partial: 34 (14%) Manubrium: 9 (34)	29 (11%) Flex: 7 Rigid: 8 aP = NS 7 of 10 deaths	Wound infection 14 (5.3%) Flex: 3 Rigid: 9a Remove prosthesis Flex: 4 (4.1%) Rigid: 5 (4.5%)	Mortality: 3.8% Morbidity: 33.2% CWR + lung rsxn: mortality 5.6% • Pneumonectomy 44% Multivariate: Age (10-y increments) Lobe/pneumonectomy Size of defect
Mansour et al,[56] 2002, Annals	200	Flex: 82 Rigid: 11 None: 43	Ribs - Mean 4 (2-9) Sternal rsxn: 56 pts Total: 16 (8%) Hemi: 18 (9%)	38 pts (20%) Combo lung rsxn: 34%	Wound infection: (5%) • Remove prosthesis: 5%	Mortality: 7% Morbidity: 24% Immediate closure: 195
Walsh et al,[58] 2001, JTCVS	51	Flex: 16 Rigid: 18 None: 17	Ribs—avg 3.8 (1-9) Sternal resection: Total: 6 Partial: 5	4 pts (7.8%)	Wound infection: 3 (5.8%) Remove prosthesis: 2	Mortality: 0% Morbidity: 24%
Lardinois et al,[77] 2000, Annals	26	Flex: 0 Rigid: 2 None: 0 Flap: 17 (65.4%)	Rib rsxn—mean 4 (3-8) Sternal rsxn: 10 pt Total: 4 Partial 6	1 pg (3.8%) Combo lung-CWR: 12 (46%) • Pneumonectomy 2 Concordant chest movement: 92%	Wound infection: 2 (8%) Remove prosthesis: 2 (8%)	Mortality: 0% Morbidity: 22%

(continued on next page)

Table 1 (continued)					
	# Pts	Prosthesis Flexible/ Rigid/ None	Skeletal Rsxn Rib Rsxn Sternal Rsxn	Pulmonary Complications	ID Complications
Deschamps et al,[55] 1999, JTCVS	197	Flex: 197 Rigid: 0 None: 0	Rib rsxn—Median 3 (1–8) Sternal rsxn Total: 7 Partial: 46	48 pts (24.4%) Combo lung rsxn: 58 pts (29.4%) • Pneumo- nectomy: 13 pts, 4 of 8 deaths (50%)	Wound infection: 9 (4.6%) • Remove prosthesis: 3 pts (2.5%) (no subsequent recon) • 3 w/contaminated wound preop	Mortality: 4.1% Morbidity: 46.2% • Lung rsxn sig assoc with mortality ($P = .0002$) • 4 of 8 deaths after pneumonectomy
Arnold & Pairolero,[54] 1996, Plast Recon Surg	500	Flex: 171 Rigid: 14 None: 315	Ribs avg: 3.9 Sternal rsxn: 231 pts	Tracheostomy: 23 pt (4.6%)	Remove prosthesis: 1 pt (only with MMA)	Mortality: 3.0%

Abbreviations: Avg, average; CWR, chest wall resection; ID, infectious disease; MMA, methyl methacrylate; Preop, preoperative; Rsxn, resection.
[a] Rigid higher wound versus non, $P = 0.05$.
Data from Refs.[54–59,75–77]

Table 2
Prosthetic options for chest wall reconstruction

	Flexible	Rigid
Porous	Polypropylene • Marlex; Davol & Bard, Cranston, RI • Prolene; Ethicon Inc, Sumerville, NJ Polyglactin • Vicryl; Ethicon Inc, Somerville, NJ	Titanium mesh
Nonporous—synthetic	Polytetrafluoroethylene (PTFE)	Methyl methacrylate Titanium plates
Nonporous—Biologic	Acellular dermis • Cadaveric human • Porcine • Bovine Acellular pericardium • Bovine	Cadaveric homografts

methacrylate with porous mesh permits customized solutions. Similar to PTFE, methacrylate does not incorporate into the surrounding tissue and thus is at increased risk of wound seroma and infection. Wound complications are reported in 10% to 20% of patients with methacrylate prostheses; 5% ultimately require removal of the prosthesis.[63] The rigidity of methacrylate furthermore can be problematic in the environment of dynamic chest wall. This can lead to stress fractures and pain with breathing. Titanium mesh plate remains are gaining popularity as alternatives for rigid chest wall reconstruction. Of note, these applications remain "off label" and should be approached with caution. Rib plating systems, for instance, generally are restricted to traversing fairly small unsupported gaps in bone. The long-term stability and durability of plates over large bone gaps is unknown.

Use of muscle flaps

Most of the investigators advocate for ensuring that reconstruction of a chest wall defect includes the use of well-vascularized, myocutaneous tissue. This can be in the form of local advancement flaps (eg, pectoralis muscle for sternal defects) or distant transfer using pedicled, rotational, propeller, or free flap techniques.[64,65] The goals are to provide complete cutaneous coverage, obliterate dead space, prevent development of seromas, and optimize tissue ingrowth and mesh incorporation to minimize risk of infection.[54,66] Myocutaneous flap selection needs to be carefully planned with consideration for operative positioning, flap viability, and available conduits following radical tumor resection.

ADJUVANT RADIATION THERAPY

Radiation treatment can be considered as an adjuvant therapy for chest wall sarcomas. A 2020 review of the National Cancer Database of 1215 patients with primary chest wall sarcoma suggested a 20-month improvement in survival in those patients who received adjuvant radiotherapy, with high-grade tumors seeing the most benefit.[67] Local recurrence rates have generally been thought to be positively affected with radiation used in soft tissue sarcoma, allowing for potentially closer margins.[68,69] More controversy surrounds the role of radiotherapy with bone sarcoma. With Ewing sarcoma, radiotherapy has not shown consistent benefit in improving local control in the setting of a negative margin.[36] In a heterogenous population of 65 chest wall sarcoma patients, radiotherapy was associated with improved disease-free survival, with improved trends in mortality within patients undergoing chemoradiation + surgery as compared with surgery alone.[30]

ADJUVANT SYSTEMIC THERAPY

Despite numerous clinical trials and meta-analyses of these trials, the role of adjuvant chemotherapy in patients with soft tissue sarcoma of the extremity and chest wall has not been established, particularly with overall survival as the endpoint. Specific to chest wall literature, a single-institution 20-year experience, looking back at 65 patients with chest wall soft tissue sarcoma (only one BS included in the series), the authors showed 5- and 10-year disease-free survival improvement with the addition of chemotherapy, radiation therapy, or a combination of both to an index surgical operation.[30] Given the small numbers and heterogeneity of the histologies, definitive regimen recommendations could not be made. There is no proved role for chemotherapy in the treatment of chondrosarcoma. Ewing sarcoma has perhaps the strongest insight into systemic therapy. A pediatric oncology group review of 98 patients aged 30 years or older with Ewing sarcoma of the chest treated in 2 multiinstitutional trials concluded that neoadjuvant multiagent chemotherapy improved the likelihood of obtaining an R0 excision and decreased the likelihood for needing adjuvant radiotherapy.[70] Prior studies have shown the risk of radiation-associated malignancy higher in the child and adolescent population.[71] Osteosarcoma, as Ewing sarcoma, has shown improved survival with the addition of multiagent therapy as a gold standard, although clear margin resection of axial location skeletal osteosarcomas continues to be important for prognosis.[72] No chest wall location–specific recommendations for chemotherapy exist.[13]

REFERENCES

1. Available at: https://www.cancer.org/cancer/bone-cancer/about/key-statistics. html. Key Statistics for Bone Cancer. Accessed April 27, 2020.
2. Available at: https://www.cancer.org/cancer/soft-tissue-sarcoma/about/key-statistics.html. Key Statistics for Soft Tissue Sarcomas. Accessed April 27, 2020.
3. Lawrence W Jr, Donegan WL, Natarajan N, et al. Adult soft tissue sarcomas. A pattern of care survey of the American College of Surgeons. Ann Surg 1987; 205:349–59.
4. Shewale JB, Mitchell KG, Nelson DB, et al. Predictors of survival after resection of primary sarcomas of the chest wall-A large, single-institution series. J Surg Oncol 2018;118:518–24.
5. van Geel AN, Wouters MW, Lans TE, et al. Chest wall resection for adult soft tissue sarcomas and chondrosarcomas: analysis of prognostic factors. World J Surg 2011;35:63–9.
6. Thomas M, Shen KR. Primary Tumors of the Osseous Chest Wall and Their Management. Thorac Surg Clin 2017;27:181–93.
7. Schuetze SM, Rubin BP, Vernon C, et al. Use of positron emission tomography in localized extremity soft tissue sarcoma treated with neoadjuvant chemotherapy. Cancer 2005;103:339–48.
8. Kopp LM, Hu C, Rozo B, et al. Utility of bone marrow aspiration and biopsy in initial staging of Ewing sarcoma. Pediatr Blood Cancer 2015;62:12–5.
9. Newman EN, Jones RL, Hawkins DS. An evaluation of [F-18]-fluorodeoxy-D-glucose positron emission tomography, bone scan, and bone marrow

aspiration/biopsy as staging investigations in Ewing sarcoma. Pediatr Blood Cancer 2013;60:1113–7.

10. Salamon J, Mautner VF, Adam G, et al. Multimodal Imaging in Neurofibromatosis Type 1-associated Nerve Sheath Tumors. Rofo 2015;187:1084–92.

11. Treglia G, Taralli S, Bertagna F, et al. Usefulness of whole-body fluorine-18-fluorodeoxyglucose positron emission tomography in patients with neurofibromatosis type 1: a systematic review. Radiol Res Pract 2012;2012:431029.

12. Van Der Gucht A, Zehou O, Djelbani-Ahmed S, et al. Metabolic Tumour Burden Measured by 18F-FDG PET/CT Predicts Malignant Transformation in Patients with Neurofibromatosis Type-1. PLoS One 2016;11:e0151809.

13. Biermann JS, Chow W, Reed DR, et al. NCCN Guidelines Insights: Bone Cancer, Version 2.2017. J Natl Compr Canc Netw 2017;15:155–67.

14. von Mehren M, Randall RL, Benjamin RS, et al. Soft Tissue Sarcoma, Version 2.2018, NCCN Clinical Practice Guidelines in Oncology. J Natl Compr Canc Netw 2018;16:536–63.

15. Schwab JH, Healey JH. FDG-PET Lacks Sufficient Sensitivity to Detect Myxoid Liposarcoma Spinal Metastases Detected by MRI. Sarcoma 2007;2007:36785.

16. Hanna SA, Qureshi YA, Bayliss L, et al. Late widespread skeletal metastases from myxoid liposarcoma detected by MRI only. World J Surg Oncol 2008;6:62.

17. Lin S, Gan Z, Han K, et al. Metastasis of myxoid liposarcoma to fat-bearing areas: A case report of unusual metastatic sites and a hypothesis. Oncol Lett 2015;10: 2543–6.

18. Sakamoto A, Fukutoku Y, Matsumoto Y, et al. Myxoid liposarcoma with negative features on bone scan and [18F]-2-fluoro-2-deoxy-D-glucose-positron emission tomography. World J Surg Oncol 2012;10:214.

19. Stevenson JD, Watson JJ, Cool P, et al. Whole-body magnetic resonance imaging in myxoid liposarcoma: A useful adjunct for the detection of extra-pulmonary metastatic disease. Eur J Surg Oncol 2016;42:574–80.

20. Beltrami G, Ristori G, Scoccianti G, et al. Hereditary Multiple Exostoses: a review of clinical appearance and metabolic pattern. Clin Cases Miner Bone Metab 2016;13:110–8.

21. O'Neill AC, Tirumani SH, Do WS, et al. Metastatic Patterns of Solitary Fibrous Tumors: A Single-Institution Experience. AJR Am J Roentgenol 2017;208:2–9.

22. Barrientos-Ruiz I, Ortiz-Cruz EJ, Serrano-Montilla J, et al. Are Biopsy Tracts a Concern for Seeding and Local Recurrence in Sarcomas? Clin Orthop Relat Res 2017;475:511–8.

23. Blay JY, Honore C, Stoeckle E, et al. Surgery in reference centers improves survival of sarcoma patients: a nationwide study. Ann Oncol 2019;30:1407.

24. Blay JY, Soibinet P, Penel N, et al. Improved survival using specialized multidisciplinary board in sarcoma patients. Ann Oncol 2017;28:2852–9.

25. Hoekstra HJ, Haas RLM, Verhoef C, et al. Adherence to Guidelines for Adult (Non-GIST) Soft Tissue Sarcoma in the Netherlands: A Plea for Dedicated Sarcoma Centers. Ann Surg Oncol 2017;24:3279–88.

26. Chintamani. Soft tissue sarcomas-the pitfalls in diagnosis and management!! Indian J Surg Oncol 2011;2:261–4.

27. David EA, Marshall MB. Review of chest wall tumors: a diagnostic, therapeutic, and reconstructive challenge. Semin Plast Surg 2011;25:16–24.

28. King RM, Pairolero PC, Trastek VF, et al. Primary chest wall tumors: factors affecting survival. Ann Thorac Surg 1986;41:597–601.

29. Scarnecchia E, Liparulo V, Capozzi R, et al. Chest wall resection and reconstruction for tumors: analysis of oncological and functional outcome. J Thorac Dis 2018;10:S1855–63.

30. Burt A, Berriochoa J, Korpak A, et al. Treatment of chest wall sarcomas: a single-institution experience over 20 years. Am J Clin Oncol 2015;38:80–6.

31. Gerrand CH, Wunder JS, Kandel RA, et al. Classification of positive margins after resection of soft-tissue sarcoma of the limb predicts the risk of local recurrence. J Bone Joint Surg Br 2001;83:1149–55.

32. O'Donnell PW, Griffin AM, Eward WC, et al. The effect of the setting of a positive surgical margin in soft tissue sarcoma. Cancer 2014;120:2866–75.

33. Provost B, Missenard G, Pricopi C, et al. Ewing Sarcoma of the Chest Wall: Prognostic Factors of Multimodal Therapy Including En Bloc Resection. Ann Thorac Surg 2018;106:207–13.

34. Fong YC, Pairolero PC, Sim FH, et al. Chondrosarcoma of the chest wall: a retrospective clinical analysis. Clin Orthop Relat Res 2004;184–9.

35. Lenze U, Angelini A, Pohlig F, et al. Chondrosarcoma of the Chest Wall: A Review of 53 Cases from Two Institutions. Anticancer Res 2020;40:1519–26.

36. Bedetti B, Wiebe K, Ranft A, et al. Local control in Ewing sarcoma of the chest wall: results of the EURO-EWING 99 trial. Ann Surg Oncol 2015;22:2853–9.

37. Saenz NC, Hass DJ, Meyers P, et al. Pediatric chest wall Ewing's sarcoma. J Pediatr Surg 2000;35:550–5.

38. Chapelier AR, Bacha EA, de Montpreville VT, et al. Radical resection of radiation-induced sarcoma of the chest wall: report of 15 cases. Ann Thorac Surg 1997;63:214–9.

39. Kara HV, Gandolfi BM, Williams JB, et al. Multidisciplinary approach to treatment of radiation-induced chest wall sarcoma. Gen Thorac Cardiovasc Surg 2016;64:492–5.

40. Chandrasekar CR, Wafa H, Grimer RJ, et al. The effect of an unplanned excision of a soft-tissue sarcoma on prognosis. J Bone Joint Surg Br 2008;90:203–8.

41. Fiore M, Casali PG, Miceli R, et al. Prognostic effect of re-excision in adult soft tissue sarcoma of the extremity. Ann Surg Oncol 2006;13:110–7.

42. Lewis JJ, Leung D, Espat J, et al. Effect of reresection in extremity soft tissue sarcoma. Ann Surg 2000;231:655–63.

43. Venkatesan M, Richards CJ, McCulloch TA, et al. Inadvertent surgical resection of soft tissue sarcomas. Eur J Surg Oncol 2012;38:346–51.

44. Alamanda VK, Delisca GO, Mathis SL, et al. The financial burden of reexcising incompletely excised soft tissue sarcomas: a cost analysis. Ann Surg Oncol 2013;20:2808–14.

45. Mesko NW, Wilson RJ, Lawrenz JM, et al. Pre-operative evaluation prior to soft tissue sarcoma excision - Why can't we get it right? Eur J Surg Oncol 2018;44:243–50.

46. Angelini A, Mavrogenis AF, Rimondi E, et al. Current concepts for the diagnosis and management of eosinophilic granuloma of bone. J Orthop Traumatol 2017;18:83–90.

47. Desmoid Tumor Working G. The management of desmoid tumours: A joint global consensus-based guideline approach for adult and paediatric patients. Eur J Cancer 2020;127:96–107.

48. Kasper B, Baumgarten C, Garcia J, et al. An update on the management of sporadic desmoid-type fibromatosis: a European Consensus Initiative between Sarcoma PAtients EuroNet (SPAEN) and European Organization for Research and

Treatment of Cancer (EORTC)/Soft Tissue and Bone Sarcoma Group (STBSG). Ann Oncol 2017;28:2399–408.

49. Griffin MO, Kulkarni NM, O'Connor SD, et al. Magnetic Resonance-Guided Focused Ultrasound: A Brief Review With Emphasis on the Treatment of Extra-abdominal Desmoid Tumors. Ultrasound Q 2019;35:346–54.

50. Redifer Tremblay K, Lea WB, Neilson JC, et al. Percutaneous cryoablation for the treatment of extra-abdominal desmoid tumors. J Surg Oncol 2019;120:366–75.

51. Reddy KI, Sinnaeve F, Gaston CL, et al. Aneurysmal bone cysts: do simple treatments work? Clin Orthop Relat Res 2014;472:1901–10.

52. Shiels WE 2nd, Mayerson JL. Percutaneous doxycycline treatment of aneurysmal bone cysts with low recurrence rate: a preliminary report. Clin Orthop Relat Res 2013;471:2675–83.

53. Woon JTK, Hoon D, Graydon A, et al. Aneurysmal bone cyst treated with percutaneous doxycycline: is a single treatment sufficient? Skeletal Radiol 2019;48: 765–71.

54. Arnold PG, Pairolero PC. Chest-wall reconstruction: an account of 500 consecutive patients. Plast Reconstr Surg 1996;98:804–10.

55. Deschamps C, Tirnaksiz BM, Darbandi R, et al. Early and long-term results of prosthetic chest wall reconstruction. J Thorac Cardiovasc Surg 1999;117: 588–91 [discussion: 91–2].

56. Mansour KA, Thourani VH, Losken A, et al. Chest wall resections and reconstruction: a 25-year experience. Ann Thorac Surg 2002;73:1720–5 [discussion: 5–6].

57. Weyant MJ, Bains MS, Venkatraman E, et al. Results of chest wall resection and reconstruction with and without rigid prosthesis. Ann Thorac Surg 2006;81: 279–85.

58. Walsh GL, Davis BM, Swisher SG, et al. A single-institutional, multidisciplinary approach to primary sarcomas involving the chest wall requiring full-thickness resections. J Thorac Cardiovasc Surg 2001;121:48–60.

59. Spicer JD, Shewale JB, Antonoff MB, et al. The Influence of Reconstructive Technique on Perioperative Pulmonary and Infectious Outcomes Following Chest Wall Resection. Ann Thorac Surg 2016;102:1653–9.

60. LeRoux BTS DM. Resection of tumors of the chest wall. Curr Probl Surg 1983;20: 345–86.

61. Khullar OV, Fernandez FG. Prosthetic Reconstruction of the Chest Wall. Thorac Surg Clin 2017;27:201–8.

62. Rocco G. Chest wall resection and reconstruction according to the principles of biomimesis. Semin Thorac Cardiovasc Surg 2011;23:307–13.

63. Sanna S, Brandolini J, Pardolesi A, et al. Materials and techniques in chest wall reconstruction: a review. J Vis Surg 2017;3:95.

64. Crowley TP, Atkinson K, Bayliss CD, et al. The surgical management of sarcomas of the chest wall: A 13-year single institution experience. J Plast Reconstr Aesthet Surg ;73(8):1448-1455;August 01,2020.

65. Merritt RE. Chest Wall Reconstruction Without. Prosthetic Mater Thorac Surg Clin 2017;27:165–9.

66. Losken A, Thourani VH, Carlson GW, et al. A reconstructive algorithm for plastic surgery following extensive chest wall resection. Br J Plast Surg 2004;57: 295–302.

67. Rehmani SS, Raad W, Weber J, et al. Adjuvant Radiation Therapy for Thoracic Soft Tissue Sarcomas: A Population-Based Analysis. Ann Thorac Surg 2020; 109:203–10.

68. Ahmad R, Jacobson A, Hornicek F, et al. The width of the surgical margin does not influence outcomes in extremity and truncal soft tissue sarcoma treated with radiotherapy. Oncologist 2016;21:1269–76.

69. Gundle KR, Kafchinski L, Gupta S, et al. Analysis of margin classification systems for assessing the risk of local recurrence after soft tissue sarcoma resection. J Clin Oncol 2018;36:704–9.

70. Shamberger RC, LaQuaglia MP, Gebhardt MC, et al. Ewing sarcoma/primitive neuroectodermal tumor of the chest wall: impact of initial versus delayed resection on tumor margins, survival, and use of radiation therapy. Ann Surg 2003;238:563–7 [discussion: 7–8].

71. Paulussen M, Ahrens S, Lehnert M, et al. Second malignancies after ewing tumor treatment in 690 patients from a cooperative German/Austrian/Dutch study. Ann Oncol 2001;12:1619–30.

72. Smeland S, Bielack SS, Whelan J, et al. Survival and prognosis with osteosarcoma: outcomes in more than 2000 patients in the EURAMOS-1 (European and American Osteosarcoma Study) cohort. Eur J Cancer 2019;109:36–50.

73. Demicco EG, Park MS, Araujo DM, et al. Solitary fibrous tumor: a clinicopathological study of 110 cases and proposed risk assessment model. Mod Pathol 2012;25:1298–306.

74. Gold JS, Antonescu CR, Hajdu C, et al. Clinicopathologic correlates of solitary fibrous tumors. Cancer 2002;94:1057–68.

75. Kachroo P, Pak PS, Sandha HS, et al. Single-institution, multidisciplinary experience with surgical resection of primary chest wall sarcomas. J Thorac Oncol 2012;7:552–8.

76. Hanna WC, Ferri LE, McKendy KM, et al. Reconstruction after major chest wall resection: can rigid fixation be avoided? Surgery 2011;150:590–7.

77. Lardinois D, Muller M, Furrer M, et al. Functional assessment of chest wall integrity after methylmethacrylate reconstruction. Ann Thorac Surg 2000;69:919–23.

Current Indications for Pulmonary Metastasectomy

Monisha Sudarshan, MD, MPH*, Sudish C. Murthy, MD, PhD

KEYWORDS

- Metastases • Metastasectomy • Pulmonary nodule • Oligometastases
- Lung resection

KEY POINTS

- Eligibility for pulmonary metastasectomy includes confirming operative candidacy, complete resection of metastases with surgery, and control of the primary cancer.
- Positive prognostic factors include longer disease-free interval, lack of lymphadenopathy, single metastatic nodule, and certain primary histologies, such as nonseminomatous germ cell tumor.
- Parenchymal preserving techniques (wedge resection and segmentectomy) via minimally invasive surgery is the preferred method for surgical metastasectomy if feasible.
- Nonoperative techniques include stereotactic body radiation therapy, radiofrequency ablation, and microwave ablation.

INTRODUCTION

With its large surface area and blood flow, it is not surprising that the lung is one of the most common site of metastases. Accordingly, pulmonary metastasectomy has been long practiced in the field of oncology ,with one of the first reports from 1882[1] reviewing the removal of lung sarcoma metastases. Since initial reports, the field has advanced, with the International Registry of Lung Metastases in 1991 reporting on 5206 metastasectomy cases, with an overall 5-year survival of 13% to 36%, depending on primary tumor biology.[2] More recently a European Society of Thoracic Surgeons (ESTS) international work group evaluated the outcomes of pulmonary metastasectomy[3] and reported similar results. Definitive recommendations are limited due to lack of robust studies and randomized controlled trials. Selection bias among retrospective studies, variable adjuvant therapies, and variable follow-up length are consistent limitations.[4] The absence of a standard-of-care approach underscores the importance of multidisciplinary review and case-by-case consideration when evaluating a patient for pulmonary metastasectomy (**Fig. 1**).

General Thoracic Surgery, Thoracic and Cardiovascular Surgery, Cleveland Clinic, 9500 Euclid Avenue, J4-1, Cleveland, OH 44195, USA
* Corresponding author. 9500 Euclid Avenue, J4-1, Cleveland, OH 44195, USA.
E-mail address: SUDARSM2@ccf.org

Surg Oncol Clin N Am 29 (2020) 673–683
https://doi.org/10.1016/j.soc.2020.06.007
surgonc.theclinics.com

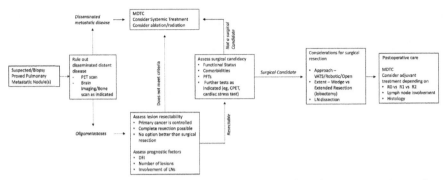

Fig. 1. Approach to the pulmonary metastases. CPET, cardiopulmonary exercise testing; MDTC, multidisciplinary tumor conference; PFTs, pulmonary function tests.

This review explores work-up of pulmonary metastases, principles for resection eligibility, outcomes of different primary histology, and alternatives to surgical resection. The goal is to attempt to create evidence-based guidelines to help guide management.

PATIENT ASSESSMENT

Evaluation of the patient with pulmonary metastases begins with a targeted history and physical examination. Generally, pulmonary metastases are asymptomatic and specific symptoms may well indicate advanced disease. However, 15% to 20% of patients can present with symptoms that include cough, hemoptysis, chest pain, or postobstructive pneumonia.[5,6] Symptoms and signs of distant metastatic disease also must be elicited. Smoking history and use of pertinent medications, including anticoagulants and steroids, are critical part of the medical history, specifically, prior history of venous thromboembolism—a frequent comorbid disease in this population.

Physical examination should focus on overall status, cardiopulmonary assessment, lymph node (LN) basin examination, and abdominal examination focusing on hepatospenomegaly.

A subjective impression of the patient's functional status can be achieved by enquiring about activities of daily living (ADLs) and instrumental activities of daily living. Scores, such as the Eastern Cooperative Oncology Group Performance Status, and Karnofsky performance scale, originally validated for suitability of systemic therapy, also can be used to complement assessment of performance status in the oncology patient.[7] Formal testing, such as 6-minute walk, shuttle walk, and stair climb, provide objective measurements for performance status, lung resection reserve, and a real-time objective assessment of physiologic reserve.[8]

RADIOLOGIC STUDIES

Pertinent imaging includes high-resolution computed tomography (CT) scan with 1-mm to 2-mm slices for assessment of pulmonary nodules and a PET scan to rule out other distant metastases. The sensitivity of PET scan varies according to histology of pulmonary metastasis. In a series by Fortes and colleagues,[9] PET scan was found positive for two-thirds of pulmonary metastases. This varied from 44% for sarcoma to 71% for renal cell carcinoma.[9,10] In general, approximately 3 out of 4 patients with pulmonary metastatic disease have other distant metastasis.[11] Completion of staging for metastatic disease in addition to PET scan can be supplemented with bone scan. Additional brain imaging, such as CT brain or magnetic resonance imaging brain, can be tailored to the histology of pulmonary disease.

The presence of hilar or mediastinal LN metastases is associated with poor prognosis. Presence of lymphadenopathy should prompt invasive mediastinal staging (mediastinoscopy or endobronchial ultrasound-guided fine-needle biopsy). Preoperative confirmation of malignant metastatic LNs does not necessarily preclude surgical resection of the pulmonary tumor(s) but the additional metastatic burden reduces the chance for a complete resection and requires careful multidisciplinary consideration before proceeding.[12]

Standard criteria used for pulmonary resection should be applied in the setting of pulmonary metastasectomy (adequate spirometry and gas exchange). Most metastasectomies are nonanatomic resections, although, depending on location, some may require lobectomies or other extended resections. Postoperative predictive forced expiratory volume in the first second of expiration and diffusion capacity for carbon monoxide above 60% generally are satisfactory to proceed with resection. Values between 30% and 60% should prompt further testing, such as shuttle walk or stair climb tests and/or perfusion-ventilation scan, for further evaluation. Values less than 30% should employ cardiopulmonary exercise testing for further evaluation.[13] Thorough risk stratification becomes increasingly important as a patient's fitness declines.

ELIGIBILITY FOR PULMONARY METASTASECTOMY

Although there is a lack of strict criteria in selecting for pulmonary metastases resection, there are a few agreed-on tenets.[14] (1) First and foremost, the patient should be a fit candidate to undergo surgical resection. (2) Once surgical eligibility is confirmed, the primary cancer must be either controlled or controllable. (3) Ideally, there should be no extrathoracic metastasis; however, if present it also must be resectable or already resected successfully. (4) Surgery should completely resect the pulmonary metastases. Patients with R1 or R2 resection have poor longer-term prognosis and an incomplete resection subjects patients to the unnecessary risk of surgery with no benefit.[12] (5) Furthermore, there should be no better proved treatment option than operative intervention existing to treat the metastasis. In current times of evolving targeted, immune, and chimeric T-cell therapy, this is perhaps the most important consideration.

PROGNOSTIC FACTORS

Primary tumor histology is the most important prognostic factor for overall survival (OS) after pulmonary metastasectomy. Germ cell tumor metastases are associated with excellent long-term outcomes, reflected by approximately 70% 5-year survival and approximately 60% 10-year survival.[2]

Disease-free interval (DFI) between primary tumor control and emergence of metastasis is an important but somewhat confounded risk factor. Several studies indicate that a longer DFI interval is associated with improved outcomes after resection. It is unclear if the indolent nature of the tumor biology associated with a longer DFI is truly responsible for the better outcomes rather than the actual disease-free time frame. In addition, the definition of DFI is somewhat variable among studies, making simple comparisons challenging. There is no consensus on minimum DFI to rule in or rule out metastasectomy. Very short intervals or synchronous metastases warrant consideration of systemic therapy and a period of observation to rule out emergence of other distant metastases. Increasing numbers of metastatic nodules and in some studies the laterality can portend a poor prognosis. Incomplete resection or positive surgical margins are nearly universally associated with poorer survival,[12] as discussed later.

OPERATIVE TECHNIQUES FOR PULMONARY METASTASECTOMY

Initial limitations of imaging propagated the need for open surgery and bimanual palpation of pulmonary nodules. McCormack and colleagues[15] performed initial video-assisted thoracoscopic surgery [VATS] resections based on the preoperative radiological evaluation; then, a thoracotomy was performed with bimanual palpation for completeness. They found that 56% of patients had additional metastatic lesions detected after VATS on bimanual palpation.[15] Other studies have demonstrated 16% to 46% of lesions identified on palpation that were not evident on preoperative CT scans.[16,17] Long and colleagues[18] have attempted bilateral hand-assisted thoracoscopy through a single sternocostal incision. They found 53% of patients with bilateral metastases were noted to have only unilateral disease on preoperative staging.

In all of these studies, however, not all additional lesions are malignant, and, in addition, there is no proved survival benefit with the resection of small lesions undetected by CT scan. Furthermore, modern high-resolution CT scanning with 1-mm slices has vastly improved detection of subcentimeter nodules, with sensitivity of 97% and negative predictive value of 96%,[19] obviating bimanual palpation.

Current studies demonstrate comparable rates in survival and cancer recurrence between VATS and open techniques of between 30.6% and 69%.[20,21] Given no apparent survival difference, the clinical significance of resection of radiologically undetected metastases is questionable. Thoracoscopic methods have demonstrated improved pain scores and shorter length of stay. Minimally invasive methods also aid in resection of bilateral lesions, and may simplify future re-resection, and generally are the standard of care for pulmonary metastasectomy.

Preservation of uninvolved pulmonary parenchyma is a key consideration. To this end, nonanatomic (wedge) resection to negative margins is the most common intervention. For patients with several foci that are being targeted, multiple stapled wedge resections within the same lobe can lead to significant distortion of the lobar architecture and consume a significant amount of uninvolved parenchyma. Consequently, fine-tip electrocautery resection is an alternative that is commonly considered during open techniques for patients with higher-burden (resectable) disease when stapled resection may not be ideal. The small parenchymal defects created can be suture repaired after hemostasis is obtained.[22] Central lesions or multiple metastases in 1 lobe may warrant a lobectomy. The indication for a more extensive resection, however, requires review in a multidisciplinary manner. The need for a pneumonectomy is not an absolute contraindication; however, it is associated with significant risk and is accompanied by variable long-term survival. Careful patient selection is key and may be considered in a patient with a soft tissue or bone tumor primary, a long DFI, and a central tumor.[23]

The need for routine lymphadenectomy during pulmonary metastasectomy is debatable and the practice of thoracic surgeons is variable.

In the International Registry of Lung Metastases published in 1997, only 5% of the patients had LN metastases reported, but LN dissection was performed in a minority of patients.[2] Recent single-institution reports have challenged these numbers. Hamaji and colleagues[24] described 500 pulmonary metastasectomy patients, of whom 319 received LN dissection. Positive LN metastases were found in 12.5% (40/319).[24] In another study of 270 resections by Seebacher and colleagues,[25] the incidence of LN involvement was 17%. Unexpected LN involvement was found in 36% of patients with breast cancer, in 21% with renal cell carcinoma, and in 9.2% with colorectal cancer. In an ESTS survey, 55% of surgeons indicated they sampled LNs, 13% completed a lymphadenectomy, and 3.2% did not remove any LNs.[26]

LN metastases clearly can complicate pulmonary metastatic disease. The specific risks for concomitant LN disease are difficult to quantify aside from primary histology. How the number and size of the metastases are associated with risk of LN involvement is unclear.[27] LN involvement is a risk factor for worse survival; positive LN sare associated with a 0% to 24% 5-year survival, whereas negative LNs have a 24.7% to 50% 5-year survival.[28] The prognostic value of specific LN station is unclear. One study demonstrated an approximately 64-month survival with N1 disease, approximately 33-month survival with N2 disease, and an approximately 21-month survival with N3 disease.[29] Other studies, however, demonstrate no survival differences between involvement of any of these stations.[30]

The remaining question when investigating LNs in the context of pulmonary metastasectomy is performing a lymphadenectomy or LN sampling. Extrapolating results from the lung cancer study by American College of Surgery Oncology Group Z0030 showing no difference between the 2, most clinicians would agree that LN sampling might be sufficient for diagnostic information, although therapeutic implications remain nebulous.[31]

TUMOR-TYPE SPECIFIC OUTCOMES

Several studies on pulmonary metastasectomy combine histologies. Tumor type, however, exerts significant influence on outcomes after metastasectomy. First-time metastasectomy is established but recurrent pulmonary metastasis, which meets resection eligibility, also should be treat surgically.[32] Overall, the true survival benefit from resection of pulmonary metastasis is debatable due to lack of controls. Some experts may argue that prolonged survival after metastasectomy is observed due to a favorable patient selection (better tumor biology and patient characteristics).

Germ Cell Tumors

Pulmonary metastasectomy for germ cell tumor, specifically nonseminomatous germ cell tumor (NSGCT), is associated with excellent, if not one of the best, outcomes among primary histology. NSGCT pulmonary metastases are initially treated with systemic therapy because they are chemosensitive.[33] Persistent disease results in approximately 10% of these lesions progressing to surgical resection. A recent series by Kesler and colleagues[34] examining 159 pulmonary resections demonstrated a 68% 5-year OS. Residual disease was an important factor in decreased survival. Overall, almost 75% of patients had a benign transformation (52.7% of patients had a teratoma and 21.5% necrosis) and 25% had persistent malignancy (15% residual NSGCT and 10.1% degenerative non–germ cell cancer).[34]

Colorectal

Metastatic colorectal cancer has significant organ tropism for the lungs. This, combined with the high prevalence of colorectal cancer, makes pulmonary metastasectomy a common indication. Hepatic metastasectomy in selected patients has been well established in the literature. Pulmonary metastasectomy for colorectal metastases has also been widely practiced, although the survival benefit is debated. Estimated 5-year survival is 32% to 54%.[35] Studies of prognostic markers are ongoing in order to select patient who will receive the most benefit. KRAS and mBRAF mutations are associated with poorer outcomes, such as early pulmonary recurrence, more diffuse pulmonary disease, and decreased survival.[36]

Sarcomas

Sarcomas are histologically diverse and survival comparisons of pulmonary metastasectomy remains controversial among each subtype. Smaller series do not demonstrate significant survival difference[37,38] yet other series show a comparable median survival of 27 months for patients with osteosarcoma and approximately 42 months for patients with soft tissue sarcoma.[39] In 62% of patients with metastatic sarcoma, the lung was the sole metastatic site,[40] and, because sarcoma is relatively resistant to chemotherapy or radiotherapy, resection often becomes the principal treatment of patients. Outcomes for osteogenic sarcoma metastasectomy range from 35% to 50% 5-year survival. A recent study by Kim and colleagues[38] demonstrated 5-year OS of 50%. DFI less than 12 months, positive margin, and more than 2 lesions of size greater 3 cm were associated with worse survival.

In soft tissue sarcomas, a large series of 225 patients demonstrated a 5-year survival of 38%,[41] although up to 50% survival with careful patient selection has been noted.[42] Again longer disease-free survival and fewer nodules were associated with better survival.

Breast

Pulmonary metastasis is found in approximately 7% to 24% of breast cancer patients.[43] In addition to short DFI, fewer metastatic lesions, and complete resection, patients with hormone receptor–positive disease appear to have a more favorable outcomes (77% 5-year survival vs 12% in receptor-negative patients).[44] A large meta-analysis of 1937 patients yielded a 5-year survival of 46% after pulmonary metastases resection[45] versus 16% in patients with limited metastasis to lung treated with systemic therapy.[46] Similar to other studies, a direct comparison is challenging due to selection bias.

Melanoma

Lung is the most common visceral site for melanoma metastasis, and isolated metastases is associated with significantly higher survival in comparison to other visceral sites (liver and brain).[47] Survival at 5 years after metastasectomy is up to 40% in selected patients with small tumors (<2 cm) and a single metastatic lesion.[48] The advent of checkpoint inhibitors has drastically improved the outcomes of metastatic melanoma. In this context, pulmonary metastasectomy also can be considered for residual pulmonary metastasis after immunotherapy.[4]

Head and neck

The challenge in head and neck cancer metastases to the lung is distinguishing true metastasis from primary squamous lung cancer. With similar risk factors, histology, epithelial cell origin, and a lack of definitive techniques to differentiate the 2 different cancers, the outcomes of pulmonary metastasectomy for head and neck squamous cell cancers (HNSCCs) often is confounded with a primary lung squamous cell cancer.[49] A DFI less than a year is of especially poor prognosis, with 0% 5-year OS in some series.[50,51] In well-selected patients, 5-year OS up to 59% is reported.[52]

Retrospective studies matching surgical and nonsurgical treatment of HNCC metastasis demonstrate a survival advantage with longer median survival (19.4 months vs 5 months, respectively[53]). Therefore, HNSCC metastasis with DFI more than a year and other general favorable characteristics, including lack of LN involvement, should be considered for surgical resection.[4]

NONOPERATIVE TECHNIQUES FOR PULMONARY METASTASECTOMY

Surgery is the first-line approach for patients who can tolerate the resection and meet metastasectomy criteria. For those who are not deemed surgical candidates, however, ablative therapy presents an alternative option. Stereotactic body radiation therapy (SBRT), radiofrequency ablation (RFA), and microwave ablation (MWA) are the principal nonoperative ablative interventions.

Traditionally, radiation therapy has been employed in a palliative therapy role for lung metastases.[54] Retrospective reports, however, demonstrate a good control rate for stereotactic radiation in the pulmonary metastases setting as well with lesion control, observed in 75% to 90% patients[55] at 3 years. Direct comparisons between studies is difficult due to different histologies, varying total radiation doses, and fractions. Interpretation of OS also is challenging due to the selection bias within the cohort. One retrospective comparison[56] of 27 patients with 70-Gy SBRT and 31 resections for osteosarcoma metastasis demonstrated comparable OS between the 2 groups. No significant differences in OS and disease-free survival have been found when comparing SBRT and surgical metastasectomy.[57–59] Most institutions use certain criteria to consider SBRT for pulmonary metastases, such as poor surgical candidate, central lesions, and short DFI.

RFA utilizes an alternative current to cause coagulative necrosis. Pneumothoraces are a frequent complication reported in 25% to 40% of patients,[60,61] when applied to lung metastases. RFA is employed very selectively in lung tumors. Masses greater than 3 cm and those near blood vessels generally are avoided.[62,63] MWA uses much higher frequencies and hyperthermia to effect tumor ablation. As with SBRT, RFA and MWA are alternative options when eligibility for metastasectomy are satisfied but the patient is not a surgical candidate. Furthermore, these 2 ablative options can be used in a previously radiated field.

FUTURE DIRECTION

The only randomized controlled trial conducted (Pulmonary Metastasectomy versus Continued Active Monitoring in Colorectal Cancer[64]) was closed early due to recruitment issues. Although it was underpowered, the estimated 5-year survival rate was 38% for metastasectomy patients and 29% in the well-matched controls.[64] Prospective studies and trials that compare systemic and targeted therapies to ablation and surgical resection will be key in advancing the field. As the use of immunotherapy becomes more prevalent in locally advanced and metastatic cancer, its role in treatment of isolated lung metastases and oligometastases will become prominent, and treatment paradigms no doubt will need to be adjusted.

REFERENCES

1. Weinlechner JW. Tumoren an der brustwand und deren behnadlung resection der rippeneroffnung der brusthohle und partielle entfernung der lunge. Wien Med Wochenschr 1882;32:589–91.

2. Pastorino U, Buse M, Friedel G, et al. Long term results of lung metastasectomy: prognostic analyses based on 5206 cases. J Thorac Cardiovasc Surg 1997;113: 37–49.

3. Van Raemdonck D, Friedel G. The European Society of Thoracic Surgeons lung metastasectomy project. J Thorac Oncol 2010;5:S127–9.

4. Handy JR, Bremner RM, Crocenzi TS, et al. Expert consensus document on pulmonary metastasectomy. Ann Thorac Surg 2019;107:631–49.

5. Ripley RT, Downey RJ. Pulmonary metastasectomy. J Surg Oncol 2014;109:42–6.

6. Kon Z, Martin L. Resection for thoracic metastases from sarcoma. Oncology 2011;25:1198–204.

7. Kelly C, Shahrokni A. Moving beyond Karnofsky and ECOG performance status assessments with new technologies. J Oncol 2016;2016:6186543.

8. Ha D, Mazzone PJ, Ries AL, et al. The utility of exercise testing in patients with lung cancer. J Thorac Oncol 2016;11(9):1397–410.

9. Fortes DL, Allen MS, Lowe VJ, et al. The sensitivity of 18F- flurodeoxyglucose positron emission tomography in the evaluation of metastatic pulmonary nodules. Eur J Cardiothorac Surg 2008;34:1223–7.

10. Mayerhoefer ME, Prosch H, Herold CJ, et al. Assessment of pulmonary melanoma metastases with 18 F-FDG PET/CT: which PET-negative patients require additional tests for definitive staging? Eur Radiol 2012;22:2451–7.

11. Erhunmwunsee L, Tong B. Preoperative evaluation and indications for pulmonary metastasectomy. Thorac Surg Clin 2016;26:7–12.

12. Murthy SC, Kim K, Rice TW, et al. Can we predict long term survival after pulmonary metastasectomy for renal cell carcinoma? Ann Thorac Surg 2005;79: 996–1003.

13. Datta D, Lahiri B. Preoperative evaluation of patients undergoing lung resection surgery. Chest 2003;123(6):2096.

14. Kondo H, Okumura T, Ohde Y, et al. Surgical treatment for metastatic malignancies. Pulmonary metastasis: indications and outcomes. Int J Clin Oncol 2005;10(2):81–5.

15. McCormack PM, Bains MS, Begg CB, et al. Role of video-assisted thoracic surgery in the treatment of pulmonary metastases: results of a prospective trial. Ann Thorac Surg 1996;62(1):213–6 [discussion: 216–7].

16. Kayton ML1, Huvos AG, Casher J, et al. Computed tomographic scan of the chest underestimates the number of metastatic lesions in osteosarcoma. J Pediatr Surg 2006;41(1):200–6.

17. Cerfolio RJ, McCarty T, Bryant AS. Non-imaged pulmonary nodules discovered during thoracotomy for metastasectomy by lung palpation. Eur J Cardiothorac Surg 2009;35(5):786–91.

18. Long H, Zheng Y, Situ D, et al. Hand-assisted thoracoscopic surgery for bilateral lung metastasectomy through sternocostal triangle access. Ann Thorac Surg 2011;91:852–9.

19. Kang MC, Kang CH, Lee HJ, et al. Accuracy of 16-channel multi-detector row chest computed tomography with thin sections in the detection of metastatic pulmonary nodules. Eur J Cardiothorac Surg 2008;33(3):473–9.

20. Carballo M, Maish MS, Jaroszewski DE, et al. Video-assisted thoracic surgery (VATS) as a safe alternative for the resection of pulmonary metastases: a retrospective cohort study. J Cardiothorac Surg 2009;4:13.

21. Gossot D1, Radu C, Girard P, et al. Resection of pulmonary metastases from sarcoma: can some patients benefit from a less invasive approach? Ann Thorac Surg 2009;87(1):238–43.

22. Perentes JY, Krueger T, Lovis A, et al. Thoracoscopic resection of pulmonary metastasis: current practice and results. Crit Rev Oncol Hematol 2015;95(1): 105–13.

23. Pairolero PC. Invited commentary: pneumonectomy for lung metastases: indications, risks, and outcomes. Ann Thorac Surg 1998;66:1930–3.

24. Hamaji M, Cassivi SD, Shen KR, et al. Is lymph node dissection required in pulmonary metastasectomy for colorectal adenocarcinoma? Ann Thorac Surg 2012; 94:1796–801.

25. Seebacher G, Decker S, Fischer JR, et al. Unexpected lymph node disease in resections for pulmonary metastases. Ann Thorac Surg 2015;99:231–7.

26. Internullo E, Cassivi SD, Van Raemdonck D, et al. Pulmonary metastasectomy a survey of current practice amongst members of the European Society of Thoracic Surgeons. J Thorac Oncol 2008;3:1257–66.

27. Bolukbas S, Sponholz S, Kudelin N, et al. Risk factors for lymph node metastases and prognosticators of survival in patients undergoing pulmonary metastasectomy for colorectal cancer. Ann Thorac Surg 2014;97:1926–32.

28. Reinersman JM, Wigle D. Lymphadenectomy during pulmonary metastasectomy. Thorac Surg Clin 2016;26:25–40.

29. Pfannschmidt J, Muley T, Hoffman H, et al. Prognostic factors and survival after complete resection of pulmonary metastases from colorectal carcinoma: experience in 167 patients. J Thorac Cardiovasc Surg 2002;74:1653–7.

30. Renaud S, Falcoz PE, Alifano M, et al. Systematic lymph node dissection in lung metastasectomy of renal cell carcinoma; an 18 years of experience. J Surg Oncol 2014;109:823–9.

31. Darling GE, Allen MS, Decker PA, et al. Randomized trial of mediastinal lymph node sampling versus complete lymphadenectomy during pulmonary resection in the patient with N0 or N1 (less than hilar) non-small cell carcinoma. Results of the American College of Surgery Oncology Group Z0030 Trial. J Thorac Cardiovasc Surg 2011;141:662–70.

32. Burt BM, Ocejo S, Mery CM, et al. Repeated and aggressive pulmonary resections for leiomyosarcoma metastases extends survival. Ann Thorac Surg 2011; 92(4):1202–7.

33. Liu D, Abolhoda A, Burt ME, et al. Pulmonary metastasectomy for testicular germ cell tumors: a 28-year experience. Ann Thorac Surg 1998;66(5):1709–14.

34. Kesler KA, Kruter LE, Perkins SM, et al. Survival after resection for metastatic testicular nonseminomatous germ cell cancer to the lung or mediastinum. Ann Thorac Surg 2011;91(4):1085–93.

35. Lo Faso F, Salaini L, Lembo R, et al. Thoracoscopic lung metastasectomies: A 10 year experience. Surg Endosc 2013;27:1938–44.

36. Dickinson KJ, Blackmon SH. Results of pulmonary resection. colorectal carcinoma. Thorac Surg Clin 2016;26:41–7.

37. Suzuki M, Iwata T, Ando S, et al. Predictors of long term survival with pulmonary metastasectomy for osteosarcomas and soft tissue sarcomas. J Cardiovasc Surg 2006;47:603–8.

38. Kim S, Ott HC, Wright CD, et al. Pulmonary resection of metastatic sarcoma: prognostic factors associated with improved outcomes. Ann Thorac Surg 2011; 92:1780–6.

39. Younes RN, Fares AL, Gross JL. Pulmonary metastasectomy; a multivariate analysis of 440 patients undergoing complete resection. Interact Cardiovasc Thorac Surg 2012;14:156–61.

40. Kager L, Zoubek A, Potschger U, et al. Primary metastatic osteosarcoma: presentation and outcome of patients treated on neoadjuvant cooperative osteosarcoma study group proocols. J Clin Oncol 2003;21(10):2011–8.
41. Van Gael AN, Pastorino U, Jauch KW, et al. Surgical treatment of lung metastases, The European organization for research and treatment of cancer – soft tissue and bone sarcoma group. Study of 255 patients. Cancer 1996;77(4):675–82.
42. Predina JD, Puc MM, Bergey MR, et al. Improved survival after pulmonary metastasectomy for soft tissue sarcoma. J Thorac Oncol 2011;6(5):913–9.
43. Kennecke H, Yerushalmi R, Woods R, et al. Metastatic behavior of breast cancer subtypes. J Clin Oncol 2010;28(20):3271–7.
44. Welter S, Jacobs J, Krbek T, et al. Pulmonary metastases of breast cancer. When is resection indicated? Eur J Cardiothorac Surg 2008;34(6):1228–34.
45. Fan J, Chen D, Du H, et al. Prognostic factors for resection of isolated pulmonary metastases in breast cancer patients: a systematic review and meta-analysis. J Thorac Dis 2015;7(8):1441–51.
46. Diaz-Canton EA, Valero V, Rahman Z, et al. Clinical course of breast cancer patients with metastases confined to the lungs treated with chemotherapy. The University of Texas M.D. Anderson Cancer Center experience and review of the literature. Ann Oncol 1998;9(4):413–8.
47. Balch CM, Soong SJ, Murad TM, et al. A multifactorial analysis of melanoma. IV. Prognostic factors in 200 melanoma patients with distant metastases (stage III). J Clin Oncol 1983;1(2):126–34.
48. Tafra L, Dale PS, Wanek LA, et al. Resection and adjuvant immunotherapy for melanoma metastatic to the lung and thorax. J Thorac Cardiovasc Surg 1995; 110(1):119–29.
49. Shiono S, Kawamura M, Sato T, et al. Pulmonary metastasectomy for pulmonary metastases of head and neck squamous cell carcinomas. Ann Thorac Surg 2009; 88(3):856–60.
50. Finley RK 3rd, Verazin GT, Driscoll DL, et al. Results of surgical resection of pulmonary metastases of squamous cell carcinoma of the head and neck. Am J Surg 1992;164(6):594–8.
51. Adachi H, Yamamoto T, Saito S, et al. Therapeutic outcome after resection of pulmonary metastases from oral and/or head and neck cancers: complete republication of the article published in Jpn J Chest Surg. Gen Thorac Cardiovasc Surg 2015;63(8):459–64.
52. Wedman J, Balm AJ, Hart AA, et al. Value of resection of pulmonary metastases in head and neck cancer patients. Head Neck 1996;18(4):311–6.
53. Winter H, Meimarakis G, Hoffmann G, et al. Does surgical resection of pulmonary metastases of head and neck cancer improve survival? Ann Surg Oncol 2008; 15(10):2915–26.
54. Bezjak A. Palliative therapy for lung cancer. Semin Surg Oncol 2003;21(2): 138–47.
55. Zhang Y, Xiao JP, Zhang HZ, et al. Stereotactic body radiation therapy favors long-term overall survival in patients with lung metastases: five year experience of a single institution. Chin Med J (Engl) 2011;124(24):4132–7.
56. Yu W, Tang L, Lin F, et al. Sterotactic radiosurgery, a potential alternative treatment for pulmonary metastases from osteosarcoma. Int J Oncol 2014;44(4): 1091–8.
57. Lodeweges JE, Klinkeberg TJ, Ubbels JF, et al. Long term outcomes of surgery or stereotactic radiotherapy for lung oligometastes. J Thorac Oncol 2017;12: 1442–5.

58. Filippi AR, Guerrera F, Badellino S, et al. Exploratory analysis on overall survival after either surgery or stereotactic radiotherapy for lung oligometastases from colorectal cancer. Clin Oncol (R Coll Radiol) 2016;28:505–12.

59. Lee YH, Kang KM, Choi HS, et al. Comparison of stereotactic body radiotherapy versus metastasectomy outcomes in patients with pulmonary metastases. Thorac Cancer 2018;9:1671–9.

60. de Baere T, Palussiere J, Auperin A, et al. Midterm local efficacy and survival after radiofrequency ablation of lung tumors with minimum follow-up of 1 year: prospective evaluation. Radiology 2006;240(2):587–96.

61. Lencioni R, Crocetti L, Cioni R, et al. Response to radiofrequency ablation of pulmonary tumors: a prospective intention-to-treat multicentre clinical trial (the RAPTURE study). Lancet Oncol 2008;9(7):621–8.

62. de Baere T, Auperin A, Deschamps F, et al. Radiofrequency ablation is a valid treatment option for lung metastases: experience in 566 patients with 1037 metastases. Ann Oncol 2015;26(5):987–91.

63. Gilliams AR, Lees WR. Radiofrequency ablation of lung metastases: factors influencing success. Eur Radiol 2008;18(4):672–7.

64. Treasure T, Farewell V, Macbeth F, et al. Pulmonary Metastasectomy versus Continued Active Monitoring in Colorectal Cancer (PulMiCC): a multicentre randomised clinical trial. Trials 2019;20:718.

UNITED STATES POSTAL SERVICE ®

Statement of Ownership, Management, and Circulation
(All Periodicals Publications Except Requester Publications)

1. Publication Title	2. Publication Number	3. Filing Date
SURGICAL ONCOLOGY CLINICS OF NORTH AMERICA	012 – 565	9/18/2020

4. Issue Frequency	5. Number of Issues Published Annually	6. Annual Subscription Price
JAN, APR, JUL, OCT	4	$309.00

7. Complete Mailing Address of Known Office of Publication (Not printer) (Street, city, county, state, and ZIP+4®)

ELSEVIER INC.
230 Park Avenue, Suite 800
New York, NY 10169

Contact Person
Malathi Samayan

Telephone (Include area code)
91-44-4299-4507

8. Complete Mailing Address of Headquarters or General Business Office of Publisher (Not printer)

ELSEVIER INC.
230 Park Avenue, Suite 800
New York, NY 10169

9. Full Names and Complete Mailing Addresses of Publisher, Editor, and Managing Editor (Do not leave blank)

Publisher (Name and complete mailing address)

DOLORES MELON, ELSEVIER INC.
1600 JOHN F KENNEDY BLVD. SUITE 1800
PHILADELPHIA, PA 19103-2899

Editor (Name and complete mailing address)

JOHN VASSALLO, ELSEVIER INC.
1600 JOHN F KENNEDY BLVD. SUITE 1800
PHILADELPHIA, PA 19103-2899

Managing Editor (Name and complete mailing address)

PATRICK MANLEY, ELSEVIER INC.
1600 JOHN F KENNEDY BLVD. SUITE 1800
PHILADELPHIA, PA 19103-2899

10. Owner (Do not leave blank. If the publication is owned by a corporation, give the name and address of the corporation immediately followed by the names and addresses of all stockholders owning or holding 1 percent or more of the total amount of stock. If not owned by a corporation, give the names and addresses of the individual owners. If owned by a partnership or other unincorporated firm, give its name and address as well as those of each individual owner. If the publication is published by a nonprofit organization, give its name and address.)

Full Name	Complete Mailing Address
WHOLLY OWNED SUBSIDIARY OF REED/ELSEVIER, US HOLDINGS	1600 JOHN F KENNEDY BLVD. SUITE 1800 PHILADELPHIA, PA 19103-2899

11. Known Bondholders, Mortgagees, and Other Security Holders Owning or Holding 1 Percent or More of Total Amount of Bonds, Mortgages, or Other Securities. If none, check box. ▶ ☐ None

Full Name	Complete Mailing Address
N/A	

12. Tax Status (For completion by nonprofit organizations authorized to mail at nonprofit rates) (Check one)
The purpose, function, and nonprofit status of this organization and the exempt status for federal income tax purposes:
☒ Has Not Changed During Preceding 12 Months
☐ Has Changed During Preceding 12 Months (Publisher must submit explanation of change with this statement)

PS Form 3526, July 2014 [Page 1 of 4 (see instructions page 4)] PSN 7530-01-000-9931 PRIVACY NOTICE: See our privacy policy on www.usps.com

---

13. Publication Title	14. Issue Date for Circulation Data Below
SURGICAL ONCOLOGY CLINICS OF NORTH AMERICA	JULY 2020

15. Extent and Nature of Circulation		Average No. Copies Each Issue During Preceding 12 Months	No. Copies of Single Issue Published Nearest to Filing Date
a. Total Number of Copies (Net press run)		102	98
b. Paid Circulation (By Mail and Outside the Mail)	(1) Mailed Outside-County Paid Subscriptions Stated on PS Form 3541 (Include paid distribution above nominal rate, advertiser's proof copies, and exchange copies)	41	36
	(2) Mailed In-County Paid Subscriptions Stated on PS Form 3541 (Include paid distribution above nominal rate, advertiser's proof copies, and exchange copies)	0	0
	(3) Paid Distribution Outside the Mails Including Sales Through Dealers and Carriers, Street Vendors, Counter Sales, and Other Paid Distribution Outside USPS®	32	34
	(4) Paid Distribution by Other Classes of Mail Through the USPS (e.g. First-Class Mail®)	0	0
c. Total Paid Distribution (Sum of 15b (1), (2), (3), and (4))	▶	73	70
d. Free or Nominal Rate Distribution (By Mail and Outside the Mail)	(1) Free or Nominal Rate Outside-County Copies included on PS Form 3541	13	11
	(2) Free or Nominal Rate In-County Copies Included on PS Form 3541	0	0
	(3) Free or Nominal Rate Copies Mailed at Other Classes Through the USPS (e.g. First-Class Mail)	0	0
	(4) Free or Nominal Rate Distribution Outside the Mail (Carriers or other means)	0	0
e. Total Free or Nominal Rate Distribution (Sum of 15d (1), (2), (3) and (4))	▶	13	11
f. Total Distribution (Sum of 15c and 15e)	▶	86	81
g. Copies not Distributed (See Instructions to Publishers #4 (page #3))	▶	16	17
h. Total (Sum of 15f and g)	▶	102	98
i. Percent Paid (15c divided by 15f times 100)		84.88%	86.41%

* If you are claiming electronic copies, go to line 16 on page 3. If you are not claiming electronic copies, skip to line 17 on page 3.

16. Electronic Copy Circulation		Average No. Copies Each Issue During Preceding 12 Months	No. Copies of Single Issue Published Nearest to Filing Date
a. Paid Electronic Copies	▶		
b. Total Paid Print Copies (Line 15c) + Paid Electronic Copies (Line 16a)	▶		
c. Total Print Distribution (Line 15f) + Paid Electronic Copies (Line 16a)	▶		
d. Percent Paid (Both Print & Electronic Copies) (16b divided by 16c × 100)	▶		

☒ I certify that 50% of all my distributed copies (electronic and print) are paid above a nominal price.

17. Publication of Statement of Ownership

☒ If the publication is a general publication, publication of this statement is required. Will be printed in the OCTOBER 2020 issue of this publication. ☐ Publication not required

18. Signature and Title of Editor, Publisher, Business Manager, or Owner

Malathi Samayan

Malathi Samayan - Distribution Controller

Date 9/18/2020

I certify that all information furnished on this form is true and complete. I understand that anyone who furnishes false or misleading information on this form or who omits material or information requested on the form may be subject to criminal sanctions (including fines and imprisonment) and/or civil sanctions (including civil penalties).

PS Form 3526, July 2014 (Page 3 of 4) PRIVACY NOTICE: See our privacy policy on www.usps.com

Moving?

Make sure your subscription moves with you!

To notify us of your new address, find your **Clinics Account Number** (located on your mailing label above your name), and contact customer service at:

Email: journalscustomerservice-usa@elsevier.com

800-654-2452 (subscribers in the U.S. & Canada)
314-447-8871 (subscribers outside of the U.S. & Canada)

Fax number: 314-447-8029

Elsevier Health Sciences Division
Subscription Customer Service
3251 Riverport Lane
Maryland Heights, MO 63043

*To ensure uninterrupted delivery of your subscription, please notify us at least 4 weeks in advance of move.

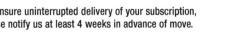

Printed and bound by CPI Group (UK) Ltd, Croydon, CR0 4YY

03/10/2024

01040402-0020